Critical Food Issues: Problems and State-of-the-Art Solutions Worldwide

Critical Food Issues: Problems and State-of-the-Art Solutions Worldwide

Volume 2: Society, Culture, and Ethics

Edited by

Lynn Walter

PRAEGER

An Imprint of ABC-CLIO, LLC

A B C ⬥ C L I O

Santa Barbara, California • Denver, Colorado • Oxford, England

Copyright 2009 by Lynn Walter

Library of Congress Cataloging-in-Publication Data
Critical food issues : problems and state-of-the-art solutions worldwide.
      p. cm.
   Includes index.
   ISBN 978-0-313-35444-1 (set: hard copy: alk. paper)—ISBN 978-0-313-35446-5 (vol. 1:
hard copy: alk. paper)—ISBN 978-0-313-35448-9 (vol. 2: hard copy: alk. paper)—
ISBN 978-0-313-35445-8 (set: ebook)—ISBN 978-0-313-35447-2 (vol. 1: ebook)—
ISBN 978-0-313-35449-6 (vol. 2: ebook)
1. Food supply. 2. Food consumption. 3. Food—Social aspects.
4. Agriculture. 5. Produce trade. 6. Nutrition policy. I. Phoenix, Laurel E.
II. Walter, Lynn, 1945-
   HD9000.5.C733 2009
   363.8—dc22   2009018999

13   12   11   10   9   1   2   3   4   5

This book is also available on the World Wide Web as an eBook.
Visit www.abc-clio.com for details.

ABC-CLIO, LLC
130 Cremona Drive, P.O. Box 1911
Santa Barbara, California 93116-1911

This book is printed on acid-free paper ∞

Manufactured in the United States of America

Contents

Foreword

Lynn Walter and Laurel E. Phoenix

Eating is one of the first things we do in life and one of the last things we do. In between our first and last bite, food sustains us, orders our days, celebrates our lives, stimulates our senses, brings us together, and sets us apart. Food is so central to our individual and collective experience that we are intimately familiar with it. But, even with all we know about food, we need to know much more; and this is as true of gourmet "foodies" as it is of those who consider food a trifle. First, we need to identify how the way that food is produced, distributed, and consumed affects human well-being as well as that of our environment and communities. *Critical Food Issues: Problems and State-of-the-Art Solutions Worldwide* examines many of the problems that derive from our prevailing agrifood system—from environmental degradation, resource depletion, and disordered eating, to declining rural livelihoods, food insecurity, unjust labor practices, and animal mistreatment.

Second, we need to know how to address these critical food issues, which is the key question of this collection. Each chapter focuses on strategies and practices that will enhance the synergy between sustainable agrifood systems and a sound environment, healthy people, and equitable communities, locally and globally. As befits the scope of the problems, the solutions are wide-ranging—from local markets, appropriate technologies for pest management and soil improvements, and policies for better working conditions for agricultural workers to social movements for land equity and environmental quality, political consumerism, and creative and scholarly work in the arts and sciences.

The critical food issues are examined by specialists from many academic disciplines who analyze the current state of research on both specific problems and potential solutions. They bring authoritative depth to their analysis of the current literature based in their specific disciplinary specializations, from environmental, nutritional, soil, and agricultural sciences; public health and dietetics; education; literature; history; philosophy; economics; sociology; anthropology; and gender studies. Most of the chapters examine case studies from around the world, wherever problems are being addressed effectively; others concentrate on the United

States, where the research in agrifood studies is growing in concert with the rapidly increasing number of communities, schools, farms, agencies, and businesses working on sustainable agrifood projects.

Each chapter is written in jargon-free language to inform citizen and consumer engagement in the future of food and agriculture and to advance interdisciplinary agrifood studies. The breadth of the problems and solutions is examined in two volumes, generally divided into more bioenvironmental issues or more sociocultural ones. Volume 1 covers *Environment, Agriculture, and Health Concerns*, while Volume 2 focuses on *Society, Culture, and Ethics*. To an extent, the partitions between the volumes and among the sections within them are simply paper ones, because addressing the problems and solutions requires integrating knowledge from the natural sciences with the social sciences and humanities. As farmer and writer Wendell Berry observed, "Eating is an agricultural act."[1] Because eating links our bodies to the Earth, developing strategies to sustain agriculture requires considering nature in relationship to the ways humans transform it into culturally appropriate foods through social processes.

Therefore, while the contributors analyze specific problems and solutions with the depth that comes from their specialization in one of the many academic disciplines represented in this collection, they share an overarching interdisciplinary problem-focus that integrates their work as a whole. That focus is on strategies to promote a sustainable symbiosis among viable agrifood systems, a sound environment, healthy people, and equitable communities. Scholars of "agro-ecology" and "the ecology of food" have conceptualized the holistic, interdisciplinary character of agrifood studies with various ecological models. The value of ecology as a framework for agrifood studies is that it takes the long-term sustainability of natural resources, the economy, and human health into consideration. As it is understood here, the ecology of agrifood framework also includes values, tastes, traditions, and an ethic of equity and justice. Because an ecology of food links health, economy, environment, community, culture, and ethics, strategies based on it should (1) provide food security for all, (2) renew and sustain the natural resource base and the biodiversity of the environment to ensure future food security, (3) build viable agrifood systems that provide for decent rural livelihoods, and (4) promote democratic access to agrifood decision-making as a basis for just and equitable communities.

Encompassing all of these factors in the creation of sustainable agrifood systems will take serious thought on all our parts and knowledge of the models, ideas, and information with which to consider the problems and solutions. Whenever we think seriously about food, we evoke the past millennia during which times turning soil, water, and sunshine into sustenance was understood to depend on prayer, since food was such a precious and precarious thing. The rising call to return food to its central place in our imaginations and our politics indicates that we are once again uncertain about the future of food. *Critical Food Issues: Problems and State-of-the-Art Solutions Worldwide* examines the bases of our fears and ways that we might address them.

NOTE

1. Wendell Berry, "The Pleasures of Eating," in *American Food Writing*, ed. Molly O'Neill (New York: Library Classics of the United States, 2007), 551–58, 552.

Preface

Lynn Walter and Laurel E. Phoenix

A project of the scope of *Critical Food Issues: Problems and State-of-the-Art Solutions Worldwide* requires a collaborative effort. Especially critical has been the work of the forty-one university researchers from around the country and around the world who have provided their academic expertise to this collection. They were asked to present complex information and ideas in a way that not only revealed the complexity of their subjects but also communicated it across the disciplinary boundaries. Communication among the many different disciplinary specialists depended on their commitment to the goals of the project as a whole—first, to provide the public with the information necessary to address the critical foods issues confronting the world today; and second, to contribute to the development of a new interdisciplinary field of food studies. Given the range of disciplines represented here—from environmental, nutritional, and agricultural sciences, to literature, history, philosophy, economics, sociology, anthropology, and psychology—this was no easy task.

The knowledge integration process has been institutionally supported by the fact that the editors and some of the contributors are faculty members at the Center for Food in Community and Culture at the University of Wisconsin–Green Bay. The mission of the center is reflected in the central interdisciplinary problem-focus of this collection, which is to promote "interdisciplinary scholarship to enhance the synergy between sustainable food systems and a sound environment, healthy people, and equitable communities, locally and globally." Its work is reinforced by the innovative, interdisciplinary structure of the university's mission, in which the faculty is encouraged to cross the traditional boundaries of knowledge within the broad frameworks of ecology and engaged citizenship.

We are indebted to Debora Carvalko and Elizabeth Potenza from Praeger and Rebecca L. Edwards of Cadmus Communications for their editorial support. At the University of Wisconsin–Green Bay, we relied on Katie Stilp for editorial assistance with the manuscript production. We are grateful for their efforts, their talents, and their encouragement.

Lynn Walter personally thanks her friends and colleagues Katherine Hall, Diane Legomsky, and Judy Martin for reading and reviewing her work throughout the process.

Finally, none of this would have been possible if it were not for the fact that people around the world, farmers and farmworkers, chefs, family cooks, gardeners, artisan food producers, community activists, journalists, and scientists, are awakening us to the critical food issues and to ways that we might learn from their experience. We recognize their work in ours and hope we have done it justice.

Introduction to Volume 2

Lynn Walter

Food security is the critical food issue with the most immediate impact on human well-being—on who lives and who dies, on who thrives and who withers. Even though the right to food was proclaimed by the Universal Declaration of Human Rights in 1948, the United Nations reports that there were 963 million hungry people in the world in 2008, most of them from the poorer countries of the global south, but many from wealthy ones as well.[1] Because the main cause of hunger is poverty,[2] in the future, even more people may be at risk if food prices rise in response to the depletion of natural resources tied to environmentally destructive agricultural practices.[3] Countering this dismal scenario are alternatives promoting a positive synergy between sustainable agrifood systems, socioeconomic equity, and food security through active citizen engagement in the process. The contributors to Volume 2 of *Critical Food Issues: Problems and State-of-the-Art Solutions Worldwide* bring their expertise in society, culture, and ethics to bear on an assessment of both potential futures with the intention of fostering the brighter one.

THE NATURE OF THE PROBLEMS AND THE SOLUTIONS

The complex nature of contemporary critical food issues is rooted in long-term, global processes of change, including urbanization, increased consumption levels and population growth, and the development of industrialized, commodified agrifood systems that have intensified the pressure on the natural resource base. Unsustainable levels of consumption of water and fossil fuels, soil degradation, pesticide contamination, and loss of biodiversity along with predicted global warming impacts do not bode well for our future food security.[4] At the same time, the consolidation of agricultural production, food processing, and distribution into fewer and fewer firms, and their concentrated political influence, have made it increasingly difficult for local communities, regions, or even states, to enact more sustainable agrifood policies; and wealth inequalities within and between nations have exacerbated this democratic deficit.[5] As rural livelihoods decline and the countryside empties of people, as well as other forms of life, fewer people have a clear understanding of where our daily bread comes from, how it is made, and what it is made of.[6] Instead, we have more often taken food for granted, eaten it alone and on the run, and absorbed much of our knowledge of it from the consumption of highly processed food and mass marketing appeals. All of these forces constrain our ability to understand and address the problems.

Yet, because food sustains our existence, it has always been the object of human creativity in all its forms—individual and collective, cultural and practical, scientific and artistic, political and philosophical. Evincing all of these forms of creativity, strategies to address critical food issues have developed in every corner of the world and from every angle. The problems and creative responses to them are the focus of the new field of *Food Studies*, which critically examines the linkages between topics as varied as organic agriculture, celebrity chefs, commodity chains, hunger, culinary traditions, and body image. The particular contribution of *Critical Food Issues: Problems and State-of-the-Art Solutions Worldwide* to food studies is that it integrates knowledge from various academic disciplinary specializations into an interdisciplinary problem-focus on ways to promote a sustainable symbiosis among a viable agrifood system, a sound environment, healthy people, and equitable communities.

The 16 chapters of Volume 2 are divided into parts—Society, Culture, and Ethics—based mostly on the disciplinary perspectives of the authors, their primary approach to the sustainable agrifood problem-focus, and the particular issue. To advance an interdisciplinary reading of their collected work as a whole, however, this introduction draws from all the chapters to develop four themes that intersect and integrate them. These are the alternative agrifood movement, communities and coalitions, the rejuvenation of agrifood knowledge, and rights and responsibilities.

THE ALTERNATIVE AGRIFOOD MOVEMENT

Many of the citizens and consumers; artists, journalists, and artisans; grassroots and transnational social movements; and indigenous and other community organizations who are working on critical food issues are doing so as part of a comprehensive mission to sustain quality food, food security, and decent livelihoods for all and a sound environment for future generations. Their effectiveness depends on securing access to natural, financial, human, and social capital; empowering ordinary people; including constituents who may hold contrary views; encouraging communication and cooperation among them; and seeking equitable and just solutions. Patricia Allen opens this volume in chapter 1 with an analysis of the roots of their struggles. She notes that at least since the early nineteenth century, individuals and social movements have been working for food safety and food security, environmental conservation, and decent livelihoods for farmers and farmworkers. The constraints they have confronted over time reveal conflicts of interest by class, race, and gender as well as by countries and regions, conflicts rooted in the structure of the prevailing agrifood systems. Allen argues that recent developments of innovative agrifood strategies such as fair trade, food policy councils, urban agriculture, organic agricultural production, and farmers markets have begun to coalesce in an alternative agrifood movement that holds promise for making the systemic changes necessary to achieve quality food, sustainable agriculture, food security, and just and equitable communities.

One of the historical precedents cited by Allen is the antislavery movement, a critical example of a nineteenth-century social movement to end an extreme form of race-based agricultural labor exploitation. Dan La Botz's chapter 3 on contemporary farmworkers and meat and poultry processing workers in the United States demonstrates that the problem of the "atrocious and shameful" working conditions of agricultural laborers is an entrenched one that, in this case, is also exacerbated by the marginalized status of Latino immigrant and African-American women workers. He sees labor organizing and labor politics as the key strategies for enforcing a living wage, fair labor practices, and better working conditions. La Botz and Allen both refer to a few recent labor victories, including those of the Coalition of Immokalee Workers who won their drive for higher wages from Taco Bell and Burger King, and their antislavery campaign to investigate and prosecute contemporary forms of farmworker slavery.[7] In general, however, the problems of low wages and unfair labor practices in agrifood production and processing persist.

The relationship between the alternative agrifood movement and labor issues is complicated by workers' employment in the commercial-industrial system. Therefore, the effectiveness of the alternative agrifood movement depends upon its capacity to support better wages and working conditions for agrifood workers and, at the same time, develop viable alternative livelihood strategies and ways of working together toward common goals of sustainable agriculture, food security, quality food, and decent livelihoods. As the power of labor unions, and even governments, has diminished in the process of the globalization of capital and agrifood systems, in chapter 6, Michele Micheletti and Dietlind Stolle argue that consumers have become more active participants in the alternative agrifood movement in support of fair labor practices. For example, they discuss the use of boycotts and *buycotts* by consumers in support of labor struggles. They identify the grape boycott in support of the United Farm Workers' strike in the 1960s and recent buycott campaigns, encouraging consumers to purchase *fair trade* coffee and chocolates to improve farm income and farmworker wages and working conditions, as examples of the ways political consumers have supported fair labor practices.

La Botz's analysis of the relationship between the disempowered status of immigrant agrifood workers and the decline of small-scale farms in Mexico, in part as a result of free trade agreements like the North American Free Trade Act (NAFTA), suggests a basis for common interests between peasant farmers and immigrant farmworkers. For example, the Farmworker Association of Florida, Inc. (FWAF), an association to empower farmworkers, is also a member of la Via Campesina, a transnational organization of rural development, farmer, and farmworker groups.[8] In his research among Mexican *campesinos*, Daniel Niles in chapter 9 identifies la Via Campesina as the largest example of a transnational organization that recognizes the link between migration and the viability of small and medium-size agricultural production. In chapter 4, William Van Lopik points out that the key elements of la Via Campesina's mission include not only agrarian reform and sustainable peasant agriculture but also migrant farmworkers' rights. This link between fairer agrifood labor practices and more equitable access to land and capital is well understood by people in the countryside and their former neighbors who have migrated to the burgeoning cities of the global south or crossed the border in search of employment. For example, Niles noticed that almost all of the men at la Via Campesina demonstration he attended in Mexico City had worked in the United States at some time in their lives.

The search for viable alternative livelihood strategies for displaced farmworkers and distressed farmers has also led to the development of alternative markets, such as CSA (community-supported agriculture) and farmers markets. E. Melanie DuPuis, in chapter 2, along with Gail Feenstra and Jennifer Wilkins, in chapter 8, point to the consolidation and distortion of conventional markets by very large, vertically integrated agrifood corporations as another reason for the development of alternative markets, especially in the United States. A third motive, as Feenstra and Wilkins explain, is the increasing demand by consumers for qualities in food that shoppers perceive are not being satisfied by the foods offered by the conventional market—qualities like healthy, fresh, flavorful, organic, fairly traded, locally grown, hormone free, cage free, sustainably caught, and grass fed. To ensure that the alternative markets for such qualities are not simply co-opted by more powerful conventional markets, as happened with organic agriculture in California,[9] and that the interests of agrifood workers, consumers, and producers are fairly represented, DuPuis calls for *civic markets*. In *civic markets* the forms of market governance are transparent and democratic, and so develop in various directions. She examines the market governance structures of several alternative markets and their governance forms, including ones supported by the European Union as part of rural development programs designed around the multifunctionality of agriculture and those to improve access to small farm producers in Europe and the global south to conventional and alternative markets.

COMMUNITIES AND COALITIONS

What distinguishes the alternative agrifood movement from earlier struggles for safe food and better working conditions is the interweaving of campaigns for just labor practices, sustainable agriculture, healthy foods, decent rural livelihoods, and sound environments, which means that consumers, producers, and workers have had to develop ways of working together as citizens and in communities. Many of their strategies focus on local communities and regional *foodsheds*[10] in efforts to reconnect regional farmers and artisans with consumers. From such locally based organizations have come grassroots coalitions at the national and global level.

This community-coalition approach to organizing has developed in the context of globalization processes that began in the 1980s. The mobility of capital markets and more capital- and resource-intensive forms of conventional agrifood production have been promoted by multinational trade and monetary agencies. In the process, multinational agrifood corporations have grown ever larger through mergers and acquisitions, decreasing market competition in agrifood production and markets and driving out small and medium-size firms and farms. It is not surprising, therefore, that as part of the processes of globalization, people also have been on the move to cities and across borders, wherever they think they might find employment and despite low wages and poor working conditions when they get there. Or, if their bodies are not moving, then their voices are, through the global spread and more equitable availability of wireless telecommunication and Internet connectivity. Only the land has not moved, although the goods produced from its natural capital are sold through a global commodity market. These global economic and communication developments have made it both easier and more urgent for people who want to address the sustainable agrifood problem to act collectively.

The fact that land does not move is important to understanding why so much of the work of the alternative agrifood movement has focused on local communities and why, to a large extent, the strength of its transnational organizations has come from the formation of grassroots coalitions among a myriad of locally based groups. In chapter 8 on "sustaining regional food systems and healthy rural livelihoods," which opens the second section of this volume, Feenstra and Wilkins provide an overview of localization strategies in the United States and the reasons behind efforts to link local producers to local consumers. They point out that as a whole the localization strategy links the health, food security, and well-being of local communities and regions to the viability of the rural livelihoods and the regional agrifood economy, the sustainability of its ecosystem, and the reduction of energy and other resource costs. They describe a rapidly growing number of communities that have developed local alternatives. Farmers markets, CSA, farm-to-school programs, community gardens, urban agriculture, and many other innovations have excited the passions of local "foodies" for fresh produce as well as those of city leaders interested in sustainable "green" growth, of farmers and processors with smaller operations looking for more profitable markets and safer agricultural practices, and of citizens who want cleaner, greener, fairer places to raise their children and grandchildren.

Predictably, this localization strategy takes different directions in different communities and even within the same community. The diverse strategies along with the sheer number of participants and programs and their swelling ranks, the deep commitment that comes from work in one's own community, and the relative ease of global coalition building are sources of organizational strength. Feenstra and Wilkins note, however, that the localization strategy does have its weaknesses, especially if community activists do not think critically about the dangers of parochialism and the pitting of interests against one another within and between communities. Feenstra and Wilkins describe the development of food policy councils as one way of bringing diverse perspectives to the table. DuPuis' case for *civic markets* within and across communities is another.

Both food policy councils and civic markets address the political question of how best to include diverse voices in the development of just and sustainable agrifood systems. The principal strategy has been to build coalitions within and across communities and countries. At the national level, Lisa Heldke in chapter 14 analyzes the U.S.-based Community Food Security Coalition as an example of a coalition that resists "us/them thinking" about food security. Internationally, la Via Campesina and Slow Food® International, analyzed by Niles (chapter 9), have built coalitions of activists in the agrifood movement around the world. They have come together in world conferences and demonstrations, through e-mail distribution lists and organizational Web sites, and through interpersonal connections between countries to form alternative agrifood movement organizations in mutual support of rural livelihoods, quality food, and sound environments.

Grassroots organizations from across the global south have responded to the problem of food insecurity by calling for *food sovereignty* as a precondition of food security. "Food Sovereignty is the right of Peoples to define their own policies and strategies for the sustainable production, distribution, and consumption of food, with respect for their own cultures and their own systems of managing natural resources and rural areas." This definition is from the Declaration of Atitlan, a 2002 consultation of indigenous peoples in Atitlan, Guatemala. From their perspective, food sovereignty builds on the principle that agrifood policy should be formed in the context of transparent democratic processes at the local, regional, and national level. In the global south, food sovereignty proponents have opposed economic development policies pushed by powerful, outside, top-down, agrifood advocates. Since the 1980s, such advocates have based their trade and foreign aid policies on the neoliberal platform that economic development proceeds when countries concentrate on expanding production of export commodities to sell in a world market. The political plank of neoliberal development limits the role of governments to enforcing private contracts and protecting private property and minimizes public expenditures in support of small and medium-size farms or social welfare programs. One critical question is whether these prescriptions increase or decrease food security in the long run. Another critical question is what role citizens should play in making decisions about their own future food security. Clearly, food sovereignty advocates are demanding a much more powerful voice in shaping their local agrifood system within a democratic process.

In the United States, some of the communities advocating food sovereignty are indigenous nations.[11] For example, programs like Tsynhehkwa in affiliation with the Oneida Community Integrated Food Systems, described by Lynn Walter in chapter 10, are part of a process of healing the wounds inflicted by their historical loss of land. The work of Tsynhehkwa focuses on the Wisconsin Oneida Nation community, but it is also connected to similar projects around the world through transnational networking. Slow Food has made developing such connections a definitive part of its mission through projects to support *food communities* and preserve heritage foods and artisanal production. According to Slow Food, a *food community* includes "people involved in the production, transformation, and distribution of a particular food, who are closely linked to a geographic area either historically, socially, or culturally."[12] For example, Slow Food has given support to the Oneidas' northern neighbors the White Earth Band of Chippewa by helping to support their defense of wild rice production. This structure—local community agrifood projects in communication with other communities across the country and around the world—is not entirely new, but its effective ability to act collectively and its need to do so are relatively recent phenomena grounded in new forms of globalization.

REJUVENATING THE KNOWLEDGE OF THE COMMONS

A key question for the alternative agrifood movement in local communities and global coalitions is how to get access to information about sustainable agrifood best practices, local food crises, and international and national policy proposals and to discuss that information among the interested groups and share the knowledge that comes from the process of discussion and debate across communities and borders. Sharing knowledge contributes to the political strength of the alternative agrifood movement by making the dimensions of the issues more transparent and, thereby, more accessible to informed democratic action.

This collection is intended to contribute to the process of sharing knowledge to support citizen engagement in democratic agrifood development. In addition to reviewing the academic literature on the sustainable agrifood problem-focus, the contributors consider the knowledge of farmers and artisans, much of it rooted in historical experience in particular ecosystems and cultures. They also evaluate the knowledge that comes from citizen and consumer engagement in efforts to promote "good, clean, and fair food"[13] as well as research invested in the development of large agrifood corporations. Exploring the implications of the *knowledge-intensification shift*, JoAnn Jaffe (in chapter 7) examines all of these ways of knowing, critically analyzing the barriers to transparency and consumer knowledge in the commercial-industrial food system, where agrifood knowledge is increasingly a highly technical, proprietary commodity in a knowledge-based economy. It is in this light that Jaffe assesses the potential of "new knowledge contexts" in which consumer demands for quality in its broad connotations of taste, health, fairness, and sustainability are linked to knowledgeable producers and publicly oriented researchers.

One of these new knowledge contexts has been developed by the political consumers who are the focus of Micheletti and Stolle's study (chapter 6). These consumer activists have led the way in establishing various labeling and certification systems for organic, fair trade, and sustainable fisheries at the global, national, or regional level. Consumer-driven certification and labeling of foods provide knowledge to consumers about a broad range of concerns from the nutritional value of specific foods, the environmental conditions of agrifood production, the use of growth hormones or genetically modified organisms, the fairness of labor practices and farmer profits, the sustainability of its wild source, and the sustainability of its ecosystem. Micheletti and Stolle point out that the labeling and certification process is a highly political one, not only because of the regulatory structure and resources needed to enforce them, but also because of the resistance to such knowledge schemes from proprietary commercial interests.

In chapter 13, Esther Katz focuses on another, much older knowledge context—traditions rooted in particular places and artisanal agrifood practices. Preserving this knowledge for the benefit of local producers is just one of the goals of *place of origin labeling* of foods, which Katz argues also includes preserving heritage varieties and promoting agrobiodiversity, protecting against *biopiracy* (the threat to the knowledge of the commons and heritage varieties through privatizing them), and improving the quality and safety of food.

Who should provide and certify the knowledge consumers and producers need as key stakeholders in agrifood knowledge? Should it be the associations of civil society, producer organizations, or governments? If the answer to building consumer knowledge and preserving producer knowledge is to establish government certification and labeling schemes, then political consumers and producers must be able to engage the state as citizens in a democratic process. In chapter 5, Larry Smith draws on the work of democracy theorist Robert Dahl to make a case for the essentiality of shared, meaningful knowledge of quality to develop *food democracy*. Among several cases of individuals and organizations promoting the sharing of such knowledge among small-scale producers and consumers, Smith highlights Indian physicist, ecologist, and publicly oriented researcher Vandana Shiva. Shiva founded the research foundation Navdanya to preserve practical knowledge of seed varieties inherited from Indian agricultural traditions as part of the knowledge of the commons that supports what she calls *earth democracy*.

As analyzed by Van Lopik (chapter 4), the Green Belt Movement in Kenya, which began as an effort to replant trees, is similar in many ways to Navdanya. Its founder, Wangari Maathai, like Shiva, exemplifies transformational leadership in the promotion of the knowledge of the agrifood commons in several ways: (1) She seeks to "rejuvenate" the indigenous knowledge of generations of local agrifood consumer/producers for the common use of future generations. As the word "rejuvenate" indicates, her goal is not only to preserve accumulated knowledge and resources but also to build on their creative potential. (2) Her understanding of the problem links agrifood knowledge to food security and to sustainable ecological systems. (3) She sees empowerment of local people, especially women, as a vital part of its environmental mission. (4) She has connected her work with other locally based organizations in a network of knowledge-sharing and power-enhancing strategies in Green Belt Movement International. Shiva and Maathai are among the most prominent of the many transformational leaders of countless grassroots organizations doing similar work around the world.

It typically has been assumed that intensified agrifood knowledge is transferred from the countries of the wealthier global north to the poorer global south through either commodified knowledge as in the case of patented genetically modified seeds or through economic development programs that rely on scientific and technical knowledge to increase agricultural production. Alternatively, Van Lopik points out that all of the many indigenous grassroots organizations he describes from the global south—from Kenya to Belize, Bangladesh, and India—are sources of rich, diverse, and profound agrifood knowledge that people in the global north can learn from, if they are "open to seeing." He credits his own experience at the Sustainable Development Institute at the College of Menominee Nation, a small tribal college in northern Wisconsin, with expanding his knowledge of sustainable practices through the numerous opportunities it has provided to share knowledge with indigenous experts from around the world.

The idea that the agrifood knowledge of local, indigenous, and artisanal producers should be valued and rejuvenated and that this goal depends on sharing knowledge and support with numerous other similar organizations worldwide is central to the organizing mission of the transnational organizations Slow Food International and la Via Campesina. Both are the subject of Niles's analysis of transnational social movement organizations as ways to support rural livelihoods (chapter 9). One aspect of his analysis of "contemporary rurality" is that the activists' goals of rural development are both *preservationist* and *prefigurative*. That is, the Mexican *campesinos* he interviewed for his study want to preserve rural livelihoods, their resource base, and artisanal knowledge but also to build on them in the light of contemporary conditions and in conjunction with other rural people as well as urban consumers. La Via Campesina and Slow Food International demonstrate that preserving cultural knowledge is served by sharing it and thereby "rejuvenating" it.

Niles's conclusion that sustaining rural livelihoods is served by sharing, and so expanding, local knowledge will not surprise students of culture who know that, as an adaptive strategy, culture is always both *preservationist* and *prefigurative*. He points out that what is actually new is that local people are better able to reach groups far from their home communities through intercommunity grassroots organizing, Internet connectivity, global conferences, and new allied intermediaries such as Slow Food International connecting the goals of small-scale producers and consumers—in the global north and global south.

That culture is preservationist with respect to accumulated knowledge is most explicitly documented in this volume by Regan A. R. Gurung, who reveals in chapter 11 the historical roots of Western, traditional Chinese, and Indian understanding and practices of the relationships between health and the foods we eat. That culture is prefigurative is also demonstrated in Gurung's discussion of the ways that immigrants carry agricultural and culinary traditions with them to their new homes where, for example, ancient prescriptions to eat foods that are in season confront the less abundant, colder, and shorter growing seasons of the north. He points specifically to a culturally prefigured adaptive response by Hmong immigrants to northeastern Wisconsin, who have become major purveyors of seasonal produce in many local farmers markets.

Artists also create works prefigured by culture, even as they "imaginatively transform [it], creating possibilities and celebrating alternatives." This quote from Aeron Haynie's chapter 12 on food and literature identifies the central purpose of her essay on several contemporary novels, including Barbara Kingsolver's *Prodigal Summer*, Ruth Ozeki's *All Over Creation*, Cormac McCarthy's *The Road*, Dave Eggers's *What Is the What*, and Louise Murphy's *The True Story of Hansel and Gretel*. She argues that these recent representations of food in literature, which focus on concerns like hunger and environmental threats to food security, reflect as well as imaginatively transform popularly recognized problems in the current agrifood system. Although her essay focuses on works of fiction, Haynie also credits contemporary journalists' accounts, especially Michael Pollan's *Omnivore's Dilemma* and Eric Schlosser's *Fast Food Nation*, for bringing greater popular awareness of critical food issues to their readers. Micheletti and Stolle (chapter 6) discuss the creative work of "culture jamming," especially with the employment of new Internet media with which culture jammers transform advertising and other popular culture images to counter mass-mediated marketing campaigns. Along with these artists and journalists, artisans have imagined innovative approaches to food and agriculture, as Smith notes in chapter 5 with reference to "grass farmer" Joel Salatin and chef Alice Waters, a pioneer in championing local, organic, and seasonal fruits and vegetables.

Their efforts to rejuvenate the knowledge of the commons by preserving, creating, and sharing it, in the context of food communities and transnational coalitions, indicate that the alternative agrifood movement has taken on the responsibility of building a just and sustainable agrifood system. In the final section, some of the ethical bases of this responsibility are considered.

RIGHTS AND RESPONSIBILITIES

In 1948, the United Nations passed the Universal Declarations of Human Rights. While most of the articles cover civil and political rights, a few declare social rights. Of particular relevance is Article 25, which states:

(1) Everyone has the right to a standard of living adequate for the health and well-being of himself and of his family, including food, clothing, housing

and medical care and necessary social services, and the right to security in the event of unemployment, sickness, disability, widowhood, old age or other lack of livelihood in circumstances beyond his control. (2) Motherhood and childhood are entitled to special care and assistance. All children, whether born in or out of wedlock, shall enjoy the same social protection.

Article 25 stands out for its call for positive action to fulfill societal responsibilities; specifically, it declares the gendered, male-breadwinner family and, ultimately, society responsible for adequately feeding, clothing, housing, and caring for one another. The second clause makes us responsible for the special social protection of motherhood and childhood, thus formally recognizing the responsibilities of the generations for one another. Inherent in Article 25 is also the "right to feed," that is the right, as stated, of the male head of household to a livelihood that permits him to feed his family, a right that marriage and the birth of children actualize. Thus, this basic human rights document recognizes kinship rights and responsibilities as well as the responsibilities of society to support kinship.

Much has changed since 1948: the *new* women's movements around the world declared enforcement of the male breadwinner family to be discriminatory, many women left the house and gained their own livelihoods, they demanded their own right to feed their families and tried to get society to fulfill its declared responsibilities for special care and assistance for mothers and children. However, notwithstanding these profound changes in gendered domestic and public life, families still have the primary responsibility for adequately feeding, clothing, housing, and caring for one another, men still have an advantage in the labor market, and women still do more of the actual feeding of their families.

Walter (chapter 10) explores the implications for the alternative food movement of the gendered, generational nexus between family and society for the right and responsibility to feed and care for one another. Specifically, she analyzes the significance of sharing food and eating together as practices that define kinship in what she calls a *relational concept of home*. Focusing on *home* as a primary locus of gendered and generational interests, she argues that specific forms of women's activism in the alternative food movement—including community kitchens and gardens—reveal conflicting and common interests in the struggles of women to feed their children. She points to women and men who are active in support of feeding their children in ways that expand the relations of home by sharing food in the wider community. Her analysis draws on Eva Feder Kittay's conceptualization of a *relational self*, a self who serves society and future generations best when those who feed and care for children and other dependent people are also cared for.[14]

In chapter 14, Heldke also builds on the concept of the relational self to make a case for her *coresponsibility* paradigm of food security. In contrast to the charity and rights paradigms, which she argues too often have an "us/them dynamic," the coresponsibility paradigm might lead us to see our own food vulnerabilities in solidarity with others. It might also help us understand how we are interdependent in the sense of being part of dependency systems, a reality that becomes obvious when these systems break down or are not appropriate for the context, such as dependence on a retail grocery chain for food in a flooded city or in a remote fishing village. Heldke intends the coresponsibility paradigm to help us recognize the connections between various forms of marginalization, in this particular case, between disability and food insecurity. Recognizing the many different ways that people are food insecure can also be the basis for the development of community food coalitions across their differences. She is careful to note that conceptualizing food security in terms of coresponsibility does not eliminate conflict, but that it reframes well-being in such a way that one person's gains do not necessarily mean another person's loss—for example, she points out that well-nourished children contribute to the community's well-being, even if they are someone else's children.

In chapter 15, Andrew Fiala, like Heldke, takes a philosopher's perspective to examine the issues of farm animal treatment from animal rights to animal welfare standpoints, from human-centered to animal-centered viewpoints, and from Aristotelian to Kantian philosophies. He concludes that the philosophical arguments about animal welfare have shaped policy. For example, he refers to recent European Union legislation based on the idea that animals are sentient beings and that they should be free from hunger, discomfort, pain, and fear and free to express normal behavior. However, he notes that factory farming, which has largely abandoned such traditional concepts of animal husbandry and stewardship, is on the increase worldwide and that philosophical arguments against the treatment of animals as nonsentient objects have encountered resistance from the immediate self-interests of producers and eaters of cheap meat.

Stewardship as a moral stance would have us be responsible for the welfare of the creatures we depend on for sustenance and consider how our treatment of them will mean that they continue to sustain us or to diminish our future well-being. Land stewardship is a concept that Eric J. Fitch traces in chapter 16 to earliest human society and in written form in Europe at least as far back as medieval times. He grounds his discussion in the relationship between scientific perspectives on land stewardship and theological and philosophical ones. He quotes appreciatively from *A Sand County Almanac* by the noted environmentalist Aldo Leopold, "A land ethic, then, reflects the existence of an ecological conscience, and this in turn reflects a conviction of individual responsibility for the health of land."[15] However, Fitch notes, as does Fiala with regard to animal welfare, that relatively recent separation of people from the land and from farming has made it difficult for most people to know what is happening to agricultural land and its resources, or to farm animals and their welfare. As a result, we must educate ourselves about the critical food issues if we are to be good stewards. Fortunately, Fitch can point to scientists working on best practices for land conservation and to many different Protestant denominations and the Catholic Church, which have produced policy statements on environmental stewardship. He concludes with the critical question of how the scientific, theological, and philosophical conceptions of land stewardship can be put into practice in "the quest to create human cultures and societies that live sustainably upon the planet." In the following chapters of *Critical Food Issues: Problems and State-of-the-Art Solutions Worldwide*, we examine efforts by people around the world who have undertaken this quest.

NOTES

1. FAO (Food and Agriculture Organization of the United Nations), "Number of Hungry People Rises to 963 Million" (Rome: FAO, 2006), http://www.fao.org/news/story/en/item/8836/ (accessed January 20, 2008).

2. FAO, World Food Summit, "Rome Declaration on World Food Security," http://www.fao.org/docrep/003/w3613e/w3613e00.HTM (accessed January 20, 2009).

3. Stanley Wood, Kate Sebastian, and Sara J. Scherr, *Pilot Analysis of Global Eco-systems: Agroecosystems* (Washington, DC: International Food Policy Research Institute and World Resources Institute, 2000).

4. David S. Battisti and Rosamund L. Naylor, "Historical Warnings of Future Food Insecurity with Unprecedented Seasonal Heat," *Science* 323 (January 2009): 240–44; USAID, "Food Security and the Global Water Crisis," http://www.usaid.gov/our_work/environment/water/food_security.html (accessed January 11, 2008).

5. Marion Nestle, *Food Politics: How the Food Industry Influences Nutrition and Health* (Berkeley: University of California Press, 2002); William Heffernan, Mary Hendrickson, and Robert Gronski, "Consolidation in the Food and Agriculture System," Report to the National Farmers Union (February 1999), http://home.hiwaay.net/~becraft/NFUFarmCrisis.htm (accessed January 12, 2009).

6. Ann Vileisis, *Kitchen Literacy: How We Lost Knowledge of Where Food Comes from and Why We Need to Get it Back* (Washington, DC: Island Press, 2008).

7. Coalition of Immokalee Workers, http://www.ciw-online.org/index.html (accessed January 19, 2009).

8. FWAF (The Farmworker Association of Florida, Inc.), http://www.farmworkers.org/fwafpage.html (accessed January 19, 2009).

9. Julie Guthman, *Agrarian Dreams: The Paradox of Organic Farming in California* (Berkeley: University of California Press, 2004).

10. Jack Kloppenburg Jr., John Hendrickson, and G. W. Stevenson, "Coming in to the Foodshed," *Agriculture and Human Values* 13, no. 3 (1996): 33–42. The term "foodshed" is used in analogy with "watershed" to focus attention on the relationship between the regional economy and ecosystem and the foods produced, marketed, and consumed within them.

11. Food and Seed Sovereignty Network, http://protectseeds.org/node/244 (accessed January 19, 2009).

12. Terra Madre, http://www.terramadre2006.org/pagine/rete/ (accessed November 2, 2008).

13. This pithy phrase, "good, clean, and fair food," comes from Slow Food International.

14. Eva Feder Kittay, *Love's Labor: Essays on Women, Equality and Dependency* (New York: Routledge, 1999).

15. Aldo Leopold, *A Sand County Almanac and Sketches Here and There* (New York: Oxford University Press, 1949), 204.

Abbreviations

AFN	alternative food networks
ALRA	Agricultural Labor Relations Act (California)
APHA	American Public Health Association
ASPCA	American Society for the Prevention of Cruelty to Animals
BMI	body mass index
BSE	Bovine Spongiform Encephalopathy
CAFO	Confined Animal Feeding Operation
CAP	Common Agricultural Policy (European Union)
CFP	Community Food Projects
CFPA	Council of Food Policy Advisors (United Kingdom)
CFS	community food security
COOL	Country of Origin Labeling
CSA	community-supported agriculture
DBCP	1,2-Dibromo-3-chloropropane (pesticide)
Defra	Department for Environment, Food and Rural Affairs (United Kingdom)
DHHS	U.S. Department of Health and Human Services
EPA	U.S. Environmental Protection Agency
EU	European Union
FAO	Food and Agriculture Organization of the United Nations
FIFRA	Federal Insecticide, Fungicide, and Rodenticide Act
FLOC	Farm Labor Organizing Committee
FLO-I	Fairtrade Labelling Organizations International
FLSA	Fair Labor Standards Act
FMNP	Farmers Market Nutrition Program (of WIC)
FPC	food policy council
FPG	food policy group
FWAF	Farmworker Association of Florida, Inc.
GATT	General Agreement on Tariffs and Trade

GMO	genetically modified organism
HFCS	high fructose corn syrup
IBT	International Brotherhood of Teamsters
IFAD	International Fund for Agricultural Development
IFOAM	International Federation of Organic Agriculture Movements
ILO	International Labour Organization
IMF	International Monetary Fund
IPC	International Planning Committee
IPHAN	National Institute of the Historical and Artistic Heritage
IUCN	International Union for Conservation of Nature
KKPKP	Kagad Kach Patra Kashtakari Panchayat
LDA	London Development Authority
MDGs	Millennium Development Goals (United Nations)
MSAWPA	Migrant and Seasonal Workers Protection Act
MSC	Marine Stewardship Council
NAFTA	North American Free Trade Act
NAWS	National Agricultural Workers Survey
NGO	nongovernmental organization
NLRA	National Labor Relations Act
NRCS	National Resources Conservation Service
NSS	Native Seeds/Search
OCA	Organic Consumer Association
OCIFS	Oneida Community Integrated Food Systems
ORBCRE	Ohio River Basin Consortium for Research and Education
OSHA	Occupational Safety and Health Administration
PARI	PARI Development Trust (Bangladesh)
PETA	People for the Ethical Treatment of Animals
PI	Peoples' Institutions
RCCQ	*Regroupement des Cuisines Collectives du Québec* (Quebec Collective Kitchens Association)
RWDWU	Retail, Wholesale, and Department Store Workers Union
SAGARPA	Secretary of Agriculture, Cattle Ranching, Rural Development, Fisheries, and Food (Mexico)
SARE	Sustainable Agriculture Research and Education
SAREP	Sustainable Agriculture Research and Education Program
SATIIM	Sarstoon-Temash Institute for Indigenous Management (Belize)
SCS	Soil Conservation Service
SFMNP	Senior Farmers Market Nutrition Program
SNDTWU	Shreemati Nathibai Damodar Thackersey Women's University (India) (SNDT)
SPCA	Society for the Prevention of Cruelty to Animals
SSHRC	Social Sciences and Humanities Research Council
STNP	Sarstoon-Temash National Park
TCM	Traditional Chinese Medicine
TFPC	Toronto Food Policy Council
TNAFA	Traditional Native American Farmers Association
UFCW	United Food and Commercial Workers
UFW	United Farm Workers [Union]

UNAC	National Farmer's Union of Mozambique
UNCTAD	United Nations Committee on Trade and Development
UNESCO	United Nations Educational, Scientific, and Cultural Organization
UNICEF	United Nations Children's Fund
UPA	urban and peri-urban agriculture
UPWA	United Packinghouse Workers of America
USDA	U.S. Department of Agriculture
UFCW	United Food and Commercial Workers
WHY	World Hunger Year
WIC	Special Supplemental Nutrition Program for Women, Infants, and Children (U.S. Nutritional Assistance Program)
WTO	World Trade Organization
WWF	World Wildlife Fund for Nature

PART I

Society

1

Roots and Roles of Alternative Agrifood Systems

Patricia Allen

The current agrifood system is in crisis in many dimensions and in many places. Impoverished farmers in India harvest meager rice crops because a Coca-Cola plant draws water the farmers formerly used to irrigate their fields. Children in Haiti eat cookies made of dirt because there is nothing else. Residents of the U.S. Midwest shop at stores and eat at restaurants of numbing sameness because the local merchants have all gone out of business.

These conditions and experiences—different as they are in geography and urgency—have been in the making for a long time, as have the efforts to change them. Today the scope and depth of the crisis has given rise to a new level of action and organizing to create sustainable food systems for everyone. In this chapter, I briefly lay out some of the key environmental and social problems in the agrifood system, discuss the roots of the alternative agrifood movement, and highlight the efforts being made to address agrifood problems.

PROBLEMS IN AGRIFOOD SYSTEMS

Modern agrifood systems have developed based on intensive resource use and social inequalities. Despite advances in science, technology, and reform efforts, people go hungry, resources are depleted, toxins enter the food chain, and food-related health problems intensify. Never before have such conditions combined to create the degree of social and environmental crisis that the world faces today. These issue areas are interconnected. For example, global climate change in the future will likely exacerbate environmental problems associated with agriculture. Weather predictability may decrease, sea levels may rise, and agricultural zones may shift. The impacts of these changes may lead to an even more skewed distribution of food resources between the rich and poor. Climate change has the potential to disproportionately affect agriculture in the global south, where most of the world's poor live.

Food Security

No other product is as essential as food. Everyone—regardless of age, gender, ethnicity, or social class—needs to eat in order to live. Yet, the food system has done a poor job of meeting the food needs of everyone. Food security, which involves both quantity and quality of food, occurs when all people are able to obtain sufficient, nutritionally adequate, and culturally acceptable food through nonemergency sources. Yet many people are not food secure.

Hunger is a growing problem—more people go hungry today than at any point in history. The Food and Agriculture Organization of the United Nations (FAO) tells us that 854 million people worldwide are chronically hungry, that 820 million of these people live in the developing world, and that a quarter of these hungry people are children.[1] Every year that hunger continues at current levels costs the lives of 5 million children. Put into perspective, this is the equivalent of ten thousand jumbo jet crashes each year, each crash with one hundred percent fatality. For the living hungry, it is not possible to have healthy, productive lives. Hungry children face stunted physical and cognitive development as well as acute and chronic health problems.

While those at greatest risk of hunger are women and children living in rural areas of Asia, Africa, and Latin America, many people in affluent nations also go hungry, where safety nets for low-income people are becoming tattered. For example, in the United States, the world's largest producer of food, nearly 36 million people were food insecure in 2006.[2] Hunger is not democratic—those most likely to be food insecure are those living in single-mother-headed households, African Americans, Latinos, the elderly, the disabled, and children. Many low-income people pay higher prices for their food, and food insecurity has been exacerbated in recent years because of the recent spike in foreclosures, increased cost of food, and increased cost of living in general. Throughout the world, more and more emergency food centers are being established to feed people, but the demand is so great that many people do not receive the assistance they need. In 2008, nearly all U.S. food banks and pantries reported an increase in the number of people seeking assistance, and most needed to reduce the amount of food they were able to distribute.

Both food insufficiency and food overabundance are major public health issues. Diseases easily treated in the industrial world, such as measles or dysentery, can kill undernourished children; undernutrition is a contributing cause to more than half of all childhood deaths.[3] For many, it is not lack of food, but too many calories that is the problem. More than 1 billion adults globally are overweight and at least 300 million of them are obese.[4] The percentage of overweight adults has more than doubled since the mid-1970s to 33 percent, and the increase is even more dramatic for children and teens. Overweight and obesity increase the risk of many diseases and health conditions, such as high blood pressure, arthritis, type 2 diabetes, heart disease, stroke, gallbladder disease, sleep apnea and respiratory problems, and some cancers.[5] For the two-thirds of Americans who neither smoke nor drink excessively, food choices influence long-term health prospects more than any other factor.[6] Overweight and physical inactivity account for more than three-hundred thousand premature deaths in the United States each year, second only to deaths related to tobacco use.[7]

Food safety scares have become regular news items, and millions of people are affected each year. The incidence of food-borne diseases is increasing worldwide due, in part, to the globalization of the food supply and chain of custody issues. The contamination often happens because of the large scale of food production and processing, with the food changing hands many times before it gets to our tables. In the meat industry, one cause of the proliferation of pathogens is the subtherapeutic use of antibiotics to increase rates of growth in livestock. This reduces the efficacy of antibiotics for fighting disease in both livestock and humans, as the pathogens develop resistance to the antibiotics. Pesticides are another source of food contamination. Even babies are exposed to pesticides and other toxins though umbilical cord blood. One study found 287 chemicals in cord blood, most of which can cause cancer, birth defects, hormone disruption, and infertility, or compromise the immune system.[8] Pesticides are also a major source of environmental degradation.

Environment

The discovery of insecticides based on synthetic organic compounds around the time of World War II greatly increased the use and consequences of pesticides in agriculture. In a very short time, they were being used on almost every crop in most countries of the world.[9] Any increased application of pesticides carries the possibility of intensifying future needs for more chemical toxins, as pests develop resistance to standard preparations. While pesticide use in the United States increased 1,000 percent between the 1940s and the 1980s, crop losses to insect pests also increased by almost 50 percent.[10] Less than 1 percent of pesticides applied in the United States actually reach the pests to which they are targeted, but pesticides end up in the bodies of wildlife or the water people drink. Agriculture is the primary cause of species endangerment in the United States, especially mammals and amphibians. Pollution from agriculture is also a major contributor to water-quality problems in U.S. surface and groundwater through agrichemical run-off and sediment deposition. Pesticide contamination can remain long after the compound is no longer used. In California, for example, the long-banned pesticide DBCP (1,2-Dibromo-3-chloropropane), one of the most potent carcinogens known, still contaminates the water of one million Californians at levels that are almost three hundred times the "safe" level for infants and children.[11]

In addition to resource degradation, resource depletion is a major problem. Approximately one-third of the original topsoil has been removed from U.S. crop-land in the past 200 years, and much of U.S. cropland erodes at rates that exceed government-established tolerance levels. The extensive use of groundwater for irrigation has meant that declining water tables have become common throughout the world. Resource depletion and degradation have caused the abandonment or threatening of farming systems because of groundwater depletion, soil salinization, and unmanageable pest problems caused by pesticide use. Worldwide, degradation of agricultural land is causing an irretrievable loss of an estimated six million hectares per year. Increasing demand for meat is a major cause of deforestation: 70 percent of deforested Amazonian rainforests have been cleared to create grazing lands for livestock. Livestock are also major contributors to global climate change, generating, for example, more greenhouse gases than all forms of transportation combined. Environmental degradation and global climate change will dramatically affect people's livelihoods in the agrifood system. For the many poor people in the system, their livelihoods are already tenuous.

Livelihoods

The modern agrifood system embodies and has depended on extremely unequal material and social relations among groups of people. For example, landless migrant farmworkers do most of the labor in the food system, for which they often are poorly paid and work in dangerous conditions. In the United States, farmworkers have the lowest family income of any occupation surveyed by the U.S. Bureau of the Census; half of these families live below the poverty line. Most of these workers are employed by the less than 2 percent of farms with the highest sales. Many farmworkers do not have adequate housing, and many still work without access to restrooms or fresh drinking water, although access to these so-called amenities was a central goal of labor-organizing efforts as far back as the early 1900s. Jobs in the farm fields are often seasonal and transitory, and this is also becoming the trend in the new flexible labor economy for those who work in food processing, retail, and service. Workers in produce and meat-processing industries are often poorly paid, seasonally terminated, receive no benefits, and work under miserable conditions. Many of these workers are new immigrants who have little bargaining power or other employment options.

One of the reasons that workers have so few options is that land ownership is so highly concentrated worldwide. In the United States, for example, only 5 percent of American landowners own 80 percent of the land and reap the lion's share of agricultural subsidies. Although many agrifood workers are doing poorly, many agrifood companies are doing well, primarily through acquisition of other companies and cornering the market. A handful of companies control global trade and retail in agrifood products. Similarly, only three companies dominate the food service industry. For many years, farmers' share of the food dollar has been decreasing. Food is becoming increasingly distant from the point of production, with the result that farmers are getting a decreasing share of the money people spend on food. Much of the price of food in the market goes toward packaging, transportation, processing, and advertising.[12]

Worker safety is also a livelihood issue. Agriculture is among the top three most dangerous industries for workers in the United States. Farmworkers are at risk from fatal or disabling injuries from machinery, falls, and livestock. Exposure to pesticides can cause acute illnesses, such as respiratory conditions and flu-like symptoms, as well as chronic conditions, such as cancer and Parkinson's disease. Injuries and illnesses are compounded by lack of adequate health care among farmworker populations.

These issues with food security, environment, and livelihoods have led people throughout the world to organize for better conditions and social systems. For the alternative agrifood movement, the focus is on creating new policies and practices to make the agrifood system more ecologically sound and socially just.

ROOTS OF THE ALTERNATIVE AGRIFOOD MOVEMENT

The alternative agrifood movement is a constellation of multiple movements that have grown from early engagements and concerns about the agrifood system dating back to the 1800s.[13] Social movements are collective efforts of people to change what they perceive to be a society-wide problem. For ordinary people who do not control major economic resources or have access to formal political power, social movements are a primary form of power. This section describes agrifood-related social movements in the areas of food security, environment, and livelihood.

Food Security

Because food is basic to all of us, it is unsurprising that movements for healthy and safe food have a long history. The integrity of the food supply and dietary rec-ommendations have been public issues for a long time. As early as the 1830s, vege-tarians protested public health recommendations for a heavily meat-based diet; and at the end of the nineteenth century, consumers protested the food adultera-tion that had become part of the industrialization of the food system. Upton Sinclair's 1906 graphic account of the meat-packing industry in his novel, *The Jungle*, caused an outcry that led to regulations aimed at improving food safety and controlling fraud. Today, in Europe and the United States, food safety problems and the development of bioengineered crops have led to active and growing move-ments to solve food safety problems and stop genetically modified organisms from entering the food supply.

The issue of hunger was first put on the international agenda in 1933, but it was not until the early 1970s that the term *food security* was coined in response to the world food crisis of the early 1970s. At that time, prices of staple foods soared, much as they have today. Food security became a clear and central policy goal of most developing countries as the 1974 World Food Conference proclaimed peo-ple's inalienable right to freedom from hunger and resolved to completely elimi-nate hunger and malnutrition.

In the 1980s, many people's economic conditions worsened in affluent nations. Low-income people lost ground they had gained, and many middle-class families joined the ranks of the poor. As a result, food security decreased. Despite these con-ditions, it was during this time that governments reduced social welfare programs. In the United States, the combination of deteriorating food security conditions, the insufficiency of private and public efforts to combat hunger, and the conceptual innovations at the international level led to the development of the concept of *community* food security in the 1990s. Community food security is an integrated approach that focuses not only on meeting people's food security needs, but also on a broad range of food-system issues, including farmland loss, agriculture-based pollu-tion, urban and rural community development, and transportation.

Environment

As early as the 1800s, the U.S. conservationist movement raised concerns about artificial fertilizers and soil depletion. As agricultural productivity began to decline dramatically in the early nineteenth century both in Europe and the

United States, technological efforts to overcome the constraints of nature included chemical and mechanical means, such as the development of artificial fertilizers and tillage equipment. These solutions, however, led to further natural resource problems and were widely recognized and criticized. In his *Lectures on Modern Agriculture* of 1859, the soil chemist Justus von Liebig considered the agricultural systems of the time to be forms of "robbery" in which the "conditions of the reproduction" of the soil were destroyed. American economist Henry Carey wrote in 1858 that "Man is but a tenant of the soil, and he is guilty of a crime when he reduces its value for other tenants who are to come after him."[14] George Perkins Marsh, one of the first Americans to understand that the condition of the land was as much a product of humanity as of nature, rejected the older idea that nature existed to be tamed and conquered.[15] It was during this period that the American transcendentalist movement, based on a rejection of materialism, brought about a renewed interest in nature.

In the early part of the twentieth century, Sir Albert Howard observed the relationship between healthy soil and healthy crops in India. He eschewed the use of agrichemicals in farming, publishing the results of his work, *An Agricultural Testament*, in 1940. Around the same time, in 1932, J. I. Rodale, concerned about the relationship between agricultural practices and people's health, started *Organic Farming and Gardening* magazine to teach and promote organic techniques. Despite these earlier efforts, it was not until Rachel Carson's 1962 publication of *Silent Spring* that the environmental movement was galvanized into action around the environmental consequences of pesticides.

The organic farming movement, which advocates farming without the use of chemical pesticides and fertilizers, developed rapidly from this point. The International Federation of Organic Agriculture Movements (IFOAM), started in 1972, is now the worldwide umbrella organization for the organic movement, with 108 member nations. In 1973, the California Certified Organic Farmers organization was formed and continues to play a leading role in promoting both organic practices and certification. Interest in and activities around sustainable agriculture grew in the early 1980s, fueled by concerns about environmental issues in agriculture. A 1980 U.S. Department of Agriculture (USDA) report, *Report and Recommendations on Organic Farming*, sparked increasing interest in alternative agriculture because it showed that organic agriculture was an effective means of producing food.

Sustainability first emerged as a major concept in the 1980s, starting with the idea of sustainable development. Most development plans for alleviating poverty and hunger were based on models that involved increased depletion or degradation of natural resources. The 1987 publication of *Our Common Future* by the World Commission on Environment and Development catalyzed a new wave of thinking and action around merging priorities of the global north and south under the rubric of sustainability. The United Nations' Agenda 21, adopted at the Earth Summit in 1992, promoted sustainable agriculture and rural development as a plan for meeting food needs without further degrading natural resources. The 2002 World Summit on Sustainable Development continued on the path of raising awareness of connections between poverty and resource degradation.

Sustainability began to be applied to agriculture with the 1983 publication of Robert Rodale's "Breaking New Ground: The Search for a Sustainable Agriculture," which sought to expand the concept of organic agriculture. Eventually, terms such as "low-input agriculture," "ecological agriculture," and "organic farming" came to describe alternatives to industrial agriculture. The term "sustainable agriculture" has emerged as the standard, due in part to its acceptance by national and international agricultural agencies. A U.S. government report framed sustainable agriculture as the fourth major era in agriculture (following the horsepower, mechanical, and chemical eras), stating that the effects of this new era could be more profound than those of previous agricultural revolutions.[16]

Livelihood

The sustainable agriculture movement also builds on the agrarian populist movement, which addressed issues of the survival of family farms in an era of economic concentration that followed the Civil War. Agrarian populism was revived during the "back to the land" movement of the late 1960s, which defended the family farm and rural communities and opposed the technological, public policy, and market advantages that large-scale, industrial agriculture enjoyed over small-scale farming. Agrarian populism surged again as a result of the 1980s economic crisis for farmers. At this time, although U.S. farm production was at its highest level in history, 1982 was the worst year for farm income since 1932. Many farmers could not make ends meet and lost their farms.

To address international issues of farmer livelihoods and end hunger, the *food sovereignty* movement began in 1996, when the term was developed at the World Food Summit by the international peasant movement, Via Campesina. The movement asserts the right of all peoples to "safe, nutritious and culturally appropriate food" as well as access to sufficient land to produce it. The food sovereignty movement is not opposed to trade, but states that trade policies and practices should be in the service of people's right to have safe, healthy, and ecologically sustainable food production. In 2007, the World Social Forum convened more than 65,000 people from more than 100 countries to discuss the food issues of the poor and advocate for change in world trade policies. At the end of the meeting, a group that included farmers, landless laborers, and environmental and human rights advocates affirmed the need for food sovereignty—that people, rather than corporations, should determine international food policies, which should focus on meeting people's food and livelihood needs rather than maximizing profits.

The fair trade movement uses market-based approaches to achieve similar goals of ending poverty and promoting ecological sustainability. In this movement, organizations work with small-scale producers in developing countries to provide market access and fair prices for their products. Starting with coffee, cocoa, and bananas, the movement has expanded to include other products and the market for fair trade goods has been expanding by almost 50 percent a year. The USA Domestic Fair Trade Working Group has launched an effort, now piloted in several states, to bring fair trade practices to the United States by working to create a third-party-certified standard that would represent social justice criteria, including a living wage.

Movements for worker rights and safety are also longstanding. The earliest agricultural labor movements, of course, were the antislavery movements. During the Great Depression, these were followed by movements that focused on migrant workers. During the Civil Rights movement, Cesar Chavez and Dolores Huerta, coming out of backgrounds as community organizers, cofounded the National Farmworkers

Association, an interethnic coalition that worked toward farmworker justice and would later become the United Farm Workers (UFW) union. During the 1970s, consumers supported the union through a boycott of table grapes and head lettuce, which was designed to both protest pesticide residues on produce and to apply pressure for legislation that would give farmworkers the right to organize without threat of retaliation. Thus, the UFW was able to organize for justice among urban consumers as well as workers in the fields. Today, the Agricultural Justice Project promotes social standards to accompany environmental standards. The Coalition of Immokalee Workers has organized boycotts to apply pressure to increase wages for farmworkers and has worked with U.S. government agencies to free more than 1,000 farmworker slaves discovered working in America's farm fields.[17]

Over the years, the food security, environmental, and labor movements have brought about significant change in the agrifood system. Food safety laws, workers' rights to unionize, and conservation and antihunger programs were brought about by the collective actions of ordinary people working through social movements to solve social problems. Throughout human history, people organizing themselves through social movements have been the main driver of social and environmental advances.

ALTERNATIVE AGRIFOOD POLICIES AND PRACTICES

The power of social movements lies in their ability to take direct actions, develop new ways of doing things, and create new ways of thinking about the world. These movements create change by providing analyses of current problems, offering alternatives, and mobilizing people to act. This section describes how the alternative agrifood movement has worked through existing channels to change public policy and through civil society to develop new food institutions and practices.

Policy Changes Initiated by Alternative Agrifood Movements

International, national, and local policies are major determinants of problems and solutions in the agrifood systems. In general, international policies and agreements such as the World Trade Organization have large impacts on agricultural production and markets, as well as the global distribution of wealth and income. For example, the "structural adjustment" programs of the World Bank and the International Monetary Fund created severe hardships in developing countries, because they resulted in cuts in public services and stalled land reform programs.

National policies also can affect the global situation. For example, a key factor in the rapid increases in global food prices is the growing market for biofuels, supported by U.S. and European biofuel programs. In most countries, national policies have supported and subsidized the current agrifood system through the allocation of resources, research, technical assistance, and management of labor supply. In the European Union, the Common Agricultural Policy sets farm subsidies, tariffs, and quotas; in the United States, equivalent programs are authorized through the federal farm bill.

Recently, however, national policies have been adopted to support alternative agrifood systems, although the size of the resulting programs is small compared with those that support conventional agrifood systems. The USDA has established programs in both sustainable agriculture and community food security. Both of these programs—the Sustainable Agriculture Research and Education (SARE) and the Community Food Projects (CFP)—fund competitive grants. In Europe, the European Council is advocating agricultural sustainability and integrating environmental and sustainable rural development goals into the Common Agricultural Policy.

Citizens have been instrumental in the establishment of these types of alternative agrifood policies. For example, the largest public response the USDA had ever received was about the proposed federal definition of organic food. Many more people will become conversant in alternative agrifood systems (thereby increasing their ability to make change) through higher education as interdisciplinary alternative agrifood programs are being established at many colleges and universities. In the United States, for example, more than 150 American agricultural universities now have sustainable agriculture programs, while there were very few even a decade ago.

At the municipal level, many cities and counties are developing food policy councils. Although the purview of these councils varies, most focus on increasing local knowledge about agrifood problems and developing policies to solve them. Food policy councils are usually public-private partnerships that include representatives of multiple sectors of a region's food system. The membership of these councils typically includes representatives from farming, hunger-prevention, retail-food, nutrition-education, food-processing, sustainable-agriculture, religious, health, government, and environmental organizations. One of the oldest of these organizations, Canada's Toronto Food Policy Council, has developed a food policy for the city that establishes the right of all residents to adequate, nutritious food, and promotes food production and distribution systems that are equitable, nutritionally excellent, and environmentally sound. This council frames food security as a health issue in which hunger and poverty are viewed as part of the larger health issue, a perspective that sees access to food as not only equitable but economical.

In the United States, the millions of low-income families who participate in the Special Supplemental Nutrition Program for Women, Infants, and Children (WIC) soon will have access to healthier food. A new program, WIConnect, will enable households to purchase fresh fruits and vegetables, whole grains, and soy products, as well as provide foods with lower amounts of fat and sugar content. Many states have policies that work to improve nutrition, plant school gardens, support farm-to-school programs, and reduce environmental pollution from agriculture. For example, in 2001 California passed a healthy foods law that sets nutritional standards for elementary schools and promotes pilot programs to increase student nutrition. Such changes in public policy create the environment in which alternative agrifood practices can develop and flourish.

Practices Developed by Alternative Agrifood Movements

Alternative food initiatives such as organic farming, farmers markets, farm-to-school programs, local label schemes, urban agriculture and gardens, and community-supported agriculture (CSA) are becoming central strategies of those working to develop ecologically sound and socially just agrifood systems. As with policy change, these efforts are driven by ordinary people who are seeking to change the agrifood system for the better.

Farmers markets, for example, serve the needs of both farmers and consumers by providing a market outlet for small farmers and by increasing consumer access to fresh produce. In the 1970s, farmers markets were organized in urban low-income communities to provide nutritious food to the urban poor. They have provided accessible markets for producers outside of the mass market and have filled an important niche for consumers who seek fresh, high-quality food. These markets provide an important sales outlet for farmers whose production is too small to participate in the conventional marketing system. The number of farmers markets has increased rapidly in the United States in the past decade, and more are opening every year.

CSA is another approach that can provide small farmers with a market, while increasing access to fresh produce for consumers. In a CSA program, a group of consumers (shareholders or members) purchase shares at the beginning of the season with the idea that they will receive a portion of the crops produced that year. Consumers pay a fee to a grower and in return receive a weekly share of fresh produce, usually harvested the same day. In many cases, consumers travel to the farm to pick up their weekly box of produce; in others, farmers may deliver the boxes to a pickup location in the community. Consumers get fresher and more varieties of produce, and the farmer has a ready market and cash flow. The vision is that farmers and nonfarmers will work together to support each other and build strong community-based economies. Almost all CSA farms use organic production methods. Like farmers markets, the number of CSAs is growing year by year.

Institutional purchasing links local farmers with public institutions that purchase large volumes of food, such as colleges and schools. Such links provide significant market outlets for growers. For example, the school food services market alone is estimated at $16 billion per year. Alternative agrifood advocates have focused their efforts primarily on farm-to-school programs. Instigated by farmers, schools, parents, and community groups, these programs are intended to address two problems concurrently: childhood nutrition problems such as obesity and lack of access to markets for small and medium-size farms. The farm-to-school initiative joins school food services with local farmers in a partnership that is intended to bring fresher, healthier produce to school meal programs, while at the same time supporting local farmers by providing an additional source of income and a relatively secure market. Farm-to-school programs may include salad bars with farm-fresh fruits and vegetables purchased at the local farmers market. In one case, a cooperative of small farmers sells produce directly to the local school district. Farm-to-college projects are also growing, often as part of the overall campus sustainability movement. Many restaurants are buying and featuring local and organic foods on their menus. One of the newest restaurant trends is the concept of "pay what you can," which is based on the idea that everyone deserves good food, but not everyone can afford to pay the same price.

These institutional efforts to serve fresh, local food are part of an overall trend to support local farmers while providing healthier food and preserving local varieties. Active in more than one hundred countries, the Slow Food® movement organizes meals, food tastings, and festivals to promote the connection between "the plate and the planet," while supporting local and artisanal food producers. In the United States, "Buy Fresh, Buy Local" organizations are springing up across the states to promote the idea of consumers supporting their local farmers. These efforts have been successful. For example, in Kansas, the Good Natured Family Farmers Cooperative, selling through a group of locally owned and operated super-markets, showed a 36 percent increase in local food sales since the chapter's inception in 2004.

In addition to these kinds of marketing initiatives that are facilitating the growth of alternative agrifood systems, changes are happening at the level of production. The number of farmers who use ecological production methods such as organic farming practices has grown significantly in the past decade. Worldwide, some 26 million hectares are under certified organic production. In the United States, certified organic crop acreage quadrupled during the 1990s, and now more than 4 million acres in the United States are certified organic. Sales of organic food have kept pace, growing significantly each year, primarily in the European Union, Japan, and the United States. This growth in sales is facilitated by the increasing availability of organic food. Once available only in natural food stores, today, organic food is sold in three out of four conventional grocery stores. Sustainability is also being supported by the annual increase in sales of vegetarian and fair trade foods.

Urban agriculture—food production on residential plots, public or vacant private land, balconies, or rooftops within a metropolitan area—is also becoming more important as food prices rise. Already, one-seventh of the world's food supply is grown in cities by eight-hundred million urban farmers.[18] The amount of food that can be produced in gardens in the United States is substantial. Worldwide, an estimated $38 million worth of food is produced from urban plots.[19] In Cuba, where twenty-six thousand hectares are cultivated within cities, urban agriculture is credited with playing a big part in Cuba's recovery from the food crisis brought on by the collapse of the Soviet Union and the U.S. embargo.[20] Home gardens and community gardens can add variety, freshness, and beauty to people's food supply, provide an important source of nutrients crucial to overall health, and reduce food costs. This will become even more important for low-income people as food prices continue to rise and the emergency food system fails to keep up with demand. Examples include Lesotho's "keyhole gardens"—small raised round garden beds surrounded by large rocks—that help hungry families survive. These gardens are also ecologically sound: the stonework protects the soil from erosion and drought in a windy, dry landscape.

CONCLUSION

The triumph of modern, industrial agriculture has been its ability to produce vast amounts of agricultural products. However, this has not solved food security problems in either the developing or industrial world, and this productivity has been at the expense of environmental quality. Food prices have risen 40 percent on average globally since mid-2007. The dramatic increase in food costs has led to increased hunger everywhere and food riots in a number of countries. For decades, people have been organizing to resolve agrifood issues. Most recently, a number of these efforts have coalesced to form the alternative agrifood movement. This movement has been successful in drawing attention to agrifood issues, changing public policies, and developing new ways of farming and marketing that are more environmentally sound and socially just. These efforts are the beginning of a large-scale change that is required to provide food security for people worldwide and to halt agriculturally related environmental destruction. Every urban garden, every fair trade purchase, and every organic farm can be a step toward a more sustainable agrifood system. To-gether with collective action and policy changes, these individual choices can cre-ate a food system that will provide healthy food for the children of the future.

NOTES

1. FAO (Food and Agriculture Organization of the United Nations), *The State of Food Insecurity in the World 2006: Eradicating World Hunger—Taking Stock Ten Years after the World Food Summit* (Rome: FAO, 2006), http://www.fao.org/docrep/009/a0750e/a0750e00.htm (accessed August 4, 2008).

2. Mark Nord, Margaret Andrews, and Steven Carlson, *Measuring Food Security in the United States: Household Food Security in the United States, 2006*, Economic Research Report No. (ERR-49) (Washington, DC: U.S. Department of Agriculture, 2007).

3. WFP (United Nations World Food Programme), *World Hunger Series 2007: Hunger and Health* (Rome: WFP, 2007).

4. WHO (World Health Organization), *Obesity and Overweight* (Geneva: WHO, 2008), http://www.who.int/dietphysicalactivity/publications/facts/obesity/en (accessed April 25, 2008).

5. CDC (Centers for Disease Control and Prevention), *Overweight and Obesity* (Atlanta: CDC, 2008), http://www.cdc.gov/nccdphp/dnpa/obesity (accessed April 25, 2008).

6. U.S. Department of Health and Human Services, Public Health Service, *The Surgeon General's Report on Nutrition and Health*, DHHS [PHS] Publication No. 88-50210 (Washington, DC: U.S. Government Printing Office, 1988).

7. CDC (Centers for Disease Control and Prevention), *Obesity Epidemic Increases Dramatically in the United States: CDC Director Calls for National Prevention Effort* (National Center for Chronic Disease Prevention and Health Promotion, 2000), http://www.cdc.gov/media/pressre/r991026.htm (accessed April 23, 2009).

8. EWG (Environmental Working Group), *Environmental Speaker Sheds Light on Toxins* (Washington, DC: EWG, 2008), http://www.ewg.org/node/26094 (accessed April 25, 2008).

9. Gordon R. Conway and Jules N. Pretty, *Unwelcome Harvest: Agriculture and Pollution* (London: Earthscan Publications Ltd., 1991).

10. David Pimentel et al., "Environmental and Economic Impacts of Reducing U.S. Agricultural Pesticide Use," *Bioscience* 41, no. 6 (1991): 402–9.

11. Environmental Working Group, "Tap Water in 38 Central California Cities Tainted with Banned Pesticide: Some Bottle-Fed Infants May Exceed 'Safe' Dose before Age 1," EWG California Policy Memorandum (Washington, DC: EWG, 1999), http://www.ewg.org/files/dbcp.pdf (accessed August 4, 2008).

12. Hayden Stewart, *How Low Has the Farm Share of Retail Food Prices Really Fallen?* Economic Research Report Number 24 (Washington, DC: USDA, 2006), http://www.ers.usda.gov/publications/err24/err24.pdf (accessed April 20, 2008).

13. For a comprehensive history of the movement, see Patricia Allen, *Together at the Table: Sustainability and Sustenance in the American Agrifood System* (University Park: Pennsylvania State University Press, 2004).

14. Ibid.

15. Benjamin Kline, *First Along the River: A Brief History of the U.S. Environmental Movement* (Oxford: Acada Books, 2000).

16. U.S. General Accounting Office, *Sustainable Agriculture: Program Management, Accomplishments, and Opportunities*, GAO/RCED-92-233 (Washington, DC: U.S. Government Printing Office, 1992).

17. In several federally prosecuted cases of tomato pickers in Florida, farmworkers were found to have been chained up, beaten, forced into debt-servitude, and charged rent for living in trailers with 8 to 10 other workers. In April 2007, the Coalition of Immokalee Workers negotiated an agreement with McDonald's and Yum! Brands (owner of Pizza Hut, Taco Bell, and KFC) in which the fast-food giants have agreed to pay a penny more per pound to workers harvesting tomatoes. For more information, see CIW (Coalition of Immokalee Workers), *U.S. Senate Hearing into Farmworker Exploitation in Florida Tomato Fields* (Immokalee, FL: CIW, 2008), http://www.ciw-online.org/Senate_hearing.html (accessed October 28, 2008).

18. Jac Smit, Annu Ratta, and Joe Nasr, *Urban Agriculture: Food, Jobs, and Sustainable Cities* (New York: United Nations Development Programme, 1996).

19. Paul Sommers and Jac Smit, *Promoting Urban Agriculture: A Strategy Framework for Planners in North America, Europe and Asia*, Cities Feeding People Report 9 (Ottawa: International Development Research Centre, 1994).

20. Peter M. Rosset, "Cuba: Alternative Agriculture during Crisis," in *New Partnerships for Sustainable Agriculture*, ed. Lori Ann Thrupp (Washington, DC: World Resources Institute, 1996), 64–74.

RESOURCE GUIDE

Suggested Reading

Allen, Patricia. *Together at the Table: Sustainability and Sustenance in the American Agrifood System.* University Park, PA: Pennsylvania State University Press, 2004.

Allen, Patricia, ed. *Food for the Future: Conditions and Contradictions of Sustainability.* New York: John Wiley and Sons, 1993.

Belasco, Warren James. *Appetite for Change: How the Counterculture Took on the Food Industry, 1966–1988.* New York: Pantheon Books, 1989.

Carson, Rachel. *Silent Spring.* Boston: Houghton Mifflin, 1962.

Gottlieb, Robert. *Environmentalism Unbound: Exploring Pathways for Change.* Boston: MIT Press, 2001.

Guthman, Julie. *Agrarian Dreams: The Paradox of Organic Farming in California.* Berkeley: University of California Press, 2004.

Lappé, Frances Moore, and Anna Lappé. *Hope's Edge: The Next Diet for a Small Planet.* New York: Tarcher/Penguin Publishing, 2002.

Nestle, Marion. *Food Politics: How the Food Industry Influences Nutrition and Health.* Berkeley: University of California Press, 2002.

Poppendieck, Janet. *Sweet Charity? Emergency Food and the End of Entitlement.* New York: Penguin Books, 1998.

Schlosser, Eric. *Fast Food Nation: The Dark Side of the All-American Meal.* Boston: Houghton-Mifflin, 2001.

Web Sites

The Center for Agroecology and Sustainable Food Systems, http://casfs.ucsc.edu.

Coalition of Immokalee Workers/Coalición de Trabajadores de Immokalee/Kowalisyon Travaye nan Immokalee, http://www.ciw-online.org.

Farm Labor Organizing Committee, AFL-CIO, http://www.floc.com.
Food and Agriculture Organization of the United Nations, http://www.fao.org.
Food First/Institute for Food and Development Policy, http://www.foodfirst.org.
Institute for Agriculture and Trade Policy, http://www.iatp.org.
International Food Policy Research Institute, http://www.ifpri.org.
Pesticide Action Network North America, http://www.panna.org.
Small Planet Institute, http://www.smallplanet.org.
World Food Programme, http://www.wfp.org.

2

Alternative Food Market Governance: Current Research and Unanswered Questions

E. Melanie DuPuis

The failure of movements to transform the modern economic system, from the decline of cooperative organizations, the welfare state, and 1960s radicalism to the fall of the Berlin Wall, has led many social change activists to abandon strategies to reform conventional institutions. Instead, many new social-change visionaries embraced the creation of "alternative" economies, essentially parallel sets of institutions that remake the economic relationships between certain sets of producers and consumers. Today these alternative worlds include the art and journalistic institutions that are part of the youth-based "indie" movements, "open space" and other nonmainstream forms of computing, alternative energy development, and alternative healing practices often linked to new spiritual movements. In the United States, where government solutions have always been mistrusted, social movement actors have been the main organizers of these alternative economies, emerging in part from the "opt out" movements of the 1960s, particularly the creation of new (often farm-based) communities that eventually evolved into new localist communitarian movements. In contrast, the establishment of alternative market institutions in Europe has become part of European Union rural development policy.

The most evident and developed form of alternative economy, and the one that has been most studied by social scientists, is the alternative food movement. Transforming and diversifying modern food provisioning in Western Europe, North America, and many other parts of the world, social change actors have created new economic and cultural spaces for alternative food markets, whose products—organic, fair trade, local, and quality foods—are different from those typically furnished by mainstream food manufacturers and retailers. These new alternative markets are particularly diverse, involving many types of outlets and strategies, the dynamics of which are poorly understood. Therefore, several social scientists are now studying community-supported agriculture (CSA), fair trade, and other alternative food market institutions to answer the question: "What makes these markets work?" This chapter will provide an overview of current research on alternative food economies. More than a decade of such research has yielded valuable insight into how alternative economic systems work. Added to this will be a few anecdotal examples from the author's own work with local food policy organizations in Upstate New York and on the Central California Coast.

Mainstream economics tend to see efficient markets as "free"—that is, private and asocial, moving buyers and sellers beyond the strictures of bureaucratic regulation or social norms. However, other social scientists have shown that no market functions without set rules of behavior.[1] From this perspective, markets simply do not exist outside of social contexts. Society sets the rules and procedures by which markets work. These rules are commonly referred to as market governance.

Social science research has expanded the understanding of market governance in general and alternative food markets in particular, especially organic markets. Drawing on this research, as well as personal experience, this section provides an overview of some basic social science insights on alternative market governance, as well as unanswered questions about this new form of exchange. As this overview will demonstrate, social scientists agree that alternative food markets tend to be even more embedded in social and political relationships than conventional markets are.[2]

THE NATURE OF GOVERNANCE

Governance is "the inter-firm relationships and institutional mechanisms through which non-market co-ordination of activities in the [marketing or 'value'] chain is achieved."[3] In other words, "markets" here do not necessarily mean just buyers and sellers; they are networks of actors that affect the "non-market co-ordination" involved in the exchange of commodities along the "value chain," including government, nongovernmental organizations (NGOs), business and citizen activists, and other consumers, organized or not. Needless to say, some actors in these networks are more powerful than others. Some social scientists study the unequal power relationships in alternative marketing systems, in particular, pointing to the control or power that large buyers have over the system, enabling them to gain most of the value (profit) from the system.[4] In particular, they note the increasing supermarket control of food purchasing, which enables these actors to have increasing control over value and profits.[5] Ten large food retailers are responsible for half of all food sold in the United States today, and these large economic actors are increasingly calling the shots in the purchase of fresh produce.[6] Studies of alternative market governance, therefore, involve a focus on issues of power, both economic and political.

Other social scientists have studied the ability of alternative food economies to provide some countervailing power to less-powerful actors in the conventional value chain, particularly farmers and consumers.[7] This effort is probably most prominent in European Union rural development policy.[8] EU policy sometimes involves enabling smaller organic producers to maintain their access to the conventional value chain (e.g., to regain the ability to sell to supermarkets). In other cases, the approach is to focus on selling to alternative market niches, helping those with smaller farms develop strategies to make these niche markets work for them. Strategies, however, require information and understanding of these alternative markets. This understanding of alternative markets tends to assume that market niches are "out there" simply waiting for someone to discover them. The current perspective also tends to see actors in the chain as involved primarily in a private set of bilateral—one-on-one—interactions to meet predetermined, private demands.

In fact, alternative marketing strategy is more than just a matter of producers discovering a group of consumers waiting for a new kind of cheese or carrot. The market governance perspective sees markets as a dynamic process based on social interaction. A number of recent studies of organic and alternative agriculture have found that these alternative governance systems are more "civic" in nature than conventional markets. For example, Thomas Lyson, Neva Hassenein, and Michael Bell have shown that alternative agriculture is a dynamic, interactive process that relies on civic engagement.[9] If one looks at alternative agriculture from a market governance perspective, one can also argue that alternative marketing strategies will always include public deliberation and that the vitality and growth of these markets will always depend on democratic engagement. Invisibility, loss of voice, lack of transparency, and the breakdown of public discussion (and even a degeneration in the belief in "the public" itself) will undermine civic markets as alternative economies. The creation of alternative markets therefore involves negotiations over the way commodities are made and sold, and "supply" and "demand" is the mutually constituted product of these interactions. Civic markets are those that are created through an open and public conversation. It makes sense, therefore, to think of market governance in alternative agriculture in terms of "civic markets."

The idea that civic engagement is a part of market governance combines two major sociological perspectives. First are the notions of civic engagement most prominently put forth by Robert Putnam and Robert Bellah.[10] Second is the research of social scientists who have shown that markets are "embedded"—that is, they are creations of their particular social and political context. The creation of market governance rules is therefore a social activity. Social scientists talk about civic engagement as part of "discursive democracy" that requires a "public sphere," a social arena in which people discuss possible social rules, including market rules, and implement them.[11] Studies of markets as part of the public sphere tend to look at who wins and who loses, as well as who is included and who is excluded, from the institution of particular market governance structures. In other words, social scientists are often interested in the fairness, or "social justice," of particular market governance systems. Needless to say, social scientists have found that markets formed through more democratic engagement tend to be fairer. Raynolds, for example, has shown that organic farmers in the less-developed world are often not equal participants in the creation of fair trade rules, which has affected their ability to maintain adequate incomes through these markets.[12]

The implication here is that civic engagement can create markets and that a number of potential markets can come out of civic processes. However, little research has looked closely at the ways in which producers and consumers engage in a public conversation about the rules around alternative markets. Further research on alternative markets could benefit from looking at studies of water and electricity markets as civic markets, with rules of transaction set through public processes that are participatory.[13]

Of course, new forms of private market contracting have also arisen, as farmers become producers of custom products for niche markets controlled by large food chains.[14] These are basically private contract systems that are arranged between individual actors. Civic markets, in contrast, describe the more public forms of exchange in which the rules are transparent and are generally open and negotiable by a larger group of buyers and sellers. One question yet to be answered is whether or not private niche markets for organic or other alternative foods could survive if the civic discourse around these foods disappeared. Could large-scale organic milk companies survive without activist civic discourse against genetically engineered food, for example?

Each alternative market has its own form of governance—that is, each follows a distinct set of rules, including rules for public deliberation. The civic dynamic of a particular alternative market affects how and whether these markets will grow and remain profitable. For example, a farmers market that simply protects founding members and excludes new members grows only as its current members expand their production. Another way to grow, however, is to admit new members who add new products or who expand the consumer choice of existing products. What makes farmers market decision-makers pursue one strategy or another? The answer to that question may depend on the power of various actors to implement their ideas about fairness in a particular alternative market. A farmers market run by founding producers, for example, may tend to be more exclusive, as founding members see the fairness in terms of the risks they took to create the market in the first place. In farmers markets where consumers have a voice, however, they are more likely to advocate for the greater inclusion of new members, in order to have greater choice.

Of course, what is fair and what is not fair is also something that gets discussed and decided on in the public sphere. People tend to disagree about what is fair and what is unfair. A set of market governance structures reflects a group of people who have agreed with each other about the fairness of the system enough to participate in this system, assuming they are not being coerced. Coercion does not always entail police power: when travelers stop at a highway rest stop and cannot find what they consider to be healthy food, they may feel like they are being coerced to participate in the conventional economy of multinational fast food chains, although it is a "soft" coercion. Lack of alternatives can therefore be a form of coercion, and the creation of alternatives can be a form of agency.

ALTERNATIVE FOOD MARKETS

The rest of this chapter will review a number of current alternative food markets, and talk a bit about the governance structures of these markets and how these market rules are the product of particular civic interactions. These social contexts are the product of particular agreements between buyers and sellers in the public, civic sphere. These agreements have their own embedded controversies, their own ways in which fairnesses and unfairnesses arise. The extent to which each of these alternative markets expands is to a great extent dependent on whether or not buyers and sellers find them worth participating in because they offer a better—or what they perceive to be a fairer—deal.

Community-Supported Agriculture

CSA involves a direct relationship between farmer and consumer in which consumers agree to pay for a season's worth of produce in return for what is usually a weekly box of produce provided by the farmer over that season. Most of the rules around CSA membership are based on a private contract between two parties. However, these contracts often involve rules of behavior that affect the entire membership of the CSA. Those rules are often set by the grower or informally between the grower and the members of the CSA. In addition, according to the report "CSA Across the Nation," 28 percent of all CSAs have a kind of governing board, generally called a Core Group.[15] Therefore, consumer and producer membership depends not just on the writing of a check, but also on creating and following social rules and obligations of membership.

Some of these rules are part of a contract between the member and the farmer. Others tend be more informal. For example, according to the CSA report mentioned above, more than three-quarters of all CSAs put together member events that go beyond the provision of produce, such as festival days, farm tours, and so on. Although these events are not part of the contract, if the farmer of a CSA in New York, for example, cancelled her strawberry festival without explanation, she would get an earful from her members.

More formal CSA rules often involve things like whether or not a member is expected to put in labor hours on the farm or at the pickup points. Specific rules often are established to regulate behavior for members at pickup points, in terms of maintaining cleanliness, controlling noise, and other things such as the ability to trade unwanted produce with others. The extent to which members follow the rules necessary to maintain the functioning of a CSA or other alternative market depends to a large extent on the social capital in the system.[16] One way that members try to expand trust in the system is to encourage a more inclusive approach to membership, so that people who cannot afford membership fees are subsidized by other members. Approximately half of the CSAs have a subsidized share program so that low-income families can participate as members.[17]

Social capital, enrollment, and issues of trust also are important in the relationship between consumer members and the producers in alternative economies. Farmers who do not feel supported by their members sometimes exit these systems. In particular, the financial aspects of landownership can be especially difficult for farmers. Member-farmer commitments to acquire land have also been a part of CSA governance in some cases. Because access to quality land is difficult and costly in many places, some CSAs have become increasingly involved in gaining access to land for the CSA farmer, and sometimes share in land costs. This involves another layer of rules of behavior—and relations of trust—between the consumer-landowners and the farmer.[18]

Another governance aspect of CSAs that have Core Groups actively involved in farm budget decisions is the issue of farmer salary. In these governance structures, the annual membership fee pays the farmer a collectively determined specific salary over the costs of growing. However, exactly what fee would maintain membership at what salary can be a constant source of worry. Many Core Groups cannot resolve such issues as health insurance, pension, and adequate salary at a reasonable membership cost. Many farmers remain committed to CSAs, despite the poor income and benefits. Clearly, health care and the need for a secure retirement are issues that farmers want to address with CSA members but often cannot.

In these various cases, decision-making, especially in those CSAs that do not have Core Groups, is often by "exit or voice." In other words, members "vote with their feet" and leave the CSA, or they choose to stay and make noise and hope the farmer listens. Farmers, in turn, if they cannot achieve their goals of health or income security or other management issues with members, also shut down their farms or move to other types of farm markets. In alternative markets with high trust, all members feel that they can express their concerns and get a fair hearing, even if the problem cannot be resolved. In addition, numerous smaller issues are a constant topic in newsletters (written by farmers or by Core Groups), with or without various forms of sanction ("please remember to . . . or we may no longer be welcome here as a pickup point next year").

More information needs to be collected on exactly how CSAs create and implement high-trust governance structures. The issue of whether or not to have a Core Group, and the extent to which that group has decision-making ability, continues to be a topic of conversation in relation to CSA governance.

Farmers Markets

The governance issues surrounding farmers markets are dauntingly large and generally not adequately understood. There has been very little generalized research around the governance structures of farmers markets, and this is a potentially rich field of study. In part, the richness comes from the sheer variety of rules—set by municipalities, business associations, and so on—that govern farmers markets. For example, some markets have rules about how far away a farm can be from the market (another issue to be addressed in the market localization section) and what can be sold. Others certify whether or not the farmers produce all the products they sell in the markets. Organic-only farmers markets rely primarily on a farm's organic certification for compliance with organic rules, but they may also certify the farm's "producer-only" status. Unlike CSAs, nearly all farmers markets have governing boards. The members of the market are the farmers, not the consumers, although consumers, along with local business members and others, are often members of the governing boards. As with CSAs, decisions about transparency, voice, honesty, inclusion, and exclusion have an effect on the extent of trust in a particular farmers market. In board-governed markets, board members have to assure both producers and consumers that rules are being followed and that they are fair. In many farmers markets, much of this responsibility rests with the farmers market director. But no comprehensive survey of how boards and directors create trust has been conducted.[19]

Farmers markets, like CSAs, are a form of food system relocalization, and the section on relocalization will continue the discussion of farmers markets.

Fair Trade and Other Ethical Marketing

Even though fair trade represents only a small fraction of the global economy, it is an arena of rapid civic markets development, in terms of production standards, prices, and the processes by which producers and consumers agree on these issues. The last ten years have seen the publication of some excellent social science research on fair trade markets.[20] This work can contribute to the understanding of alternative governance structures as civic process.

Fair trade markets generally develop their own unique market governance structures. Because "fairness" is the prevailing idea behind these markets, civic engagement is generally part of the process. Who decides and who benefits from a fair trade market, however, differs from one system to the next. In many cases, NGOs representing consumers determine what the rules of fairness will be, and then work with farmers who are willing to work within those rules. As recent studies[21] have shown, however, a "fair" market is not easy to define and is generally a topic of public conversation among actors in various fair trade commodity chains. Once again, actors participate through both voice and exit strategies; they either try to make a system that does not work for them more fair, or they leave the chain and participate in other markets. The extent to which nongovernmental actors make decisions that build trust has a great deal of influence on the maintenance and growth of these markets. Much of the research in this area has focused on whether fair trade actually helps farmers. Issues of market governance are only beginning to come to the fore, particularly in relation to coffee markets.

Civic Markets as Small and Artisanal Farm Support Policy

In some cases, especially in the European Union, alternative governance systems have worked to increase the access to markets to growers with small farms.[22] In addition, the European Union has initiated policies that enable greater market access to agriculturalists with small farms from the global south.[23] In other cases, EU policymakers have been interested in protecting artisanal and territorially based specialty food producers in Europe.[24] These are civic markets in that they involve public discussion about who deserves to participate in the EU market and what benefits they deserve from that participation. In general, the idea is to create new value chains in which actors (both consumers and producers) who have less power in conventional value chains are able to gain more power and therefore gain greater benefits from the system. These policies are meant to serve farmers in terms of gaining greater profits as well as consumers in terms of making a higher quality of food available.[25]

Some of these programs focus primarily on providing assistance to farmers to enter conventional markets, but other projects attempt to create new value chains that follow different market governance rules. These alternative value chains often meet up against government regulations, particularly those protective of sanitation. This is particularly true in the case of raw milk, artisanal cheeses, and other highly perishable products. Dairy grading, pricing, and market governance systems create different value chains out of milk. Not surprisingly, different chains enable vastly different forms of dairy production with different uses of natural resources as well.[26] British researchers Sonnino and Marsden have argued that the entry of large food retail companies as buyers of organic production has had a negative impact on alternative marketing channels.[27] One unanswered question is the extent to which civically engaged market governance processes hold the key to the survival of alternative markets that are threatened with private niche competition.

Market Localization Projects

It is almost a mantra among smaller organic farmers on the Central Coast of California to say that they are refocusing their marketing efforts to their local communities. These local marketing strategies are sometimes undertaken in the context of community support and often are organized through local food policy councils. Market strategy in California has historically been oriented toward out-of-state and export markets. The organic sector has been no exception, even for medium-size farms. However, even these midsize organic farmers in California speak of increasing difficulty finding conventional market outlets.

In response, many of these farmers state that they are turning to their local home markets to identify customers. In some cases, these farmers are now partici-pating more in farmers markets or have organized CSAs. However, many farmers markets no longer have space for new farmers, or the governance structure limits new entries. As a result, less formally organized farmers markets are on the rise, which along the Central Coast of California sometimes are referred to as "guerilla farmers markets." Some of these markets exist in neighborhoods, others may provide merely a private farm stand, and yet others are composed of a group of farmers for-mally organized in a marketing cooperative. These markets have a different gover-nance structure than the "certified" (e.g., by the State of California) farmers markets around town. In its cooperative form, farmers agree among themselves what they can sell and how they will sell their products. In certified markets, this is the provenance of a governing board made up of farmers, consumers, local nonprofits, and other participants. The guerilla market relies on a co-op membership agreement to maintain "producer-only" status, not certification from the state. In some cases, agreements are made between the co-op members to allow a member to sell the produce of another farmer (or a crafted food product, such as dried fruit or honey).

The number of private farm stands has also risen, particularly along Central Coast Route 1 in California, which has a great deal of tourist traffic. The market potential of these farm stands usually depends on access to property along a major travel route. The governance structure of these farm stands is probably the closest to "Wild West" standards. Hand-painted signs on the highway make claims about organic or "no spray" fruits and vegetables, although certification of these claims is often slim. The general governance system appears to be either community trust or, for the one-time tourist stop, "let the buyer beware." Farm stands, however, do fall under direct marketing regulations, which can include either state or county regulations.

Little research has been conducted on the social and political context in which these farm stand rules are created and implemented, the consistency of rules between regions, and the prevalence of other more formal or informal nonstate rules between farm stand sellers and buyers. However, these stands can fall under various rules about zoning and sanitation, and other city rules that apply to local businesses.

The lack of local alternative market access along the Central Coast of Califor-nia, because of the saturation of CSA, farm stands, and farmers markets, has led to new community-based efforts, led by coalitions of farmers and consumers organized in a food policy council, to create new local market opportunities. Like fair trade, social scientists have taken a critical look at food localization movements. These researchers argue that consumer movements concerned about injustice in the food system often see the relocalization of the food system as a cure-all for inequalities. In fact, local politics can be pretty unjust as well. Careful attention needs to be paid to governance structures and the types of processes by which people create and implement these structures, understanding that certain forms of governance may be more equitable than others. In a series of articles on this topic, David

Goodman and I argue that people have to approach these problems "reflexively"—that is, they need to be aware of potential unfairnesses in the ways decisions tend to get made. Although no process can be totally fair, constant and reflexive attention to issues of fairness is important, especially in situations in which people define "fair" differently.[28]

More research is needed on how these processes of relocalization take place on the ground, with real people in real places. For example, to encourage the growth of the local food system in an Upstate New York city, a food policy group (FPG) put on such events as local harvest festivals and CSA "sign-up days" for consumers to become members of established and new CSAs in the area. Formal rules were never established for the policy group to take on this responsibility, but its acceptance of responsibility for the growth and maintenance of CSAs in the area built trust among both consumers and producers (and between them). When groups of actors successfully carry out trust-creation activities, they can create a greater willingness among people to work with them to further other projects. Some social scientists talk about this kind of trust creation as "enrollment"; others see trust as a kind of economy in itself, with its own form of exchange, or capital, which they call "social capital."[29]

A local FPG in Santa Cruz County developed a kind of structured public discussion of local food issues that grew out of nonviolent communication strategies designed to promote inclusion and reflexivity as well as trust creation. During these food forums, structured public conversations give participants an equal chance to have their voices heard in a nonthreatening environment that encourages active listening and nonjudgmental behavior. Little change in local food system governance has emerged from these discussions, and the FPG is largely inactive at the moment, subsumed under the more active local food NGOs. The two food forums did create an impetus for certain actors to initiate new projects, such as farm-to-institution efforts. Yet, in a community saturated with food and farm NGOs, the FPG struggled to find an identity and mission that did not compete with more-established groups and their food policy missions.

Most communities, however, are more like the Upstate New York city, with no local food policy NGOs. In these places, the establishment of a local FPG can provide the main institutional umbrella under which projects to create local alternative markets are able to place.[30] FPGs vary greatly in their structure and activities from one place to the next. They can be organized by state, county, or city (or sometimes all three). Their missions can be different from one place to the next, with some groups more concerned about nutrition or local hunger issues than with the creation of alternative or local markets. In many cases, however, FPGs have taken as a main mission the expansion of local markets for local farmers. These projects usually are created in conjunction with consumers who are seeking to resolve a particular food issue they face in terms of lack of food choice. For example, many FPGs are involved in starting or assisting farm-to-school programs in which farmers provide produce directly to school cafeterias as a way to improve nutrition and to educate students about good eating.[31] Piecemeal communication between farmers and each school district, however, is resource intensive, and FPGs have attempted to provide an arena in which farm-to-institution efforts can be more effective. In Santa Cruz, the University of California–Santa Cruz Food Policy Working Group and other NGOs have created a consortium of farmers who provide the university with local organic food. It is expanding to work with a consortium of other local public institutions involved in institutional feeding.

Finally, the "Buy Fresh, Buy Local" advertising campaign has put a single brand face on the marketing of local food as a way to grow local alternative markets.[32]

In all of these situations, questions remain: Who will be responsible for setting up the rules of interaction between local consumers and local farmers? To what extent will these rules remain fractured between subgroups, and to what extent will that fracturing lessen the growth of the local food market?

Does an entirely devolved and local form of governance work, or are other scales of governance necessary for the creation of alternative markets? Daniel Block and I have looked at the history of local milk market orders as an example to understand the politics of scale in localization strategies. In local "milkshed" politics, the definition of what is a local market has been an intensely political decision. Historically, peri-urban farmers have vigorously defended their right to sell into city milk markets; in other words, they have defended their right to be defined as local.[33] For farmers attempting to preserve a highly risky and often marginal livelihood, the fact that some may have access to spaces in the local farmers market, while others do not, can lead to bitterness over what is a perceived injustice. Exactly how to create fair governance structures about access to limited farmers market spaces is one of the justice challenges faced by the food relocalization movement. In some cases, the following questions need to be answered: How does "local" get defined in relocalization efforts? Are the farmers who have access to the market representative of the diversity of farmers in the surrounding area? Or, do local market governance processes give access to certain less-than-representative groups of people? To what extent do founding members deserve to restrict access to protect their initial investment in what was originally a risky business venture?

Other questions that need to be asked about setting the rules of local food market governance are as follows: Who will have a say in this process? Will this commodity chain be, in the words of Gerry Gerrefi, consumer or producer driven?[34] Also, who will do the work, and will this work be conducted mainly by volunteers? Will consortiums of farmers work together or will relocalization mostly depend on the growth of individual CSAs selling to individual families? How will governance issues vary by community context? Also, importantly, who wins and who loses when particular market governance rules are put into place? For example, what happens to the farmers 101 miles away from a city that applies a 100-mile definition of "local" to its farmers market rules? In other words, the question of organic market growth at the local level is laden with governance issues that have not been adequately understood, much less resolved.

CONCLUSION

As this overview demonstrates, how market governance issues are resolved will have a significant effect on the future vitality and growth of alternative markets. Yet, this discussion has brought up many more questions than answers. Nonetheless, existing research on alternative markets leads to some tentative conclusions.

First, governance is not just a set of regulations. Governance is the process by which regulations are formed, the underlying formal (legal) and informal (community consensus) authority upon which the rules are based, who gets to form them, and how they are implemented. The social context "embedding" these markets is there-fore important and more attention needs to be paid to the civic interactions around organic markets to understand how and when they will grow and how and when civic processes and governance structures help or hinder organic market growth.

Second, fairness is an important issue in the creation of market governance structures. If people think governance is unfair, they may exit the system. Many people talk about food localization as the creation of networks of trust. However, as David Goodman and I have recently argued, "trust" tends to be "black-boxed"—that is, everyone talks about trust but no one ever says directly what trust is and how you can recognize it when it exists.[35] It is necessary to open up this box to understand the micropolitics of trust in local networks. Understanding mar-ket governance structures is one way to achieve this, to thereby understand how and when the rules of interaction are set in ways that allow fairness and trust.

In our interest to expand alternative markets, we need to recognize that the expansion alternatives will require the setting of market-expanding governance structures that will involve more public interaction between farmers and consum-ers. In many cases, the context for these civic interactions is place based, with local consumers working with local farmers to create new local markets. Unfortu-nately, for farmers, going that extra mile to schmooze with consumers can seem like yet another stress on an already overwhelmingly stress-filled life. Farmers who are interested in growing their local markets need to talk to each other to learn how to interact with local consumers in ways that are not only sane but efficient and perhaps pleasurable. Consumers need to figure out how to interact with farm-ers in ways that do not simply exhaust farmers. This may sound like an unimpor-tant point, but at many consumer-led local food policy meetings farmers, glassy-eyed with exhaustion, clearly wonder why they are in attendance. Consumers in these organizations often have day jobs, too, and personal lives. We need to come up with processes that create governance structures that are straightforward and easy, while being respectful of both diverse views and limited amounts of time.

As this overview shows, the dynamics of alternative food market structures are poorly understood. What current research shows is the extent to which these mar-kets are a product of social deliberation. It is clear that the vitality of organic mar-kets depends on maintaining its "civic" nature, its openness to ongoing public deliberation and decision-making. Otherwise, consumers will become doubtful as to why they are participating in alternative food markets.

In addition, the civic nature of alternative food markets makes them intrinsi-cally dynamic. A reflexive approach to alternative market governance enables market actors to maintain the civic dynamic necessary for the survival and growth of alternative food markets, as well as to maintain the continuing autonomy of these markets as "alternative" to the conventional system. Social scientists have contributed to reflexive civic processes by mapping out the dynamic alternative food market landscape. Much more, however, needs to be done.

NOTES

1. Douglas C. North, *Institutions, Institutional Change and Economic Performance* (Cambridge: Cambridge University Press, 1990); Ronald H. Coase, *The Firm, the Market and the Law* (Chicago: The University of Chicago Press, 1988); Oliver Williamson, *The*

Economic Institutions of Capitalism: Firms, Markets, Relational Contracting (New York: The Free Press, 1985); Mark Granovetter, "Economic Action and Social Structure: The Problem of Embeddedness," *American Journal of Sociology* 91 (1985): 481–510.

2. Thomas Lyson, *Civic Agriculture: Reconnecting Farm, Food and Community* (Boston: Tufts University Press, 2004); Laura B. de Lind, "Place, Work and Civic Agriculture: Common Fields for Cultivation," *Agriculture and Human Values* 19 (2002): 217–224. I was on the founding board of the Farm and Food Project in Albany, New York; I participated in the Core Group of my New York CSA; and I have more recently worked closely with the Santa Cruz County Food Policy Working Group and the University of California, Santa Cruz, Food Policy Working Group. These experiences have brought me into contact and interaction with numerous farmers, activists, extension agents, local entrepreneurs, and public officials involved in these efforts. I am fortunate to have lived in two vastly different places in terms of the dynamics of alternative food markets: my Upstate New York city had an active food-consumers co-op but in a local food producers "desert." I was part of a group of local citizens that created a Food Policy Group to create a local food system "from scratch." My current Santa Cruz County home has a concentration of alternative food NGOs and one of the highest percentages of organic farmland under cultivation of any county in the United States. Living in these places has provided me with tremendous opportunities to study the social context surrounding the governance of alternative food markets.

3. John Humphrey and Hubert Schmitz, *Governance in Global Value Chains* (Sussex, UK: Institute of Development Studies, University of Sussex, 2000); Raphael Kaplinsky and Mike Morris, *A Handbook for Value Chain Research* (Sussex, UK: Institute of Development Studies, University of Sussex, 2000).

4. Kevin Morgan, Terry Marsden, and Jonathan Murdoch, *Worlds of Food: Place, Power, and Provenance in the Food Chain* (Oxford: Oxford University Press, 2006).

5. Everard Smith and Terry Marsden, "Exploring the 'Limits to Growth' in UK Organics: Beyond the Statistical Image," *Journal of Rural Studies* 20, no. 3 (2000): 345–357.

6. Paul Kaufman, Charles Handy, and Roberta Cook, "The Changing Structure of Produce Buyers—Food Retailing and Wholesaling—and Implications for Suppliers," *Perishables Handling Quarterly* 103 (2000): 3–6.

7. Mark Lapping, "Toward the Recovery of the Local in the Globalizing Food System: The Role of Alternative Agricultural and Food Models in the US," *Ethics, Place and Environment* 7, no. 3 (2004): 141–150; Jack Kloppenburg, John Hendrickson, and G. W. Stevenson, "Coming into the Foodshed," *Agriculture and Human Values* 13, no. 3 (1996): 33–42.

8. Morgan, Marsden, and Murdoch, *Worlds of Food.*

9. Lyson, *Civic Agriculture*; Neva Hassanein, *Changing the Way America Farms: Knowledge and Community in the Sustainable Agriculture Movement* (Lincoln: University of Nebraska Press, 1999); Michael Bell, *Farming for Us All: Practical Agriculture and the Cultivation of Sustainability* (University Park: Pennsylvania State University Press, 2004).

10. Robert Putnam, *Bowling Alone: the Collapse and Revival of American Community* (New York: Simon and Schuster, 2001); Robert Bellah, *Habits of the Heart* (Berkeley: University of California Press, 1996).

11. Jurgen Habermas, "Three Normative Models of Democracy," *Constellations* 1 (1994):1–10; John Dryzek, *Discursive Democracy: Politics, Policy and Political Science* (Cambridge: Cambridge University Press, 1990).

12. Laura Raynolds, "Re-embedding Global Agriculture: The International Organic and Fair Trade Movements," *Agriculture and Human Values* 17 (2000): 297–309.

13. Carl Pechman, *Regulating Power: The Economics of Electricity in the Information Age* (Amsterdam: Kluwer, 1999); Brendt Haddad, *Rivers of Gold: Designing Markets to Allocate Water in California* (Washington, DC: Island Press, 2000).

14. Julie Guthman, *Agrarian Dreams: The Paradox of Organic Farming in California* (Berkeley: University of California Press, 2004).

15. Daniel Lass et al., "CSA across the Nation: Findings from the 1999 CSA Survey" (Madison: Center for Integrated Agricultural Systems, University of Wisconsin, 2003), http://www.cias.wisc.edu/pdf/csaacross.pdf.

16. "Social capital" describes the extra "wealth" possessed by individuals through their membership in social networks. Societies in which many people are members of many social networks are said to have higher social capital than those with fewer networks.

17. Ibid.

18. Steven McFadden, "The History of Community Supported Agriculture Part II: CSA's World of Possibilities," *New Farm* (2004), http://www.newfarm.org/features/0204/csa2/part2.shtml (accessed July 27, 2008).

19. Allison Brown, "Farmers' Market Research 1940–2000: An Inventory and Review," *American Journal of Alternative Agriculture* 17, no. 4 (2002): 167–176; Neil Hamilton, "Farmers Markets: Rules, Regulations and Opportunities," http://www.statefoodpolicy.org/.

20. Patricia Allen, *Together at the Table: Sustainability and Sustenance in the American Agrifood System* (University Park: Pennsylvania State University Press, 2004); Chris Bacon, "Confronting the Coffee Crisis: Can Fair Trade, Organic and Specialty Coffees Reduce Small-scale Farmer Vulnerability in Northern Nicaragua?" *World Development* 33 (2005): 497–511; Elizabeth Barham, "Towards a Theory of Values-based Labeling," *Agriculture and Human Values* 19 (2002): 249–260; Michael K. Goodman, "Reading Fair Trade: Political Ecological Imaginary and the Moral Economy of Fair Trade Foods," *Political Geography* 23 (2004): 891–915; Laura Raynolds, Douglas Murray, and Peter L. Taylor, "Fair Trade Coffee: Building Producer Capacity via Global Networks," *Journal of International Development* 16 (2004): 1109–1121; Aimee Shreck, "Resistance, Redistribution, and Power in the Fair Trade Banana Initiative," *Agriculture and Human Values* 22 (2005): 17–29. The Fair Trade Resource Network has an excellent list of research articles on fair trade: http://www.fairtraderesource.org/bib-journalarticles.html.

21. Ibid.

22. Perpetua McDonagh and Patrick Commins, "The Promotion and Marketing of Quality Products from Disadvantaged Rural Areas," End of Project Report, Project # 4485 (Brussels, Belgium: EU FAIR Programme, 2000). European Union studies and projects were mostly concerned with the expansion of markets for small "quality" food producers (generally producers of artisanal products like cheeses and wines) rather than organic producers.

23. Suzanne Friedberg, *Green Beans and Food Scares* (New York: Oxford University Press, 2004).

24. See, for instance, Elizabeth Barham, "Translating Terroir: The Global Challenge of French AOC Labeling," *Journal of Rural Studies* 19 (2003): 127–138; Terry Marsden and Everard Smith, "Ecological Entrepreneurship: Sustainable Development in Local Communities through Quality Food Production and Local Branding," *Geoforum* 36 (2005): 440–451.

25. E. Melanie DuPuis, David Goodman, and Jill Harrison, "Just Values or Just Value? Remaking the Local in Agrofood Studies," in *Between the Local and the Global: Confronting Complexity in the Contemporary Agri-Food Sector*, ed. Terry Marsden and Jonathan Murdoch (London: Elsevier, 2006), 241–268.

26. E. Melanie DuPuis and Daniel Block, "Sustainability and Scale: US Milk-market Orders as Relocalization Policy," *Environment and Planning* A 40, no. 8 (2008): 1987–2005.

27. Roberta Sonnino and Terry Marsden, "Beyond the Divide: Rethinking Relationships between Alternative and Conventional Food Networks in Europe," *Journal of Economic Geography* 6 (2006): 181–199.

28. C. Clare Hinrichs, "The Practice and Politics of Food System Localization," *Journal of Rural Studies* 19 (2004): 33–45; E. Melanie DuPuis and David Goodman, "Should We Go Home to Eat?: Toward a Reflexive Politics of Localism," *Journal of Rural Studies* 21 (2005): 359–371; DuPuis, Goodman, and Harrison, "Just Values or Just Value?"

29. Bruno Latour, *The Pasteurization of France* (Cambridge, MA: Harvard University Press, 1988); Putnam, *Bowling Alone*.

30. For an overview of Food Policy Councils, see publications by the Drake Agricultural Law Center: http://www.statefoodpolicy.org/.

31. Patricia Allen and Julie Guthman, "From 'Old School' to 'Farm to School': Neoliberalization from the Ground Up," *Agriculture and Human Values* 23 (2006): 401–415.

32. Patricia Allen and C. Clare Hinrichs, "Buying into 'Buy Local': Engagements of United States Local Food Initiatives," *Constructing "Alternative" Food Geographies: Representation and Practice*, ed. Damien Maye, Lewis Holloway, and Moya Kneafsey (Oxford: Elsevier, 2007), 255–272.

33. DuPuis and Block, "Sustainability and Scale."

34. Gary Gereffi, "The Organization of Buyer-Driven Global Commodity Chains: How US Retailers Shape Overseas Production," in *Commodity Chains and Global Capitalism*, ed. Gary Gereffi and Miguel Korzeniewicz (Westport, CT: Praeger, 1994), 95–122.

35. DuPuis and Goodman, "Should We Go Home to Eat?"

RESOURCE GUIDE

Suggested Reading

Allen, Patricia. *Together at the Table: Sustainability and Sustenance in the American Agrifood System*. University Park: Pennsylvania State University Press, 2004.

DuPuis, E. Melanie, and Daniel Block. "Sustainability and Scale: US Milk-market Orders as Relocalization Policy." *Environment and Planning* A 40, no. 8 (2008): 1987–2005.

DuPuis, E. Melanie, and David Goodman. "Should We Go Home to Eat? Toward a Reflexive Politics of Localism." *Journal of Rural Studies* 21 (2005): 359–71.

Hinrichs, C. Clare. "The Practice and Politics of Food System Localization." *Journal of Rural Studies* 19 (2004): 33–45.

Humphrey, John, and Hubert Schmitz. "Governance in Global Value Chains." Institute of Development Studies, University of Sussex, 2000.

Kloppenburg, Jack, John Hendrickson, and G. W. Stevenson. "Coming into the Foodshed." *Agriculture and Human Values* 13, no. 3 (1996): 33–42.

Lapping, Mark. "Toward the Recovery of the Local in the Globalizing Food System: The Role of Alternative Agricultural and Food Models in the US." *Ethics, Place and Environment* 7, no. 3 (2004): 141–50.

Lass, Daniel, G. W. Stevenson, John Hendrickson, and Kathy Ruhf. "CSA across the Nation: Findings from the 1999 CSA Survey." Madison: Center for Integrated Agricultural Systems, University of Wisconsin, October 2003. Available at http://www.cias.wisc.edu/wp-content/uploads/2008/07/csaacross.pdf.

Lyson, Thomas. *Civic Agriculture: Reconnecting Farm, Food and Community.* Boston: Tufts University Press, 2004.

McCarthy, James. "Rural Geography: Alternative Rural Economies—The Search for Alterity in Forests, Fisheries, Food, and Fair Trade." *Progress in Human Geography* 30, no. 6 (2006): 803–11.

McFadden, Steven. "The History of Community Supported Agriculture Part II: CSA's World of Possibilities." *New Farm* (2004). Available at http://www.newfarm.org/features/0204/csa2/part2.shtml.

Morgan, Kevin, Terry Marsden, and Jonathan Murdoch. *Worlds of Food: Place, Power, and Provenance in the Food Chain.* Oxford: Oxford University Press, 2006.

Raynolds, Laura, Douglas Murray, and John Wilkenson. *Fair Trade: The Challenges of Transforming Globalization.* New York: Routledge, 2007.

Web Site

Fair Trade Resource Network, http://www.fairtraderesource.org/bib-journalarticles.html (includes an excellent list of research articles on fair trade).

3

Farmwork and the Labor of Meatpacking and Poultry Processing: Another Way of Working Is Possible

Dan La Botz

Improving the lives of U.S. farmworkers, meat packers, and poultry processors—between two and three million wage earners—is an enormous challenge. The oligopolies that dominate large-scale agriculture and meat and poultry industries are enormously powerful economically and politically, and their sole concerns are productivity, market share, and profits—profits derived from the exploitation of low-wage labor. Small agricultural producers, without the economies of scale of large producers, must make the most of labor and thus may be equally exploitative. Federal and state governments have proved poor defenders of the rights, health and safety, and social well-being of workers in these industries. As a consequence, farmwork, meatpacking, and poultry processing are among the worst jobs in the United States today: physically demanding, psychologically stressful, frequently hazardous and unsafe, low paid, and low status.[1]

The social situation for these workers is often poor. Farmworkers frequently have bad housing and poor living conditions, such as dilapidated buildings, over-crowded conditions, and poor facilities that contribute to disease and illness. Both farmworkers and meat and poultry workers, many of whom are immigrants or African American, generally have low annual incomes, often lack health care, and in many cases live lives hemmed in by the racial prejudice, poverty, and social exclusion. Immigrant farmworkers may labor in areas that are politically and socially hostile. The working lives of meat- and poultry-processing workers are by and large not only oppressive and exploitative, but also inhumane. In some cases, conditions verge on a kind of *industrial torture* that cause pain and anguish and take both a physiological and a psychological toll.[2]

Employers have been able to create and to maintain such conditions because workers in these industries are often either new immigrants or citizens who form part of the country's rural poor. The rural poor of the U.S. Southeast constitute an industrial reserve army for the meat and poultry industry in areas of the country where high unemployment forces workers to accept awful jobs at near-subsistence wages. Many of the workers in the poultry industry are African American women for whom these exhausting, dirty, and dangerous low-paid jobs are the best paid jobs available. Other workers are immigrants from Latin America, Vietnam, Laos People's Democratic Republic, and the Balkans.[3]

Many workers in these industries are undocumented Latino immigrants who work under false names and social security numbers, and consequently, live a life in the shadows. About half of crop farmworkers and as much as 25 percent of meat and poultry workers were undocumented in the 1990s and early 2000s.[4] These workers are in many cases pariahs without the right to legal residence, with no civil or political rights, in many cases without even the most minimal recognition of their human rights.[5] Immigrant workers in agriculture, poultry, and meat industries are often brought into the United States by *coyotes*, smugglers of human contraband, and in agriculture a fifth of the workers are employed by labor contractors.

Nowhere else in our economy is the relationship between economic exploitation and police repression so clear. Many farm, meat, and poultry workers live in fear of the immigration authorities and of the local sheriffs and police who also engage in immigration enforcement in several states, counties, and cities.[6] Living in dread of arrest and deportation, they often hesitate to use emergency rooms and hospitals, and they may be reluctant to call the police or fire department in an emergency. Those who are foreign workers often do not know the language, culture, and laws of the country; and they often do not know their labor rights. In either case, these workers may be reluctant to demand their rights for fear of being fired or turned over to immigration authorities, imprisoned for using false identification, or deported to their home countries.

The economic structures of these industries and their workforces, and the corporate organization of work itself at the level of the field or the plant, create jobs set up to force workers to work as hard, as fast, and as intensely as possible to produce more product and higher profits. The corporations that own the factories and the factories in the fields have designed the workplaces, the processes, the tools, the work relationships, and the labor itself completely in the interest of higher productivity and greater profitability and generally without even a minimal concern for the impact of work organization on human beings.

Where this work is organized on a bureaucratic and industrial model, as it is on larger farms and in virtually all meat and poultry plants, it is alienating in the sense that all humanity has been squeezed out of it, all self-expression extinguished. The work organization is completely hierarchical, vertical, and authoritarian with a military-style command-and-control structure that gives workers virtually no latitude or input, much less opportunities to offer suggestions or make decisions. Above all, the pace of work set by the machine or driven by piece-rate payment forces these workers to give up not only their workday, but also their health and their future well-being, and in some cases their very lives for the corporations' profits. These industries are among those with the highest rates of accidents, illnesses, and deaths, and they produce high levels of stress and depression. Not surprising, worker turnover is high, sometimes reaching 100 percent in a year.

Adding insult to injury, these industries often pay below a subsistence wage. In the case of farmworkers, few of these in the United States earn a living wage.[7] In the case of meatpacking, which once paid a decent wage, employers have succeeded in two decades of industrial warfare in breaking unions or weakening contracts so that today's wages and benefits have been reduced to low levels, and conditions have deteriorated. Poultry workers, who remain largely unorganized, have wages below even those of the meatpacking industry.[8]

The employers in these industries with few exceptions do all in their power to prevent the unionization of their workforces, turning to specialized law firms and often engaging in illegal, unfair labor practices. In violation of labor law, employers have frequently punished or fired union activists, threatened workers with deportation, and in some cases have called in the immigration authorities to break union-organizing drives. Workers in these industries do not enjoy the fundamental rights that are guaranteed to workers under the law, even if they are immigrants and even if they are undocumented.[9]

The existence of such atrocious and shameful conditions in our nation for farmworkers and their families, several million people, is not only an evil in itself, but also represents a threat to other workers and to our society at large, for where the combination of corporate power and government neglect is permitted to exist, they threaten also to jeopardize the working and living conditions of others in our society. The problems in these industries are enormous and the need for change urgent, yet the tremendous investments of capital in the current structure and the economic and political power of the corporations are so great that clearly reform will not be simple, easy, or quick.

The big question in proposing reforms in the areas of agriculture and meatpacking and poultry processing is how not only to bring about reform, but also how to strengthen working people in relation to capital, so that over time the problems that arise from the existing system of exploitation can be eliminated permanently. I look at here some purported best practices in these industries, examine their real impact, and ask whether these practices are truly useful, and, if they are, how these practices might or might not be generalized and extended to improve the lives of workers.

Labor union organization and the negotiation of collective bargaining agreements could improve farm, poultry process, and meatpacking workers' lives. Social democratic legislation to provide universal health care, free kindergarten through postgraduate education, one-month vacation for all workers, and the other features of a European-style social safety net would benefit all workers. In turning to real long-term solutions, human beings ought to be able to create a system of agriculture and of agricultural labor that produces decent lives for workers, maintains and improves the environment, and produces healthy food for consumers, without the profit motive and without repression. Socialism, publicly owned industries with worker-run farms and factories in the context of a democratic government represents a humanistic alternative for these workers.

THE GLOBAL POLITICAL ECONOMIC CONTEXT

American agricultural labor, poultry processing, and meatpacking all were transformed over the last 30 years within the broader context of the transformation of the U.S. and world economy through the policies of the neoliberal economic model of deregulation and privatization accompanied by the policies of open markets, free trade, and world production in the process called globalization. Ronald Reagan and Margaret Thatcher introduced the neoliberal model at the national level beginning in 1980, and subsequently in the 1980s and 1990s, under the rubric of "The Washington Consensus," the International Monetary Fund, the World Bank, and the World Trade Organization used structural adjustment policies to impose this model on developing countries and the former Eastern Bloc nations.[10]

All of this has meant increased economic competition on a world scale, leading to the creation of rival trading blocs, in particular the completion of the European Union and the establishment of the North American Free Trade Agreement (NAFTA) in 1994 by Canada, Mexico, and the United States. These agreements have been supplemented by myriad bilateral and multilateral trade agreements. NAFTA had devastating consequences for many Mexican farmers. As millions of tons of subsidized U.S. agricultural products flooded Mexico, hundreds of thousands of small farmers failed.[11] At the same time, the Mexican government stopped subsidies to farmers and ended the country's fixed price for corn at about twice the world market price. The 1994 peso devaluation also hurt Mexican farmers. Unable to make a living in farming, many farmers and their families migrated to Mexican cities, to the border region, or to the United States in search of work. Undocumented immigrants rose from 2.5 million in 1995, to 4.5 million in 2000, to 11 million in 2005. Sixty percent or six million of these immigrants were Mexican.[12] Today, about 10 percent of all Mexicans live in the United States. Many found work on farms and in meatpacking and poultry plants.

THE POLITICAL ECONOMIC CONTEXT
IN THE UNITED STATES

These global and continental political economic transformations profoundly affected American industry, including agriculture, meat, and poultry. For agriculture, the principal change has been demographic, a change from native-born workers, many of them Mexican American, to immigrant workers, most of them Mexican and many of them undocumented. For meatpacking and poultry processes, the changes have been more thoroughgoing—that is, a complete reorganization of the industry, geographically, demographically, and in terms of industrial relations. What has happened in these industries reflects broader changes in the American economy and labor movement.

During the period between 1940 and 1980, most industries in the United States remained relatively stable, often regulated, and dominated by a few large corporations. The industrial core of most heavy industries was organized by a major industrial union, and worker wages and benefits improved until the 1970s. Beginning around 1981 with Ronald Reagan's firing of thirteen thousand unionized air traffic controllers, government and private employers launched an offensive against unions and workers with devastating consequences. Unions were broken, contracts weakened, wages stagnated, and benefits were cut.[13] Today, unions represent only 7.5 percent of the private workforce in the country, while total unionization stands at only 12.1 percent.[14]

Agriculture, however, had never been widely organized except for a brief period in the 1970s in California when the United Farm Workers (UFW) union succeeded in organizing and winning contracts for a significant number of workers.[15] After a brief period of success, growers turned to modest mechanization, the use of farm labor contractors, and the hiring of immigrant Latino workers, often undocumented. The

UFW was barely able to keep a toehold in the industry. Today less than 2 percent of California farmworkers are organized and have contracts, although there have been gains in organizing H-2A visa workers in North Carolina by the Farm Labor Organizing Committee (FLOC) and food-processing workers in California by the UFW and the Teamsters.[16] The Coalition of Immokalee Workers has won higher wages for workers in Florida through campaigns against Taco Bell and Burger King.[17]

In meatpacking, the big five packers of the period from 1890 to 1960—Swift, Armour, Morris, Wilson and Cudahy—were organized by the United Packinghouse Workers of America (UPWA), (later merged with the Amalgamated Meat Cutters and then becoming part of the United Food and Commercial Workers [UFCW]). Between the 1960s and 1990s, a new breed of packer moved plants to rural areas where land and labor were cheaper and introduced a system of boned-and-trimmed boxed beef. When rural labor was not sufficient, the companies recruited immigrants, mostly from Mexico and many of them undocumented. The corporations adopted a more aggressive attitude toward unions, forcing strikes, engaging in lockouts, breaking militant local unions, and wiping out pattern agreements (master contracts). Union density and strength declined, and so did wages. The UFCW turned to bargaining concessions in the 1980s. By the 1990s, a new Big Three of meatpackers had emerged—IBP, Excel (a subsidiary of Cargill), and ConAgra—that had increased productivity and employed a partially unionized workforce at much lower wages.

The poultry industry as we know it today has grown up in the last few decades and is almost a new industry altogether. Before the 1950s, the poultry industry had been a small farm business. During the 1960s to 1980s, a process of economic concentration began so that by the 1990s half a dozen companies dominated the industry, which employed a quarter of a million workers.[18] Concentration was accompanied by mechanization and the deskilling of jobs so that virtually all jobs are unskilled labor. Three firms, Tyson Foods, Pilgrim's Pride, and Gold Kist, control nearly 50 percent of the poultry industry. The UFCW and the RWDWU (the Retail, Wholesale, and Department Store Workers Union, which is part of the UFCW) have succeeded in organizing about 30 percent of the industry.[19]

AGRICULTURE AND FARMWORKERS

The United States had approximately two million farms in 2002.[20] Agriculture is diverse in terms of size, crops, revenues, and workforces. Some states have produced more or less the same principal crops, such as corn and wheat, for decades, and other states, particularly California, represent "a caldron of perpetual change." There are powerful trends toward horizontal and vertical integration, although they manifest themselves differently in different states with different geographies, climates, and crops. While oligopolies (a few producers) or oligopsonies (a few buyers) dominate some markets, others are more competitive. For example, four companies control 89 percent of the market in grains, whereas in vegetable crops, the market is far more diverse. However, even where producers are diverse, the market may be dominated by processors, distributors, or retail grocers. Even in California, where agriculture is most diverse and dynamic, 4,775 farms or 6 percent of all farms in the state "had sales exceeding a million dollars and accounted for 75 percent of total sales." However, fruit, vegetables, nuts, dairy, and ornamental products all remain competitive markets with few exceptions.[21] Some are large farms that employ large numbers of farmworkers on a seasonal basis, although others are midsize and have fewer workers.[22] A typical 40-acre strawberry farm in California has about $1 million in revenue and employs about 20 workers, half of whom work at least 150 days per year.[23]

The U.S. Census of 2002 reported that 927,708 hired farmworkers are working 150 days and 2.1 million are working less than 150 days.[24] Workers employed more than 150 days are often hired by farmers; those not working 150 days are usually hired by labor contractors or crew leaders.[25] The trend is toward more workers hired by farmers rather than contractors. The National Agricultural Workers Survey (NAWS), based on interviews with 6,472 crop farmworkers during the period from October 2000 to October 2002, found that 79 percent of workers interviewed were men. Only 23 percent of workers were native born, while 75 percent were born in Mexico, 2 percent born in Central America, and 1 percent born in other countries. Most are Spanish speakers (81 percent), and only 25 percent of workers are U.S. citizens. Some 53 percent of crop farmworkers lacked authorization to work in the United States, while 21 percent were legal permanent residents. Many of these workers were migrants, defined as having traveled 75 miles within the previous year to obtain a farm job. While 26 percent traveled within the United States, 35 percent came from a foreign country (usually Mexico), and 38 percent were newcomers in the United States (i.e., present for less than a year at the time of the survey). Most of these workers, 79 percent, were directly employed by growers or packing firms, while 21 percent were hired by labor contractors, a 50 percent increase since 1993–1994.[26]

Farmworkers and their families have wages so low that many can be classified as poor. Workers worked an average of 42 hours per week; and their average hourly earnings were $7.43, ranging between $6.76 and $8.05 based on tenure with their employers. Wages have fluctuated throughout the past decade. Individual income in 2001–2002 ranged between $10,000 and $12,499 per year, and total family income was between $15,000 and $17,499. Thirty percent of farmworkers had total incomes below poverty guidelines. Only 23 percent of workers report that they have health insurance. In the past two years, more than 20 percent of these workers or their families had received some sort of public assistance, including Medicaid, Special Supplemental Nutrition Program for Women Infants and Children (WIC), or food stamps. Almost half of these workers have some assets: 49 percent own a car, and 17 percent are buying a home either in the United States or their home country.[27]

Much farmwork requires skill, but many farm laborers are semiskilled or unskilled. Farm labor often involves long days of 10 to 12 hours, working outdoors under the sun and sometimes in inclement conditions. For farmworkers, overtime does not begin until after 60 hours have been worked, so the 12-hour day is common. Growers and contractors push workers to work as fast as possible, either under the orders of a foreman, pushed along by the pace of a machine, or driven by piece-rate payment. Foremen sometimes yell at, swear at, or otherwise verbally abuse workers who fall behind the pace of work. Workers in the fields and packing sheds may be exposed to fertilizers, pesticides, herbicides, and rodenticides and other chemicals in the air, on plants, or in the soil. Exposure to pesticides may result in dermatitis, cancer, eye injuries, and respiratory disease. Farm crop labor is physically demanding. Workers often engage in bending, stooping, pulling, twist-ing, lifting, throwing, climbing, reaching, and stretching, and repetitive motions sometimes result in musculoskeletal disorders. "Backaches and pain in the should-ers, arms, and hands are the most common symptoms that farmworkers report." These injuries can be disabling. Farmwork is one of the most hazardous industries for occupational injuries and deaths. Workers are endangered by potential acci-dents and injuries resulting from lifting and from exposure to tractors or other farm machinery, or by accidents such as falling from a truck. The living conditions of farmworkers may lead to alcoholism or to depression or result in child abuse.[28] Heat exposure is a health hazard and in 2008 resulted in worker deaths in North Carolina and California.[29]

Crop workers themselves offer their own critique of the industry and work organization. They complain of growers or contractors who treat them disrespect-fully. They also find the pace of work, often driven by piece-rate payment, to be too fast, and the wages too low. Most would like year-round employment, which not all have. Health insurance, which three-quarters of farmworkers lack, is a priority for these workers. Health and safety concerns are further down the list for farmworkers, although these issues are serious. These workers would like to have a pension plan, something most of them do not enjoy. Most would also like involvement in deci-sion-making processes and clear and effective grievance procedures.[30]

Federal law should protect farmworkers, but federal labor laws that protect workers' rights do not cover most farmworkers. Farmworkers were specifically excluded from the National Labor Relations Act (NLRA) that protects the rights of other workers. Nor are they covered by the Fair Labor Standards Act (FLSA), which establishes maximum hours and minimum wages for other workers. Because the Occupational Safety and Health Administration (OSHA) inspects only farms with more than 10 workers, 90 percent of U.S. farms are exempt.[31] Some states such as California have more progressive laws. California's Agricultural Labor Relations Act (ALRA) and CalOSHA regulations apply to all farms. Still, under California law, overtime applies to farm laborers only on the seventh day after six consecutive 10-hour days.[32] Throughout the country, children as young as 12 and 13 may work with parents' consent. Some federal laws are intended to offer special protection to farmworkers, such as the Federal Insecticide, Fungicide, and Rodenti-cide Act (FIFRA), which has worker health and safety provisions enforced by the U.S. Environmental Protection Agency (EPA). The Migrant and Seasonal Agri-cultural Workers Protection Act (MSAWPA) governs the recruitment, hiring, and provision of services (such as housing and transportation) by labor contractors and crew leaders. The act is enforced by the Department of Labor's Wages and Hours Division.[33] Although most federal labor laws do not cover farmworkers, even where such laws exist, they are not always aggressively enforced; and seldom are employers jailed or fined for violations of the law.

ANOTHER KIND OF FARMWORK

How might we reorganize farmwork to make it not only a human but also a humane occupation—that is, one in which human beings not only make a living, but also express themselves through their creativity? Researchers and scholars, some growers and farmworkers, and union organizers have suggested different models of reform for making farmwork more humane, more economically rewarding, and sustainable. Philip L. Martin, professor at the University of California–Davis and a leading researcher on agricultural labor, suggests that farm labor can be reformed by changing immigration policy. He argues that more restrictive immigration policies will result in higher labor costs, leading growers to mechanize agriculture. Such changes, he suggests, might make unionization more likely among the remaining, more skilled workers. In any case, he believes that in the long run such developments will lead to a smaller, more stable, and more highly skilled workforce that will be better paid and live a life more like that of other U.S. workers.[34]

Researchers at the California Institute for Rural Studies, collaborating with both growers and farmworkers, have put forward a different strategy for the humanization of farmwork. They suggest short- and long-term strategies for improving farmwork that revolve around several key ideas: treating workers with dignity; paying a living wage; providing workers adequate housing; creating stable, year-long employment; pursuing immigration reform to ensure that workers have legal status; providing access to health care; making farmwork safe and healthy; codifying workers' rights and creating a grievance procedure; giving workers a voice in decision-making; and providing for older workers. These researchers and their collaborators have identified several farms, most of them smaller or niche crop farms engaged in sustainable agriculture, that implement some of these policies, and they have identified programs in several communities that encourage and support such developments.[35]

Finally, the UFW and other farmworker organizations organize workers to force employers to do many of the things mentioned above, from paying a living wage and providing decent housing to making work safe and creating a grievance procedure. The UFW and other farmworker organizations also pressure government to reform immigration policy, generally by providing legal status for workers and by creating opportunities for legal permanent employees and guest workers. The unions take the position that the workers' collective self-organization as expressed through the union will win contracts and legislation that will make farmwork humane and farmworker communities viable. The UFW has seen these goals as being achievable through collaboration with the liberal wing of the Democratic Party.

These three alternatives can be characterized as (1) the corporate agricultural industry position, (2) the small farm or niche crop position, and (3) the organized labor position. All three positions offer the hope of change, but all are fraught with problems. Fundamentally, Martin wants to make agriculture just another American industry, but he does so at a moment in history when U.S. manufacturing hardly provides a humane model. In fact, manufacturing corporations have been imitating agriculture and its worst practices. Corporations have pared back their permanent, full-time workforce through practices pioneered in agriculture, such as subcontracting. Manufacturers have turned to unskilled immigrant workers from Mexico and Central America. Through such changes in production, they have been able to cut wages, reduce health care benefits, and increase the intensity of work. Why would one think that if agricultural producers made more modern factories in the fields that they would treat the workforce in mechanized agriculture any differently than they treat industrial and service workers? In fact, the pressures of competition in the global marketplace would tend to pressure them to reduce wages and benefits while speeding up production.

The California Institute for Rural Studies and its grower and worker collabora-tors envision boutique agriculture as the road to more humane agricultural work, mostly smaller sustainable farms producing high-quality products for upscale niche markets. Some owners of these farms believe in environmentally sound and socially just agriculture. But this is a vision of best practices on the margins of the industry, among niche crop growers in specialized organic products. Some of the practices they propose would be easy to implement and, in some cases, cost noth-ing. In the Institute's survey of twelve California farms, they found that one, for example, had a "no yell" policy—that is, foremen and supervisors were not permit-ted to yell at workers. Many tried to promote personal contact between farm own-ers, supervisors, foremen, and the workers, and they found that farmworkers appreciated having a "personal relationship with farmers." Most of these farms gave their workers some paid days off (at least the public holidays). Several farms offered workers free or subsidized housing, but only for some workers. Several offered housing and others paternalistic benefits, such as personal loans, and access to food from the farm, even free farm food in some cases.

Yet, even among such a relatively prosperous and successful group of growers, it is hard to point to models. Wages are among the top two considerations of workers. One exceptional farm pays its permanent workers $24,000 per years plus a productivity bonus. Yet among all twelve farms examined in the study by the California Institute for Rural Studies, the investigators found that "it was difficult to find a farm that offered a living wage." Nor did any farm provide an annual wage for all of their field staff, although most of the farms provided year-round work for at least some of their workers. And half of the sustainable farms used farm labor contractors at least for short time periods. Most of these farms recruit workers' family and friends, but when necessary, they also turn to the farm labor contractors, although some attempt to use contractors whose practices are more humane. While these growers emphasize that they treat workers with dignity, some remarks from both growers and workers have the ring of paternalism. In any case, the growers have the last word in all questions, and the workers are depend-ent on them.[36]

No doubt, at least for the privileged permanent workforce, labor on these farms would be much preferable to work in factory fields of agribusiness. Yet these can-not be solutions for most workers in agriculture because they are based on mostly small farms or niche crop growers selling high-end products. The greatest problem for niche farms is that their products become more popular and therefore of inter-est to large-scale corporate agribusiness. When corporate agriculture takes an inter-est in these products, it introduces factory-style production, mechanized, paid by piece rate, and based on low-wage workers. Those new megafarms then compete with the boutique producers. If the boutiques do not change their production, they succumb; if they change their production methods and survive and grow, they become large-scale corporate producers with all the attendant problems; and others will be bought out or merge with big producers. Of course, given the protean char-acter of agriculture and its markets, new niche groups and boutique producers will emerge, but that only proves the marginal nature of these producers.[37]

Finally, the labor union model has its own problems. César Chávez, the charis-matic leader of the UFW, succeeded in building a union and leading victorious strikes in the late 1960s. With the support of Democratic Party Governor Jerry

Brown and the passage of the California ALRA in 1975, the UFW succeeded in organizing a significant portion of the mostly Mexican American farmworkers of California, and the union reached a membership of 40,000 to 50,000 by 1980. Workers' wages rose substantially as the union signed scores of contracts in several crops. Nevertheless, the union could not hold on to its success for several reasons. Divisions within the UFW, an inability to deploy union workers as needed, and unrealistic demands in negotiations in the 1970s all weakened the union.[38] When Republican George Deukmejian became governor of California, ALRA ceased to be effective for the UFW. Employers turned to farm labor contractors and new immigrant workers or to H-2A visa workers and escaped the union and its contracts. The immigrant amnesty of 1982 led former farmworkers to seek work in higher-paying industries, thinning the union's ranks. In addition, when union wages in some crops became too high, growers turned to mechanization, reducing the number of farmworkers. By the 1990s, most farmworkers in California were unauthorized workers from Mexico and Central America, and the UFW had lost most of its contracts, being reduced to representing less than 2 percent of the state's farmworkers.

Labor union organization among farmworkers is highly desirable because it gives workers' unions the power to negotiate contracts that can improve workers' wages, better their conditions, protect their health and safety, and gain health and pension benefits. Farmworker unions should negotiate the right to control the introduction of new technologies and operations in the fields, something other unions have won in a factory setting, so that they have some control over the threat to the replacement of workers by agricultural mechanization. Farmworker unions also play an important role in organizing for political candidates who support labor and social legislation of benefit to farmworkers.

In Western European countries, a majority of agricultural workers are represented by labor unions, have collective bargaining agreements, and often enjoy the same social benefits as other workers, such as health care and pensions. Although wages may be only two-thirds of that of industrial workers, farmworkers share in other social benefits that guarantee their security and well-being in the society.[39] Some agricultural unions have taken steps to protect the rights of migrant workers. German and Polish unions cooperate to educate Polish migrant workers about labor rights in Germany.[40] With labor unions, workers have a vehicle for improving their conditions and defending themselves from abuse.

Each of these models offers some vision of improving lives for farmworkers, but in many respects these are utopian solutions. The interconnectedness of finance, industry, and agriculture in the United States makes it difficult to envision lasting changes in our political economy in anything less than the system as a whole. Only the labor union organizing model offers some suggestion of a long-term solution by increasing the power of labor in relation to capital.

THE MEATPACKING AND POULTRY-PROCESSING INDUSTRIES

More than 500,000 workers are employed in slaughtering and processing industry in approximately 5,700 plants in the United States. The workers are young (43 percent under age 35), usually male (63 percent), and Hispanic (42 percent), and an estimated 26 percent are foreign-born noncitizens.[41] Workers in many of these plants are represented by the UFCW or in a few cases by the International Brotherhood of Teamsters (IBT), but many plants remain unorganized.

In meatpacking and poultry plants, no model companies or plants exemplify best practices. These industries might be improved in the following three ways: (1) by corporate initiative, (2) by government regulation, and (3) by union control.

What have corporations done to improve workers' lives? Donald D. Stull and Michael J. Broadway found in their study of the meatpacking industry that,

> Machines now work alongside people on meat and poultry lines, but jobs remain tedious, monotonous, and risky. And workers who fill them rarely earn a "living wage," one sufficient to feed, clothe, and shelter themselves and their families.[42]

Although some corporations and plants do establish safety programs, very often their actual practices vitiate them. Stull and Broadway found that in the meatpacking industry productivity takes precedence over other concerns, such as quality and safety. Improvements in the industry are complicated by the tendency of supervisors to pass the buck and avoid taking responsibility, making change difficult. Also, many Anglo supervisors have racist attitudes toward Mexicans and other immigrant workers, discriminate against them, and mistrust them. Supervisors often have cultural and linguistic difficulties in communicating with their subordinates and generally do not attempt to deal with these issues.[43]

Poultry-processing work often exposes workers to extreme temperatures, it distorts the body or wears it out through repetitive motions, it deafens workers with loud noises, and it disgusts and repulses them with its blood and guts. Workers suffer frequent lacerations and amputations. The rapid line speed drives workers to their physical and mental breaking point. The working conditions, often accompanied by low wages and consequently poor living conditions, combine to cause depression in many of these workers. One group of researchers described poultry management practices as "benign neglect," and said there was "little evidence of coercive or abusive supervisory practices" nor of any "commitment on the managers for workers' safety."[44] But "benign neglect" is clearly the wrong term because *the system is intentional and rational*, run to produce profit by employers well aware of the human cost but with no concern for it. A better term would be "malign intent." The combination of physical pain and mental anguish produced by the system constitutes the recognized definition of torture, and this should be called "industrial torture." At present, poultry workers even where unionized often have no defense against such institutionalized mistreatment and abuse.[45]

The best practices in the area of safety and health might be OSHA's voluntary standards.[46] These standards are meant to protect workers from illness or injury in their work by describing hazards and precautions for each job. For example, one of the jobs in a poultry plant is the Neck Breaker. OSHA describes the job as follows: "The neck breaker uses a knife to cut the neck of the bird. Most companies have eliminated this position by installing an automatic neck breaking machine. Employees serve as backup to this machine." The hazards Neck Breakers face are listed as follows: "Standing for a long time, reaching to the shackles, and ergonomic hazards from use of knives." To take an example of the standards for just one of these areas: "Neck Breakers perform various tasks by reaching repeatedly to

the shackles. Reaching creates stress on the arms, shoulders, neck, and back."
Therefore, OSHA makes the following recommendation:

- Lower shackles and/or move them closer to employees so they can perform the task with elbows in close to body.
- Install height-adjustable stands so employees can properly position themselves.
- Install automatic machines and ensure they are working properly.

OSHA describes dozens of such tasks, pointing out the potential hazards and describing safe practices that might make poultry workers safer.[47]

Despite such recommendations as these, several problems persist. The biggest is that most of these are *voluntary*, not *mandatory*, standards, that is, employers are not required by law to enforce them and are not liable for fines, jail time, or other penalties. Second, there is *no ergonomic standard*. Although many of workers' health and safety problems—such as those of the Neck Breaker—are musculoskeletal issues that arise from ergonomic issues, OSHA *has no ergonomic standards*; and the industry has strenuously opposed not only the standards but even attempts to do the studies that might lay the basis for such standards. Where mandatory standards do exist in these industries, under recent administrations, OSHA has not acted vigorously to protect workers' health and safety. Rather than using its existing police powers, OSHA has often preferred to create partnerships with employers and to establish voluntary guidelines rather than enforce regulations and impose penalties. Even when OSHA uses its police powers and fines corporations for violating one of its mandatory standards, it seldom takes legal action to prosecute and jail corporate chief executives, plant managers, supervisors, or foremen when workers are killed, maimed, injured, or suffer unhealthy or unsafe work situations. Corporate executives in this country may and do kill workers with no repercussions, with few exceptions.

The election of an administration in Washington that was more concerned about workers' issues might make a considerable positive difference.[48] To do so, it would have to make OSHA standards mandatory not voluntary, it would have to create ergonomic standards and also enforce them, and it would have to use its police powers and cooperation with the courts to not only fine corporations but also to jail executives, supervisors, managers, and foremen responsible for violations regulations that harm workers. It is doubtful that it would solve the problems of the industry without an increase in the power of workers and their unions.

LABOR UNION ORGANIZATION

Labor union organization would be the most effective way to improve conditions in these industries.[49] Labor union organization would have to be achieved through strikes that would give workers a sense of power and break the company's absolute control over the industry and the workplace. The unions would then be in a position to negotiate collective bargaining agreements that might achieve a living wage, health and pension benefits, rules governing workplace conditions, and a grievance procedure to enforce the contract. The unions would be in a position to demand that federal OSHA and state OSHAs enforce the law. Equally important, if workers had unions that built workplace strength, workers could stop abuses and even control line speed.

Corporations in the poultry industry could improve conditions through practices suggested by researchers, such as job rotation, slowing the line speed, and avoiding abusive and coercive supervisory tactics.[50] They have not done so because such practices would cause them to lose out in national and world competition and thus reduce their corporations' stock value and profits. Only government regulation and union power will force corporations to improve worker conditions. When unions were strong in the meatpacking industry, workers often simply stopped the line when necessary to protect their health and safety, to force a slowdown in the pace, or simply to take a break. Where unions have become strong enough to dominate an industry, as they have sometimes in mining, they have introduced contract language that gives the union the right to refuse unsafe work or even to shut down the entire operation. If meat packers and poultry workers had such language, they might use it to force management to reduce line speed and the resultant repetitive motion traumas that cripple workers. Clearly, unions able to win longer lunch periods, more breaks, rotation of workers to different jobs, and slower line speeds would go a long way toward humanizing fieldwork, slaughtering, butchering, and packing.

Labor Politics

Labor unions would not only benefit workers as economic organizations, but also could use their political clout to back legislation that benefits workers. If the meatpacking and poultry industries were organized, presumably within the context of a resurgence of the American labor movement that would return unions to some significant level of unionization, they would have more political leverage. We might see unions play a stronger role in the Democratic Party or even see the creation of a labor party that would put forward a program for industrial regulation and social democratic reforms, such as those adopted in Europe during the postwar period (from 1945 to 1980). For this to happen, workers would have to transform the existing bureaucratic labor unions into more democratic and militant organizations.[51]

Imagining democratic socialism as representing the best way to improve the lives of workers may seem utopian, but it is certainly no more utopian than imagining that the answer lies with a government dominated by corporations, employers driven by profits, or labor unions locked into a capitalist economy. Workers would be better off if they had control over the workplace, the industry, and the government. When workers in Europe in the nineteenth and twentieth centuries gained power through unions and political parties, they not only organized unions but also created workplace councils of various sorts. Labor and socialist parties promoted these notions under the name of workplace democracy or economic democracy. At various periods, workers succeeded in establishing factory committees in which workers participated in running the factory. Through the power of the labor unions in the postwar period, a more conservative version of this notion became institutionalization in Germany under the name of *Mitbestimmung* or codetermination. Some U.S. unions have seats on company boards of directors, a yet weaker version of codetermination.

Labor unions and a labor party to fight for legislation to defend workers on the job and to give them a decent life in society would transform agricultural labor. Still, while we live in a system of private property in the means of production, free markets, economic competition, and the profit motive, neither farmworkers, meatpacking workers, nor poultry workers will be able to have safe and healthy jobs, or secure employment at a living wage. Nor will anyone's job and life be secure while society is subject to capitalism's boom-and-bust economic cycles. The best chance for farmworkers, for poultry process and meat workers, and for the rest of us is strong labor organization, a political party of working people, and the revolutionary transformation of our societies leading to democratic socialism.

NOTES

Thanks to Sherry Baron, Hester Lipscomb, Roni Neff, Jackie Nowell, and particularly Don Villarejo for comments, suggestions, and other views. I alone am responsible for the views presented in this article.

1. GAO (U.S. Government Accountability Office), *Safety in the Meat and Poultry Industry, while Improving Could Be Further Strengthened* (Washington, DC: GAO, 2005), http://www.gao.gov/new.items/d0596.pdf.; Don Villarejo and Sherry L. Baron, "The Occupational Health Status of Farm Workers," in *Occupational Medicine: State of the Art Reviews* 14, no. 3 (1999): 613.

2. I use the term "torture" advisedly. In 2004, acting Assistant Attorney General Daniel Levin said torture is defined as physical suffering or lasting mental anguish. The discussion of torture has led to recognition that stress positions, extreme temperatures, and loud noises constitute torture. In a series of studies of poultry workers, Hester Lipscomb and her colleagues have found that such conditions as well as an inhuman line speed lead to both physical disabilities and to depression. Hester Lipscomb's articles are cited below in a more detailed discussion of poultry workers.

3. William G. Whittaker, *Labor Practices in the Meatpacking and Poultry Processing Industry: An Overview* (Washington, DC: Congressional Research Service of the Library of Congress, October 27, 2006), http://www.nationalaglawcenter.org/assets/crs/RL33002.pdf. This paper describes many of these conditions.

4. For farmworkers see, U.S. Department of Labor, *National Agriculture Workers Survey, Executive Summary*, http://www.doleta.gov/agworker/naws.cfm; for meat and poultry workers see, GAO, *Safety in the Meat and Poultry Industry*.

5. Dan La Botz, "The Immigrant Rights Movement: Between Political Realism and Social Idealism," *New Politics* 11, no. 3 (2007), http://www.wpunj.edu/~newpol/issue43/LaBotz43.htm.

6. April Clark et al., "2007 National Survey of Latinos: As Illegal Immigration Issue Heats Up, Hispanics Feel a Chill" (Pew Hispanic Center, December 13, 2007), http://pewhispanic.org/files/reports/84.pdf.

7. There is no commonly accepted formula to figure a living wage. The federal poverty guidelines can be found at http://www.census.gov/hhes/www/poverty/threshld/07prelim.html, where it should be clear that those do not constitute a living wage. Economic Policy Institute, "Basic Family Budget Calculator," http://www.epi.org/content.cfm/datazone_fambud_budget, constitutes another better measure of a living wage. (Thanks to Stephanie Luce for suggesting those sources.) Beyond calculations, the reader might ask what wage he or she would need or accept as a minimum. Presumably, this could be called a living wage, unless the reader thinks these workers and their families deserve less than others earn.

8. National Agriculture Workers Survey, Executive Summary, at http://www.doleta.gov/agworker/naws.cfm; Whittaker, *Labor Practices*. This paper describes many of these conditions.

9. Lance Compa, *Blood, Sweat, and Fear: Workers' Rights in U.S. Meat and Poultry Plants* (New York: Human Rights Watch, 2004). This documents the violation of workers' rights in meat and poultry plants.

10. David Harvey, *A Brief History of Neoliberalism* (New York: Oxford University Press, 2005). Harvey gives the best overview and explanation of neoliberalism.

11. Ana de Ita, "Fourteen Years of NAFTA and the Tortilla Crisis" (Americas Program Special Report, January 10, 2008), http://americas.irc-online.org/am/4879; Public Citizens, "The Ten Year Track Record of the North American Free Trade Agreement: The Mexican Economy, Agriculture and Environment," http://www.citizen.org/documents/NAFTA_10_mexico.pdf.

12. Philip Martin, "NAFTA and Mexico-US Migration" (December 16, 2005), http://giannini.ucop.edu/Mex_USMigration.pdf.

13. Kim Moody, *An Injury to All: The Decline of American Unionism* (New York: Verso, 1988).

14. U.S. Department of Labor, *Bureau of Labor Statistics for 2007* (Washington, DC: Government Printing Office, 2007).

15. Philip L. Martin, *Promise Unfulfilled: Unions, Immigration and the Farm Workers* (Ithaca, NY: Cornell University Press, 2003), chapter 3, 57–89.

16. The U.S. government issues H-2A visas to temporary or seasonal agricultural workers.

17. "The Price of a Tomato," *The Economist* June (2008): 38–39. The article reports, "The extra cent a pound [won by the COIW from Burger King] is the first pay increase in 30 years. Even with it, a picker would have to fill fifteen 32-pound buckets an hour to earn Florida's minimum wage [for nonfarmworkers] of $6.79—a tall order in the broiling sun."

18. Whittaker, *Labor Practices.*

19. Correspondence from Jackie Nowell of the UFCW, May 28, 2008.

20. USDA, NASS (National Agricultural Statistics Service), http://www.nass.usda.gov/Charts_and_Maps/graphics/data/fl_frmwk.txt.

21. Don Villarejo, personal communication, May 2008.

22. For two papers that look at different aspects of current developments, see Democratic Staff of the Committee on Agriculture, Nutrition, and Forestry, U.S. Senate, "Economic Concentration and Structural Changes in the Food and Agriculture Sector: Trends, Consequences and Policy Options" (October 28, 2004), Tom Harkin, Iowa, Ranking Democratic Member; Giannini Foundation of Agricultural Economics, University of California, "Whither California Agriculture: Up, Down or Out? Some Thoughts about the Future" (September 2007). The first paper reflecting the Iowa experience points to increasing concentration in grain and meat, while the second paper from California notes that "[d]espite perceptions of increased concentration of production among a few large-size farms, U.S. census data do not reveal strong evidence of increased concentration over the past several decades." The quotation "caldron of perpetual change" comes from the Giannini Foundation paper.

23. Villarejo, personal communication, May 2008.

24. USDA NASS 2002, at http://www.nass.usda.gov/research/2002mapgallery/hiredlabor.html.

25. I do not discuss livestock workers in this paper. More than 900,000 livestock workers are working an excess of 150 days per year. Their jobs are often more dangerous than those of agricultural workers.

26. U.S. Department of Labor, Employment and Training Administration, "National Agriculture Workers Survey, Executive Summary," http://www.doleta.gov/agworker/

naws.cfm; The NAWS is an ongoing survey process, but 2002 is the last set of study results available.

27. Ibid.

28. Sherry Baron et al., *Simple Solutions* (Cincinnati, OH: National Institute for Occupational Safety and Health, 2001); Villarejo and Baron, "The Occupational Health Status of Hired Farm Workers."

29. Associated Press, "San Joaquin Coroner Says Young Farm Worker Died of Heat Stroke," June 19, 2008; Dan Glaister, "Migrant Farmworker's Death in U.S. Highlights Poor Labour Conditions," *Guardian* (United Kingdom), June 5, 2008. The victim was a 17-year-old pregnant girl. Glaister writers, "Since 2005 there have been 23 suspected heat-related fatalities among California's 450,000 seasonal agricultural workers." The Centers for Disease Control and Prevention report: "During this 15-year period [1992–2006], 423 workers in agricultural and nonagricultural industries were reported to have died from exposure to environmental heat; 68 (16%) of these workers were engaged in crop production or support activities for crop production. The heat-related average annual death rate for these crop workers was 0.39 per 100,000 workers, compared with 0.02 for all U.S. civilian workers" (*Morbidity and Mortality Weekly Report*, June 20, 2008, http://www.cdc.gov/mmwr/preview/mmwrhtml/mm5724a1.htm).

30. Ron Strochlic and Kari Hamerschlarg, "Best Labor Management Practices of Twelve California Farms: Toward a More Sustainable Food System," *California Institute for Rural Studies* December (2005): 1–28, 15. The authors list 16 things workers would most appreciate: "respectful treatment, slower pace of work, fair compensation (through wages and other forms of supplementing incomes), year-round employment, health insurance, personal loans, food from the farm, healthy and safe work environment, paid time off, flexible work schedule, housing, opportunities for advancement and professional development, diversity of tasks, involvement in decision making processes, clear and effective grievance procedures, and retirement plans." I would question whether all of these really would be desirable. For example, there is a long history of employers using personal loans as a way to keep farmworkers dependent and even of holding agricultural workers captive in poor conditions, that is, of creating a system of debt peonage.

31. USDA, *Census of Agriculture 2002*, U.S. and State Data (Washington, DC: USDA, 2002), Table 7, 281.

32. Villarejo and Baron, "The Occupational Health Status of Hired Farm Workers," 618–20.

33. GAO, "Child Labor in Agriculture: Changes Needed to Protect Health and Educational Opportunities" (Washington, DC: GAO, 1998), 30, http://www.gao.gov/archive/1998/he98193.pdf.

34. Martin, *Promise Unfulfilled*, 180–96.

35. Strochlic and Hamerschlarg, "Best Labor Management Practices"; Martha Guzman et al., "A Workforce Action Plan for Farm Labor in California: Toward a More Sustainable Food System," *California Institute for Rural Studies* June (2007): 1–21; see also, for an example of sustainable farm, The Farm, http://www.swantonberryfarm.com.

36. Strochlic and Hamerschlarg, "Best Labor Management Practices," 4–15.

37. I remember that in 1999 while working for Global Exchange as director of its California Program, I led a group on a tour of Northern California and Central Valley agricultural areas. We visited former immigrant farmworkers who had established an organic farm and been successful for a while, until the big grocery chains and agricultural producers became interested in organic vegetables and they came into competition with new, large-scale organic farms. They feared they would be driven out of business soon.

38. Dan La Botz, *César Chávez and La Causa* (New York: Longman, 2005), chapters 8, 9.

39. "Industrial Relations in Agriculture," *Eironline: European Industrial Relations Observatory On-Line* (September 2005), http://www.eurofound.europa.eu/eiro/2005/09/study/tn0509101s.htm.

40. "German and Polish Unions Cooperate over Seasonal Workers in Agriculture," *Eironline: European Industrial Relations Observatory On-Line* (October 2003), http://www.eurofound.europa.eu/eiro/2003/10/inbrief/de0310204n.htm.

41. GAO, *Safety in the Meat and Poultry Industry*, 1.

42. Donald D. Stull and Michael J. Broadway, *Slaughterhouse Blues: The Meat and Poultry Industry in North America* (Belmont, CA: Wadsworth/Thomson Learning, 2003), 74.

43. Ibid., 82–98.

44. Joseph G. Grzywacz et al., "The Organization of Work: Implications for Injury and Illness among Immigrant Latino Poultry-Processing Workers," *Archives of Environmental & Occupational Health* 62, no. 1 (2007): 19–26, 24.

45. H. J. Lipscomb et al., "Musculoskeletal Symptoms among Poultry Processing Workers and a Community Comparison Group: Black Women in Low-Wage Jobs in the South," *American Journal of Industrial Medicine* 50 (2007): 327–38; H. J. Lipscomb et al., "Upper Extremity Musculoskeletal Symptoms and Disorders among a Cohort of Women Employed in Poultry Processing," *American Journal of Industrial Medicine* 51 (2008): 2–36; H. J. Lipscomb et al., "Depressive Symptoms among Working Women in Rural North Carolina: A Comparison of Women in Poultry Processing and Other Low-Wage Jobs," *International Journal of Law and Psychiatry* 30, no. 4, 5 (2007): 284–98; H. J. Lipscomb et al., "Are We Failing Vulnerable Workers? The Case of Black Women in Poultry Processing in Rural North Carolina," *New Solutions* 17, no. 1, 2 (2007), 17–40.

46. OSHA (Occupational Safety and Health Administration) poultry standards and guides can be found at http://www.osha.gov/SLTC/etools/poultry/user_guide.html.

47. Ibid.

48. The Clinton administration created the "No Sweats" policy at the Department of Labor in 1995, which included more frequent and serious inspections, but its standards were still voluntary.

49. Workers cannot be successful in union organizing, winning contracts, and building workplace power as long as many of them do not enjoy the legal right to live and work in the country. The AFL-CIO and Change to Win, the two major labor federations in the United States, as well as the Catholic Church and many Protestant and Jewish organizations, have supported calls for what they call "comprehensive immigration reform." Dan La Botz, "If Not Now When?" *New Labor Forum* Spring (2008), http://www.newlaborforum.org/html/2008/spring/abstracts.html#ifnotnow.

50. Grzywacz et al., "The Organization of Work," 25.

51. Kim Moody, *US Labor in Trouble and Transition: The Failure of Reform from Above, the Promise of Revival from Below* (New York: Verso, 2007). Moody addresses the need for the democratic transformation of unions in this book.

RESOURCE GUIDE

Suggested Reading

Bacon, David. *Illegal People: How Globalization Creates Migration and Criminalizes Immigrants*. Boston: Beacon Press, 2008.

Compa, Lance. *Blood, Sweat, and Fear: Workers' Rights in U.S. Meat and Poultry Plants.* New York: Human Rights Watch, 2004.

Fink, Leon. *The Maya of Morganton: Work and Community in the Nuevo South.* Chapel Hill: The University of North Carolina Press, 2007.

La Botz, Dan. *César Chávez and la Causa.* New York: Longman, 2005.

Martin, Philip L. *Promise Unfulfilled: Unions, Immigration, and the Farm Workers.* Ithaca, NY: Cornell University Press, 2003.

Pew Hispanic Center. *Annual Labor Report—2008.* Available at http://pewhispanic.org/reports/report.php?ReportID=88.

Southern Poverty Law Center. "Close to Slavery." Available at http://www.splcenter.org/legal/guestreport/index.jsp.

Stull, Donald D., and Michael J. Broadway. *Slaughterhouse Blues: The Meat and Poultry Industry in North America.* Belmont, CA: Wadsworth/Thomson Learning, 2003.

U.S. Government Accountability Office. *Safety in the Meat and Poultry Industry, while Improving Could Be Further Strengthened.* Washington, DC: GAO, 2005, http://www.gao.gov/new.items/d0596.pdf.

Web Sites

Farm Labor Organizing Committee (FLOC), http://www.floc.com/.

Farm Worker Justice Fund, Inc., http://www.fwjustice.org/.

Philip Martin, University of California–Davis, http://martin.ucdavis.edu/.

Migration News, http://migration.ucdavis.edu/mn/.

National Agricultural Workers Survey (NAWS), http://www.doleta.gov/agworker/naws.cfm.

National Institute for Occupational Safety and Health (NIOSH), http://www.cdc.gov/niosh/topics/agriculture/.

United Farm Workers (UFW), http://www.ufw.org/.

United Food and Commercial Workers (UFCW), http://www.ufcw.org/.

4

Equity in Access to Land, Human Rights, and Capital: Food Security Movements from the Global South

William Van Lopik

Equity in access to land, human rights, and capital historically has been a contentious issue in the poor regions of the world. This chapter describes and analyzes the effectiveness of a rapidly expanding number of local, regional, international, and global initiatives that are addressing issues of hunger, poverty, and inequity. Movements of various scale and motive are developing in the global south in response to the failed economic and development agendas from the global north that have not benefited them. Whether it is farmers in Latin America, churches in Africa, or indigenous people in Belize, groups are organizing to meet their food security needs according to their agenda. Gender inequality has led women activists in Sub-Saharan Africa and India to advocate for equal rights in addressing their poverty issues in organizations like the Green Belt Movement in Kenya and the Wastepickers Association in India. The leadership map of developmental geography has shifted significantly to the south. Indigenous and grassroots organizations outside of North America and Western Europe are now on the cutting edge of effective programs in sustainable development.

INTRODUCTION

In the summer of 2007, the College of Menominee Nation through the leadership of its Sustainable Development Institute sponsored a week-long conference entitled "Sharing Indigenous Wisdom: An International Dialogue on Sustainable Development." The conference was held to foster dialogue on traditional indigenous knowledge being utilized and incorporated as models and methods of sustainable practices. Traditional or indigenous knowledge refers to the wisdom, embodied within the indigenous communities, that is utilized to preserve and protect resources vital to the continuity of that community. This was the second such conference that the small tribal college located in rural northeast Wisconsin had sponsored in the past four years.

The intent of the conference was to bring together indigenous researchers from different parts of the globe to create a dialogue on a wide variety of issues from land rights, to the empowerment of women in community development, to communities managing and building their own natural and capital assets. The key word that was used throughout the week was "sovereignty." The interpretation of the word in the context of the conference addressed the fundamental question of "who has control over the decisions that are made in a community pertaining to its assets?" These assets include land, human, economic, and natural resources. The presentations resonated strongly with me and echoed the stories I had heard while living for seven years in Central America and visiting dozens of poor rural villages. That is, poverty and hunger issues are directly tied to the question of who controls the resources. Examples of lack of control over resources include farmers who are dependent on renting only marginal land from rich landowners, who then siphon off any profits, and local markets that are flooded by cheap imported food that undermines the locally grown food. Examples of lack of sovereignty are found when poor countries use their foreign aid to pay off interest payments to rich countries for bad loans that seem to benefit only the elite. Examples of lack of control over destiny emerge when poor women are forced to sacrifice their own health and basic human rights because they are not entitled to own land, acquire a bank loan, or hold individual financial assets. It is when people are able to build up, manage, and acquire land and capital assets that they are able to combat hunger and alleviate extreme poverty. Economist Hernando de Soto says that the poor

> lack the process to represent their property and create capital. They have houses but not titles; crops but not deeds; businesses but not statutes of incorporation. . . . This explains why people have not been able to produce sufficient capital to make their domestic capitalism work.[1]

The examples discussed here will demonstrate various processes by which poor people are addressing these problems and gaining capital assets.

Much of the inspiration to write this chapter came out of these two conferences sponsored by the College of Menominee Nation. The initiatives mentioned in this chapter range in scale, geography, and visibility. All of them provide much-needed hope and have been successful in no small measure at alleviating hunger and poverty in the lives of poor families. Six organizations are highlighted in this chapter. Via Campesina and the Micah Network are global campaigns addressing poverty and hunger issues through global advocacy. The Green Belt Movement is working on environmental and women's rights issues in East Africa. The Sarstoon-Temash Institute for Indigenous Management (SATIIM) is a regional program in southern Belize that addresses indigenous rights. The Wastepickers Association is a local initiative in the city of Pune, India, in which the empowerment of marginalized women is the key objective. Finally, the PARI Development Trust in Bangladesh (PARI) focuses on building capital assets in communities through a unique community savings program.

LA VIA CAMPESINA

Sustainable development requires simultaneous attention to economic growth, environmental protection, and social equity to meet the needs of present generations without compromising those of the future. The World Resources Institute has said secure tenure over land and resources by all segments of society, and particularly by the poor, has been identified as a critical enabling condition for sustainable development to occur.[2]

Land tenure is a key asset for the rural poor that provides an important foundation for the economic and social development of a community. Without secure tenure, it is unlikely that a farmer will invest either financially or physically in the conservation of their land. Tenure is vital for transferability of land, access to credit markets, and investment in sustainable farming practices. Land tenure offers the potential to the rural poor to adjust to the unpredictability of globalization and ensure their own food security. Extensive research has shown that most development organizations are in agreement about the importance of land tenure to the development process in alleviating poverty, although few devote significant financial resources to the issue.[3]

La Via Campesina (from Spanish, "the peasant farmer way") is an initiative that describes itself as "an international movement which coordinates peasant organizations of small and middle-scale producers, agricultural workers, rural women, and indigenous communities from Asia, Africa, America, and Europe."[4] It is an international movement of peasants, small- and medium-size producers, landless rural women, indigenous people, rural youth, and agricultural workers. Their purpose is to defend the values and the basic interests of their members. Now in its sixteenth year, Via Campesina includes 142 member organizations from 56 countries in Asia, Africa, Europe, and the Americas. It was formally constituted in 1993 during a conference held in Mons, Belgium, when a group of forty-six farm leaders gathered to define a progressive alternative to the further liberalization of agriculture and food reflected in the Uruguay Round of the General Agreement on Tariffs and Trade (GATT).

The principal objective of Via Campesina is to develop solidarity and unity among small farmer organizations to promote gender parity and social justice in fair economic relations. This objective includes issues pertaining to the preservation of land, water, seeds, and other natural resources, as well as food sovereignty and sustainable agricultural production based on small producers. Via Campesina focuses its work on seven key issues affecting peasants and farmers everywhere: the need for genuine agrarian reform, food sovereignty and trade liberalization, biodiversity and genetic resources, gender relations in the countryside, sustainable peasant agriculture, migration and migrant farmworkers' rights, and human rights.[5]

The main goal of Via Campesina is to build a peasant-based alternative model of agriculture. To reach this goal, Via Campesina organizations work together to achieve the following:

- Organize exchanges of information, experiences, and strategies
- Develop connections among farm organizations
- Build solidarity and unity among farm organizations
- Strengthen the participation of women at all levels of farm organizations
- Articulate joint positions and policies
- Engage in collective action

Since its inception, farming peoples around the world have marched together in the streets of Paris, Geneva, Seattle, Rome, Genoa, Porto Alegre, and Quebec

City, among other cities. With its members chanting slogans, wearing dark green caps, bandannas, and white T-shirts, and waving green flags decorated with the movement's logo, Via Campesina has become an increasingly visible actor and audible voice of radical opposition to the globalization of a neoliberal and corporate model of agriculture.

Food sovereignty has always been a fundamental issue of particular concern for Via Campesina especially given the global crisis of rising food prices. Peter Rosset, former executive director of the Institute for Food and Development Policy, says that now is a critical time to listen to directives of the movement. Some of these directives include the need to stimulate the recovery of a country's national food-producing capacity, specifically that capacity located in the peasant and family farm sectors. It means stopping the dumping of artificially subsidized cheap food from rich countries on poor countries, which then undercuts the market share of local farmers. Via Campesina also calls for genuine agrarian reform. Land reform is urgently needed in many countries to rebuild the peasant and family farm sectors, whose vocation is growing food for people, because the largest farms and agribusinesses seem to produce only biofuel for cars and export crops for insatiable appetites in the global north. Via Campesina advocates for national governments to implement export controls and to stop the forced exportation of food desperately needed by their own populations.

Finally Rosset points out,

> [W]e must change dominant technological practices in farming, toward an agriculture based on agroecological principles, that is sustainable, and that is based on respect for and is in equilibrium with nature, local cultures, and traditional farming knowledge. It has been scientifically demonstrated that ecological farming systems can be more productive, can better resist drought and other manifestations of climate change, and are more economically sustainable because they use less fossil fuel.[6]

Subsistence farmers have many years of experience in relying on their locally available resources. They are capable of producing the optimal quantity and quality of food with few external inputs. They do well when they grow food for family consumption and domestic markets and are not competing against artificially supported transnational agribusinesses.

Via Campesina sees food sovereignty as a right of peoples, countries, and state unions to define their own agricultural and food policy. This view is based on Article 25 of the United Nations Declaration of Human Rights that "everyone has the right to a standard of living adequate for the health and well-being of himself and of his family, including food, clothing, housing and medical care."[7] Food sovereignty organizes food production and consumption according to the needs of local communities, giving priority to production for local consumption. Food sovereignty includes the right to protect and regulate the national agricultural and livestock production and to shield the domestic market from the dumping of agricultural surpluses and low-price imports from other countries. Landless people, peasants, and small farmers must get access to land, water, and seed as well as productive resources and adequate public services. Food sovereignty and sustainability must take a higher priority than trade policies.[8]

Ismael Ossemane, a farmer and founding member of the National Farmer's Union of Mozambique (UNAC), in a public speech given at a Via Campesina conference on August 17–18, 2007, in Mozambique, said, "[We] must . . . Focus on food for the people; Give the due value to food producers; Establish local food systems; Strengthen local control; Develop local knowledge; Work with nature."[9]

THE MICAH NETWORK

In September 2000, at the United Nations Millennium Summit, world leaders agreed to a set of time-bound and measurable goals and targets for combating hunger, disease, illiteracy, environmental degradation, and discrimination against women. Placed at the heart of the global agenda, they are now called the Millennium Development Goals (MDGs). Eight goals were agreed on by the 189 United Nations member states to try to achieve by the year 2015. The first of those eight goals is to "Eradicate extreme poverty and hunger." The two target areas that pertain to this goal are as follows:

(a) Halve, between 1990 and 2015, the proportion of people whose income is less than $1 a day.
(b) Halve, between 1990 and 2015, the proportion of people who suffer from hunger.[10]

The world is making progress toward the MDGs, but this progress is uneven and too slow. A large majority of nations will reach the MDGs only if they get substantial support, including advocacy, expertise, and resources, from outside their countries. The challenges for the global community, in both the industrial and developing world, are to mobilize financial support and political will, reengage governments, reorient development priorities and policies, build capacity, and reach out to partners in civil society and the private sector.[11]

Jeffrey Sachs, the main architect of the United Nations Millennium Project, says that a "global compact" must be established between rich and poor nations. He says,

> The poor countries must take ending poverty seriously, and will have to devote a greater share of their national resources to cutting poverty rather than to war, corruption, and political infighting. The rich countries will need to move beyond the platitudes of helping the poor, and follow through on their repeated promises to deliver more help.[12]

The Micah Challenge campaign is an international antipoverty campaign organized by the World Evangelical Alliance, which represents more than 3 million congregations around the world and the Micah Network, a coalition of more than 270 Christian relief and development groups. Chapters have formed in the Andean region, Australia, Bangladesh, Canada, India, and the United Kingdom. The purpose of this global campaign is to mobilize Christians against the extreme poverty that is pervasive in many countries. It aims to deepen Christian engagement with impoverished and marginalized communities, and to influence leaders of rich and poor nations to fulfill the promises they made to achieve the MDG of halving absolute global poverty by the year 2015. The goals of the Micah Challenge are summed up in its global petition, the Micah Call. They are twofold: (1) within the church, to deepen connections to and solidarity with the poor, and (2) in society at large, to call on national and international decision-makers to fight poverty. It calls on Christians to lobby and advocate on behalf of and with the poor to increase and improve aid, drop the unfair debt burden on the poorest countries, and achieve a more just trading system.[13]

The lobbying and advocacy efforts are aimed at the national governments in the global north and south, as well as international organizations such as the World Bank and transnational corporations. On a national level in Peru, for example, that means encouraging the government not to concentrate all its resources on the middle class or the urban population of Lima, but to take real steps for economic development in rural communities, especially indigenous ones. In wealthier countries, likely actions include pushing for debt relief as well as more and better-targeted foreign aid.[14]

Each country campaign is in charge of defining its own strategies for meeting the MDGs. In places like Malawi in southeastern Africa, the Micah Challenge has translated into initiatives such as the following:

- The development of contextual stewardship and discipleship Bible study and sermon outline materials for churches to respond to the MDGs
- District visitations of 367 church leaders to the collective congregations of more than 30,000 people to discuss the campaign
- Production and presentation on national radio programs regarding the Micah Challenge to raise awareness, education, and advocacy
- Training of twenty-four church leaders throughout Malawi in the utilization of a Constituency Development Fund tool to monitor the governance, institutions, processes, and promises of the national government[15]

The Micah Challenge has united groups that traditionally have not worked together. Ban Ki-Moon, the secretary general of the United Nations and one of the world's most influential leaders, did the unimaginable in the fall of 2007. He was invited to speak at a dinner of the National Association of Evangelicals. He met with a diverse group of 400 evangelicals near Washington, D.C., and asked for help from the church. Speaking on behalf of 192 nations that have committed themselves to cutting global poverty in half by 2015, Ban told evangelicals,

> We cannot do it alone. We need good allies such as you. We need . . . the faith community to help be a voice to the voiceless people. Your engagement can push governments to push through on their commitments. Do not underestimate your power. With faith and the will, we can make a difference.[16]

This campaign, uniting two hundred million to four hundred million evangelical Christians around the world, has the potential to make a significant impact. It definitely should be noticed and appreciated as this group follows a prophetic call to bring the issues of poverty to political leaders of the world and seeks to influence them to achieve justice for the poor and rescue the needy.[17] The success of the Micah Challenge in addressing critical food issues is still unknown, but the desire and commitment is a positive and laudable initiative.

THE GREEN BELT MOVEMENT

For most of the world, the Green Belt Movement remained in relative obscurity outside of environmental circles until the year 2004 when its founder and director, Wangari Maathai, was awarded the Nobel Peace Prize. Even though the organization had been in existence since 1977, it was not until 2004 that the general public noticed this grassroots environmental organization, which has assisted women and their families in planting more than forty million trees across Kenya. Since then, Wangari Maathai has been thrust onto the world stage in her call for people to recognize that for peace to exist resources need to be sustainably and equitably distributed. While much attention has deservedly been put on Wangari Maathai as an advocate of sustainable development, this chapter will focus on the positive aspects of the forty million trees and their role in alleviating hunger and creating healthy living environments.

A task force formed by the International Union of Forest Research Organizations reported that trees have a potential to restore degraded ecosystems and to provide food, medicinal products, health care, and meaning to people around the world. Trees provide shade, protection from air pollution and wind, soil fertility, erosion control, and groundwater recharge.[18] Forests also provide a safety net during times of environmental, political, or personal stress. During seasonal or emergency food shortages, the nuts, seeds, leaves, fruits, and tubers found in the forest can supplement a family's diet. Forest food is often rich in protein, vitamins A and C, iron, niacin, and riboflavin.[19] Medicinal forest plants and meat from wild animals are additional benefits that an emerging forest can offer a community.

In many parts of Kenya, the demand for wood has surpassed local supply, and people cannot afford other forms of energy; thus, they face an increased vulnerability to illness and malnutrition from consuming (unboiled) microbiologically contaminated water and improperly cooked food. Poor women and children in rural communities often are those most affected by a scarcity of fuel wood. Many must walk long distances searching for fuel and firewood and hauling it home. These time-consuming tasks reduce the time and energy available for tending crops, cooking meals, or attending school. Therefore, access to a sustainable source of fuel-wood is fundamental not only for economic development, but also for health and well-being.[20]

The mitigation of climate change is an additional attribute of reforestation. In Kenya, two of Africa's highest mountains (Mount Kilimanjaro and Mount Kenya) will lose their ice cover within twenty-five to fifty years, say scientists, if deforestation and industrial pollution are not stopped. Mount Kenya is one of the few places near the equator with permanent glaciers, and it has already lost 92 percent of them over the past 100 years. This is of major concern for Kenya because seven rivers in the country claim the ice cap as their headwaters. If these were to dry up, it would have devastating effects for the people of Kenya. The Green Belt Movement plans to plant 2 million trees in the coming 30 years over an area of 4,942 acres within the areas of Mount Kenya to mitigate the climate change of the area.[21]

Certainly the capacity for two million trees to offset carbon emissions are significant; however, it probably will not be sufficient to ward off the melting of the glaciers on Mount Kenya without additional conservation of carbon emissions in the rich countries. The Green Belt Movement cannot expect to do it on its own.

Much like Via Campesina, the Green Belt Movement puts emphasis on the issue of food security. Planting trees, as mentioned, plays a role in food security; but the movement also contributes by promoting sustainable farming methods and offering community education on nutrition and food production. Green Belt promoters give community training in organic farming, crop rotation, growing indigenous food crops, family gardening, and proper farming techniques.[22] Their focus is always on self and community empowerment while instilling in people a love for environmental conservation.

SARSTOON-TEMASH INSTITUTE FOR INDIGENOUS MANAGEMENT

In southern Belize, in the Toledo District of the country lies the Sarstoon-Temash National Park (STNP). It is Belize's second-largest national park, encompassing an area of forty-one thousand acres of pristine forest and coastline along the southern border with Guatemala. The park includes 16 miles of Caribbean coastline and contains 14 ecosystem types, including undisturbed mangrove, the only comfre palm forest in Belize, and the only known lowland sphagnum moss bog in Central America. The national park was declared by the Belizean government in 1994 on lands traditionally used by the Garifuna and Maya communities who live in the area. What is now SATIIM began in 1997 as the Sarstoon-Temash National Park Steering Committee, which was formed after the indigenous communities around the park came together to stake a claim in the management of the land and natural resources in and around the park.

SATIIM represents several Ketchi Maya and Garifuna indigenous communities that have traditionally inhabited the area surrounding the national park. These communities provide a buffer zone surrounding the park. Representatives from five of these communities sit on the board of directors of SATIIM.[23]

In 2003, the government of Belize signed an agreement with SATIIM giving it authority to comanage the park with the Department of Forestry, and for the last five years, SATIIM has been taking care of the management of the park. The idea of comanagement is based on the principle that those living closest to the land are best suited to care for it. The Maya and Garifuna communities living near the park possess an integral relationship with the land. Their very existence as farmers and fishermen is tied directly to the health of the environment. Their present and historical relationship to the land ensures their motivation and interest in the parks' ecological health and vitality.

The SATIIM Web site states their mission "to safeguard the ecological integrity of the Sarstoon-Temash region and employ its resources in an environmentally sound manner for the economic, social, cultural, and spiritual well-being of its indigenous people."[24] SATIIM's conservation of the SNTP is important not only for its ecological significance as a sanctuary and biological corridor, but also for its economic, cultural, and spiritual importance to the indigenous Maya and Garifuna communities living around it.

One of the key challenges that SATIIM has faced in recent years is the pressure by the government of Belize to offer logging concessions to multinational corporations who want to log in the region as well as pressure from U.S. oil companies who want to do exploratory drilling in the area and seismic testing in the national park. The government has not shown the same level of resolve in protecting the human and biological diversity of the region as SATIIM has. In 2007, two of the indigenous communities won a landmark decision in the Belizean Supreme Court through the tireless efforts of SATIIM. On October 18, 2007, the Chief Justice of the Supreme Court of Belize ruled that the indigenous villages of Santa Cruz and Conejo hold collective and individual rights to the resources and lands that they have occupied since before the Europeans ever arrived and that they have used according to Maya customary practices. This was a critically significant ruling because the communities did not have legal title to the land, even though they have been living on the land for many years under the auspices of Maya customary land rights, and because the government of Belize had issued or threatened to issue leases, grants, and concessions to these lands without respecting the traditional land tenure of the communities. This ruling states that the government of Belize will now recognize that the Maya people have rights to land and resources in southern Belize based on their longstanding use and occupancy, not based on whether the government had issued them a written lease. They now can continue to farm, hunt, and fish on their land without fear that it will be lost to outside resource extractors. Sovereignty to their land has now been won.[25]

It is the work of SATIIM that helped achieve this victory. SATIIM mounted a multifaceted advocacy campaign that involved raising awareness of the oil exploration issue through public outreach and education, coalition building, legal action, policy research, and analysis; mobilizing local supporters; lobbying government ministers; generating international political, technical, and financial support; and preparing to monitor and mitigate activities in the national park if oil exploration went ahead.

They began the campaign with ambitious objectives—to halt or mitigate the impacts of resource extraction in the STNP and to incorporate biodiversity conservation and indigenous community concerns into Belize's relevant policies and regulations. Thanks to funding from the International Union for Conservation of Nature (IUCN), the Summit Foundation, Green Grants, Conservation International, and the Oak Foundation, SATIIM has been able to carry out their advocacy activities that support these objectives in a timely and effective way.

WASTEPICKERS OF PUNE, INDIA

In the city of Pune, India, a unique university is devoted to the "Empowerment of Women through Education." It is called the Shreemati Nathibai Damodar Thackersey Women's University (SNDTWU or SNDT). It was convened in 1916 by social reformer Bharat Ratna Maharshi Karve and philanthropist Sir Vithaldas Thackersey, both of whom had radical visions, for their times, of offering women the same education advantages that were then the exclusive privilege of men. Today, the university has expanded to more than seventy thousand students spread over many states in India. In 1968, the SNDT College of Home Science was founded under the motto "An Enlightened Woman Is a Source of Infinite Strength." The university practices this motto in many ways.[26]

One of these ways is through a pilot project of training for wastepickers in Pune that was coordinated in 2007 by Dr. Gita Sundaresh, a faculty member at SNDT College of Home Science in the department of Family Resource Management. It is a project that demonstrates the objectives of the university by providing higher education to women through formal and nonformal means. It has been effective at inculcating a positive self-concept among the students, raising awareness of women's issues and rights, and instilling a sense of human values and social responsibility.

Pune is a city of 3.1 million people in the state of Maharashtra; 40 percent of the city dwellers live in slum conditions. The rapid growth of the city and increased consumption levels of its residents have led to a huge problem of solid waste management to the tune of more than one thousand tons daily. Unfortunately, the waste is not managed in a scientific and sanitary method. It is disposed of in open pits and not confined to specific landfill sites. These open-pit sites attract some of the most desperate members of Indian society belonging to the lowest, most depressed social groups in the country. They are the wastepickers, who sift through the garbage looking for recyclable items that they sell for a few pennies to recycling brokers for their livelihood. These wastepickers are mainly women and children from the marginalized sections of the society, who search for scrap paper, metal, glass, and plastics. It is a morbid existence for these women who suffer from unhealthy working conditions, harassment by police, indignity of existence, exploitation, and the poor quality of scrap collected.[27]

In 1990 SNDT's Continuing and Adult Education Department took notice of the plight of these workers while implementing the National Adult Education Program. The initiators of the program (Poornima Chikramane, Laxmi Narayan, and Shabana Diler) felt strongly motivated to fulfill the mandate of the university to even this most marginalized group of women. They realized that by having the households segregate the recyclable items at the source rather than at the landfill they could create better health conditions for the wastepickers, who could collect the segregated waste yielding better-quality scrap with higher monetary returns, and allow education time for the wastepickers.

Wastepickers, however, were not legally recognized as municipal workers and, therefore, not entitled to worker privileges, even though they actually were doing the recycling for the city. Organizers from the SNDT Women's University were instrumental in arranging public rallies that resulted in the formation of a Wastepickers' Association called the Kagad Kach Patra Kashtakari Panchayat, literally meaning an association of workers of paper (Kagad), glass (Kach), and metal (Patra) (KKPKP). The trade union has around 7,500 members, making it one of the biggest wastepickers' unions in India. It has a governing structure, registered membership, and photo-identification cards for each wastepicker. This structure finally gave them legal worker status and exemption from police harassment, not to mention a great deal of personal dignity.

The Wastepickers' Association then negotiated with the Pune Municipal Authorities to begin picking up waste directly from individual houses so that they would not have to rummage through the garbage pits. Buckets were distributed to residential homes, one to collect recyclable items and another to collect wet waste (food scraps). This doorstep method of collecting waste reduced the collection by civic authorities and facilitated the segregation of waste and its management. This method provided better working conditions for the women, enabled them to collect a higher percent of clean recyclables, and provided them dignity and freedom from social exploitation. These women were able to get a better price from the recycling brokers because they collected better-quality waste.

The fact that the workers were then recognized as legitimate civil workers entitled them to get free education for their children, provided them with access to medical insurance and municipal food rations, and helped them form credit cooperatives. This latter benefit freed them from their dependence on money lenders who would often charge interest rates of 60 percent per year. Their work hours have now gone down, allowing them time to attend basic literacy classes.

These benefits are directly attributable to an increase in the income of the wastepickers. They are getting higher prices now from the brokers because of the high quality of the recyclable scrap that they are now collecting. They also charge a nominal fee to each household for picking up the waste at the doorstep. The residents segregate garbage into dry and wet and put it in different colored bins. The wastepickers then collect the garbage, dump the wet garbage in the bins, and take the dry garbage. The wet waste that they collect is deposited in large concrete and metal receptacles that are strategically placed throughout the city. In some colonies, the wet waste is collected in pits for vermi-composting, where it biodegrades after a period of time. The fertile compost is then sold to the public for those who want to put it on their fruit and vegetable gardens. This is an additional source of income for the wastepickers, something they did not have before the formation of the association.[28]

The project has created a great example of sustainable development in action. More material is now being recycled and compost fertilizer is available to city residents, creating environmental benefits. Additionally, the quality of life is now much better for the women wastepickers and their families. Although tension still exists between the wastepickers and the Pune Municipal Corporation, which wants to mechanize all recycling efforts, the positive gains are indisputable. Mangal Gaikwad, a wastepicker by profession, was quoted as saying in the local newspaper,

> Today I earn Rs. 3,000 [US$60] from doorstep collection and the sale of scrap. Residents who used to frown at me while I was at the garbage bin now know me by my name and greet me. One of them even gave me a second-hand bicycle, which I now ride to work.[29]

COMMUNITY SAVINGS PROGRAMS IN BANGLADESH

The Grameen Bank in Bangladesh has received worldwide attention as the premier model of a successful village-level microcredit program. However, another model in the country has received sparse publicity but has proven to be even more transformational than the Grameen Bank. In Bangladesh, a consortium called "The Learning Circle" includes twelve development organizations. Besides having development programs in the standard areas of literacy training, agricultural assistance, and health care, these organizations have developed unique community savings groups that have truly transformed the lives of thousands of Bangladeshi families. One of these organizations is the PARI Development Trust, which works in rural Bangladesh. The methodology that they use is to first form a primary group composed of fifteen to twenty community members. Separate groups for men and women address the strong cultural morays against unfamiliar men and women working together. Each group has an executive committee of three to five members. Additionally, five subcommittees include community initiatives in income generation, justice and rights, adolescent development, functional education, and community-based primary health care. The second tier of the community structure is the Peoples' Institutions (PI). They are formed by approximately ten to fifteen primary groups. At this level, they include a mixed group of women and men. Each primary group elects one or two representatives to serve on the PI. PARI has 180 primary groups in the district of Mymensing, with 3,600 total participants. Forty percent of the participants in the program have increased their family income levels by more than 10 percent in the past year. This increased income allows families to meet their essential daily needs, including eating three meals a day.

The goal of the microenterprise program is to achieve the following:

- Create funds through regular savings
- Invest the funds in community income-generating projects
- Create permanent employment opportunities
- Properly monitor the funds
- Utilize the funds and local resources to effectively bring financial solvency and positive changes to families as well as in society

Primary groups are motivated to save a small amount of money every week. The groups are trained by PARI staff in effective financial management and recordkeeping. They receive training in how to open bank accounts, do basic financial audits, and invest their funds in profitable local businesses.[30]

Members of the primary group who want to start a business can request a loan from the primary group funds at reasonable interest rates. They are accountable to their fellow group members to pay the loan back on time. The funds are replenished by the continuous savings of the members as well as the accrued interest from the rotating loan fund. Each primary group then contributes a portion of their funds to the PI. The PI also establishes a rotating loan fund, which gives out loans to members who request larger loans. This methodology follows the line of a community credit union in which the poor, who might not be able to acquire a standard bank loan, now have access to a line of credit from their group. The groups manage their own funds and are the sole contributors to the fund. Most participants can contribute only a few cents per week to the fund, but now the entire program has more than $138,000 in available loan funds.[31]

In 2002, Faterna began attending the weekly meeting of one of the primary group meetings that started up in her village. She initially contributed US$.07 a week to the group, even though it was financially difficult. After attending a series of training workshops on literacy and money management, she was able to take out a small loan of US$73 to start raising poultry and ducklings, maintaining a fishpond, and cultivating a kitchen garden. Before being group members, her family monthly income was only US$10 per month. Now it has grown to US$87 per month from their many projects. Her personal savings at the group is US$32 and total group savings is US$470 as of December 2006.[32]

The community savings program of PARI has transformed the lives of many families in Bangladesh by building their personal and community assets. It differs markedly from the Grameen Bank in that community members maintain the accounting and decide themselves what microenterprise projects they choose to invest in. It is transformational in creating businesses, jobs, and a security net for the poor in these communities. It is unique in that it is based on savings from the community and does not receive outside funding except for the training they receive from PARI. Sustainable community development, after all, is based on the development of community ownership among community members.

CONCLUSION

The common theme that transects all of the examples cited in this chapter is that they are movements started from below. That is, they are not government initiatives, or United Nations initiatives, or even global philanthropic initiatives. They are movements of those who are marginalized, poor, and disenfranchised. They are people who know what they need for their communities and have designed a strategy to achieve it. They are successful movements that have been able to leverage their success to gain support and attention. The global north can learn from its friends in the global south regarding critical food issues. Access to food is an essential requirement for human survival, and if equity is one of our core values, supplies are sufficient for all. The examples cited in this chapter demonstrate in different ways how people are achieving food security by accessing the necessary land, finances, and social capital to grow and purchase their own food.

NOTES

1. Hernando de Soto, *The Mystery of Capital* (New York: Basic Books, 2000), 7.

2. Amy Cassara, "The Importance of Tenure in Sustainable Development," *World Resources Institute* (June 2007), http://earthtrends.wri.org/updates/node/212 (accessed June 12, 2008).

3. Klaus Deininger et al., "Land Policy to Facilitate Growth and Poverty Reduction," *Land Reform: Land Settlement and Cooperatives: FAO Special Edition* (Rome: Food and Agriculture Organization of the United Nations, 2003), 5; William Van Lopik, "The Response of U.S.-Based Non-Governmental Development Organizations to Inequitable Land Tenure in Latin America" (PhD dissertation, Michigan State University, 2002), 147.

4. Institute for Food and Development Policy, "Global Small-Scale Farmers' Movement Developing New Trade Regimes," *Food First News & Views* 28, no. 97 (Spring/Summer 2000): 2.

5. Annette Aurelie Desmarais, "United in the Via Campesina," *Food First Backgrounder* (Fall 2005): 2.

6. Peter Rosset, "La Hora de La Vía Campesina," *La Jornada* 24, no. 8521 (May 9, 2008): 8.

7. United Nations, "United Nations Declaration of Human Rights" (1948), http://www.un.org/Overview/rights.html (accessed June 2, 2008).

8. La Via Campesina, "What Is La Via Campesina?" http://www.viacampesina.org/main_en/index.php?option=com_content&task=blogcategory&id=27&Itemid=44 (accessed May 16, 2008).

9. Institute for Food and Development Policy, "Food Sovereignty and Agroecology: Growing Movements for Constructive Resistance," *Food First News and Views* (Winter 2007), http://www.foodfirst.org/en/node/1809.

10. United Nations Millennium Project, *Investing in Development: A Practical Plan to Achieve the Millennium Development Goals*, report to the UN Secretary General (London: Earthscan, 2005), http://www.unmillenniumproject.org (accessed May 16, 2008).

11. United Nations, "The Millennium Development Goals and the United Nations Role" (2002), http://www.un.org/millenniumgoals/MDGs-FACTSHEET1.pdf.

12. Jeffrey Sachs, *The End of Poverty* (New York: Penguin Group Inc, 2005), 266.

13. Lawrence Temfwe, "Micah Challenge," *Sojourners Magazine*, July 2005, 23–24.

14. Elizabeth Palmberg, "What's Right With This Picture?" *Sojourners Magazine*, March 2005, 9.

15. Micah Challenge Malawi, "Strategic Areas of Focus," http://www.micahchallenge. org/uploaded_docs/Tell%20it/MC_Malawi_update_June_2008.pdf (accessed June 15, 2008).

16. Dana Milbank, "Guess Who Came to the Evangelicals' Dinner," *Washington Post*, October 12, 2007, A02.

17. Jim Wallis, *God's Politics* (New York: HarperCollins Publishers, 2005), 204.

18. International Union of Forest Research Organizations Task Force (2007–2011), "Forests and Human Health," http://www.iufro.org/download/file/1879/3770/tf-terms-of-reference.doc (accessed June 18, 2008).

19. Carol Pierce Colfer, Douglas Sheil, and Misa Kishi, "Forests and Human Health: Assessing the Evidence" (Occasional Paper No. 45, Center for International Forestry Research, CIFOR, Indonesia, 2006), 13, 25.

20. Anthony McMichael, Simon Hales, and Carlos Corvalan, *Ecosystems and Human Well-Being: Health Synthesis* (Geneva: World Health Organization Press, 2005), 3.

21. Malkhadir Muhumed, "Group Warns That Mountains Will Lose Ice Caps," *CBS News, Sci-Tech*, October 12, 2006, http://www.cbsnews.com/stories/2006/10/12/ap/tech/mainD8KN9DQ80.shtml (accessed May 16, 2008).

22. Wangari Maathai, *The Greenbelt Movement* (New York: Lantern Books, 2006), 42–46.

23. Author unknown, "I-A Commission says GOB must protect indigenous people of Toledo," *The Reporter*, January 5, 2007, http://www.corpwatch.org/article.php?id=14293.

24. SATIIM (Sarstoon-Temash Institute for Indigenous Management), http://www.satiim.org.bz/index.php?section=2 (accessed May 27, 3008).

25. Legal Proceedings of the Supreme Court of Belize, October 18, 2007, Claim Nos. 171 and 172, 2007.

26. SNDT College of Home Science, "About Us," http://www.sndthsc.com/about%20us.htm (accessed June 28, 2008).

27. Gita Sundaresh, "Multi-focal Dimensions of Urban Domestic Solid Waste Management (Pune City)" (paper presented at the College of Menominee Nation, Keshena, WI, October 25–26, 2007).

28. Rahul Chandawarkar, "Making It Your Culture," *The Times of India*, March 15, 2002, http://timesofindia.indiatimes.com/articleshow/3895177.cms.

29. Author unknown, "Pune Union Helps Ragpickers Build Lives—Scrap by Scrap," *The Times of India*, October 31, 2007, http://timesofindia.indiatimes.com/articleshow/2504102.cms.

30. Kohima Daring, Christian Reformed World Relief Committee country consultant in Bangladesh, e-mail message to author, August 5, 2008.

31. Susan Van Lopik, Delta Team Leader for the Christian Reformed World Relief Committee, interview with the author, August 6, 2008.

32. Kohima Daring, "Empowerment Blossoms in the 'Ghardaraj' (Gardenia) Group," *The Learning Circle*, October 4, 2007, 3.

RESOURCE GUIDE

Suggested Reading

Lappé, Frances Moore, Joseph Collins, Peter Rosset, and Luis Esparza, *World Hunger: Twelve Myths*. New York: Grove Press, 1998.

Maathai, Wangari. *Unbowed: A Memoir*. New York: Vintage Books, 2007.

Web Sites

Sharing Indigenous Wisdom: An International Dialogue on Sustainable Development Conference, http://www.sharingindigenouswisdom.org/.

Food First, Institute for Food & Development Policy, http://www.foodfirst.org/.

The Micah Network, http://www.micahnetwork.org/.

World Bank, Social Capital, http://go.worldbank.org/VEN7OUW280.

Grameen Bank, http://www.grameen-info.org/.

5

Food and Democracy

Larry Smith

How can you be expected to govern a country that has 246 kinds of cheese?
—Charles de Gaulle

Democracy shares biological and cultural roots with concern for collective human well-being, grounded in accessing and sharing food. Human roots in foraging likely shaped our genetic predispositions in ways that complicate food democracy. That is, beyond simply responding to preferences, general equity in access to food among many preagrarian cultures, and clear domination of poorly nourished masses by a few better-fed elites in many agrarian cultures, the parameters of food democracy are grounded in genetic predilection for culturally supported, varied and nutrient-rich diets, and moral interaction.[1] Britain, China, India, and North Africa all provide early written legacy of food-related proto-democratic sentiments.[2]

Such food-related democratic attitudes also blossomed in eighteenth-century France based, in part, on the physiocratic understanding that agriculture was the only independently and naturally productive cultural activity. The economic theorists known as physiocrats envisioned the possibility of positive self-organizing collaboration among three freely interacting social groups: farmers (for them, the only net producers), landowners, and artisans.[3] Such ideas, summarized as *laissez faire* (let them alone), became the foundation of the "self-evident" truth of collective benefit as a result of independent "pursuit of liberty" that inspired the American Revolution. Many of the European American founders were influenced by these ideas through their contact with France and, some argue, indigenous North American collaborative management.[4] The physiocrats' agrarian productivity and freedom-grounded thought inspired some colonial American rebels as they embarked on what became modern political democracy. Subsequently, the virtue of mutually reinforcing self-interested decision-making, borrowed from the physiocrats, was reshaped by British emphasis on industry into the foundation of the classical school of economics with Adam Smith's *An Inquiry into the Nature and*

Causes of the Wealth of Nations as its seminal text. Smith's argument, related to food democracy, is best summarized in this famous passage:

> It is not from the benevolence of the butcher, the brewer, or the baker, that we expect our dinner, but from their regard to their own self-interest. We address ourselves, not to their humanity but to their self-love, and never talk to them of our own necessities but of their advantages.[5]

A long century later corporate interests outmaneuvered both the political and the cultural meanings and experience of democracy, as understood by Adam Smith and by many of the American founders, particularly Thomas Jefferson.[6] The principal tool of corporate domination remains the 1886 reinterpretation of the Fourteenth Amendment to the U.S. Constitution, promulgated to clarify the full legal personhood of just-freed slaves, to the legal "interpretation"[7] that corporations deserve the same legal status as individual persons. Additional corporate legal privileges added later include the priority of shareholder monetary considerations, the equation of purchased political communication with individual political speech, and pushing the costs of corporate actions onto others.[8] These constitutional interpretations have dominated food politics for the past century and a quarter,[9] while both the quantity of food produced and the human population have increased astonishingly under what Lang and Heasman call the productionist food paradigm.[10] But, recent assessment suggests that in the process human and planetary ecosystem health have been pushed to near failure.[11]

RECENT PERSPECTIVES

Amartya Sen gave us history's most robust empirical statement linking food and democracy with his observation that cultures with democracies supported by free and pubic sharing of information do not experience famine.[12] Sen observed the relationship between democracy and food security operating through a free press, but recently, the even less controllable Internet has sometimes moderated abusive attempts at political control.[13] However, some look anxiously at the world's food future and wonder about the durability of Sen's observation. In any event, the story of how humanity first created and later overcame famine, and today paradoxically stands challenged by both excess and inadequate nutrition, teaches much about the connections between food and democracy.[14]

Food and democracy, and her muse freedom, wend complexly through all human experience. Curiosity and freedom encourage exploration of different foods and their production and preparation. But freedom also reduces biological diversity and planetary productivity, as with overharvesting and desertification, and destroys some specific food sources, such as easy-to-hunt species, overproduction in fragile environments, heirloom plant and animal varieties overshadowed by "modern" not-quite-equivalents, and heritage foods and food skills crowded out by "easy" or "tasty" market-based alternatives and, with them, both cultural awareness and nutritionally critical dietary diversity. Restrictions on and excesses of freedom, many grounded in individual-, cultural-, policy-, and marketing-driven choices, can be problems. Such choices often express themselves in poor nutrition.[15] Examples include the following:

- Soft drinks and caffeinated beverages
- Most candy and desserts
- Nearly all "fast" and processed "convenience" foods
- Excessive salt in the American diet[16]
- Low-income-driven choice of energy-dense foods made artificially inexpensive by industrial-agriculture-favoring policy choices[17]
- Widespread hunger and forced migration, as when overly intensive land use or climate change or both degrade productivity
- Diet-related diseases, like some cancers and circulatory problems, diabetes, fetal alcohol and other nutritional syndromes, hypertension, obesity, and scurvy

Given our appetites for animal fats and sweets, probably inherited from our forager predecessors,[18] food democracy must attend to both access and restraint, not just to the provision of whatever foods seem abundant, appealing, convenient, or inexpensive. Lang calls this concern *choice editing* in relation to democratic food policy.[19] From this perspective, democracy requires not only the freedom to preserve and create food choices, but also to limit them.

DEMOCRACY

Then, what, after all, is democracy? Both Lincoln's hopeful "A government of, by, and for the people"[20] and Churchill's cynical "The worst of all political systems except for all those others that have been tried"[21] lack operational detail, while the revolutionary sentiment that "the government is best which governs least"[22] reveals physiocratic *laissez-faire* commitments. De Gaulle's question, "How can you be expected to govern a country that has 246 kinds of cheese?" suggests conflict between authority and independent food artistry, the most universally practiced and widely accessible productive activity and, perhaps, the ultimate manifestation of nascent economic democracy.

In *On Democracy* Robert Dahl, the virtual dean of democratic theorists, identifies five prerequisites for people in democratic "state" governments:

- Effective participation
- Equality in voting
- Gaining enlightened understanding
- Exercising final control over the agenda
- Inclusion of adults

He also suggests that pursuit of these ideals yields ten desirable consequences:

- Avoiding tyranny
- Essential rights
- General freedom

- Self-determination
- Moral autonomy
- Human development
- Protecting essential personal interests
- Political equality
- Peace-seeking
- Prosperity

Dahl emphasizes that his lists of democratic prerequisites and consequences are never-completely-realized ideals for governments and have never-fully-experienced consequences. Being state focused, some of these prerequisites are not directly applicable to all food issues.[23] Still, we can focus Dahl's list of prerequisites on food democracy as follows:

- Access to food (an individual biological necessity)
- Choice among foods (a cultural and, for some, genetic[24] necessity)
- Access to quality information and meaningful support, including purchasing power, for learning and participating focused on nutrition, health, and food selection and preparation (a general health and social efficiency necessity)

These prerequisites are used below to assess some food democracy-related activities that are a subset of a larger activity web sometimes collectively referenced as alternative food networks.[25]

CASE STUDIES

Food Policy Councils

World Hunger Year's (WHY) overview of food policy councils celebrates their growth and expansion since their start in Knoxville, Tennessee, in 1982. It emphasizes that "Food policy councils respond to a simple question. If food is a basic human need—on par with water, housing, and health services—why don't state and local governments have a Department of Food?" WHY also emphasizes that

> [N]o U.S. city, state, or county has a Department of Food, and food issues continue to be embedded throughout various local, state, and federal government agencies. Typically, a food policy council at the city or county level does not fully realize the vision of a Department of Food, as its resources and powers are usually quite limited.[26]

Toronto has one of the more active and visible food policy councils. In 1991 the City of Toronto Public Health created the Toronto Food Policy Council (TFPC). The TFPC partners with business and community groups to promote food security through food system awareness, equitable food access, nutrition, community development, and environmental health. The TFPC operates as a modestly funded subcommittee of the Toronto Board of Health. Members include city councilors and volunteer representatives from consumer, business, farm, labor, multicultural, antihunger advocacy, faith, and community development groups. TFPC has brought food security and food policy development to Toronto's municipal agenda by seeking to bridge the gap between producers and consumers.[27]

The TFPC recognized that durable, local solutions require more than a global market and its "mind-numbing notions of food as commodity, people as consumers, and society as marketplace. Instead advocates need to cultivate food citizenship and associated rights and responsibilities."[28] The TFPC focuses on an integrated and self-reinforcing program to encourage food democracy by offering information and experience-rich alternatives to conventional approaches.

> For example, rather than relying on the traditional charity approach their Field to Table program (one of hundreds of community food projects) sells food produced by area farmers at wholesale prices to organized groups of primarily low-income people, and trains these groups in food-related skills . . . lost with the food industry's emphasis on convenience and . . . consequent "de-skilling" of consumers.[29]

Most documentation on TFPC activities is found in reports from the late 1990s and early 2000s celebrating the first 10 years of experience. Although activity continues, it seems likely that something like policy or volunteer fatigue comparable to WHY's critique presented above and discussed below for community gardening has reduced TFPC enthusiasm and activity expansion.

Continuing activity by other interests and governments inspired by the pioneering work of early food policy councils include the 2002 formation of the Chicago Food Policy Advisory Council, which, as its title suggests, chooses to operate "outside of formal city structures" and is thus also vulnerable to volunteer fatigue. In his glowing introduction to this report, Mark Winne of the Community Food Security Coalition, and perhaps the most visible and vocal of the food policy council advocates, praises the CFPAC for

> working for several years to bring together those neighborhood and organization voices that cry out for a just and sustainable food system. They have worked closely with the City of Chicago officials to identify opportunities within city government to . . . push the food system in the right direction . . . public and private sectors are working and planning for access to healthy food for all, see food as a critical part of a sustainable environment, and recognize that food is a major driver in the region's economic engine.[30]

Still, statements from the body of the report like "There was concern if the council was run and managed by the city, participants would lose their ability to set the agenda and priorities for the council" suggest that a deep tension exists between government and people's perceptions of their own interests. Clearly, food is at the epicenter of an enduring contest between human interests and government perspectives reflected in durable policy.[31]

The London Food Board, established in 2004, and the national U.K. Department for Environment Food and Rural Affairs Council of Food Policy Advisors (CFPA), established in October–December 2008, are other efforts in the evolution of urban and national food policy that likely took cues from the TFPC among other projects.

The London Food Board seeks "to develop activities and policies which support a sustainable food system in the capital."[32] It relies on activity and individual influence of its twenty-five Food Board members, to encourage and secure the delivery of healthy and sustainable food for London. The London Development

Authority (LDA), in partnership with Go London, provides Secretariat support, and the LDA and the Department for Environment, Food and Rural Affairs (Defra) provide operational funding to the London Food Board.[33]

The Defra CFPA is the most hopeful new hybrid in the evolving development of food policy. It is new and untested, but its formative documents and membership are impressive, as is its home in a national department with food in its title.[34] The press release announcing the intent to create the department says that it will advise the government on food affordability, security of supply, and the environmental impact of food production, and will contribute to a policy for food security and supply, which is expected to be published within a year. To date, fourteen members of the still-expanding council advisory team with appropriately diverse food system experience have been appointed.[35]

The Defra CFPA is charged with providing advice on the following:

- Achieve sustainable production, distribution, and consumption of food, ensuring that it is available and affordable for all sectors of society
- Consider the effects of global trends on the above
- Advise the secretary of state on how to achieve the four objectives (economics and equity, health, safety, and environment) for food policy set out in the Strategy Unit's report *Food Matters: Towards a Strategy for the 21st Century*
- Make practical policy recommendations

One worrisome detail of the initial organization is that "The role is unpaid, but Defra will reimburse travel and associated expenses." This, of course, means the members are volunteers who must secure their livelihood elsewhere and, though officially "appointed . . . in a personal capacity, not as representatives of any sector, company, or organization" they will face problems supporting recommendations that may challenge interests within the food chain that support them. That concern would be moderated, however, if the council were to move the discussion toward what Lang and Heasman call *evidence-based policy* and away from the historic interest-based approach.[36] Fortunately, "[t]he Council will be established for two years in the first instance, with a review after 18 months. If, when the Council is reviewed, it is decided that a more permanent body is required, a formal appointments process will be followed."[37] Ideally, these recommendations will include the possibility that representatives of critical food chain interests who lack economic security can serve in a paid capacity.

Just as the U.S. political response to climate change has grown primarily from city initiatives, the two newest major urban models of democratic action, which are now followed by a new British national model, may foretell a food policy future—like that called for by WHY, in which departments of food exist at all levels of government.[38] While it is too soon to assess the outcome of these initiatives, it not too soon to suggest that national governments everywhere, including and especially the new U.S. administration, consider similar initiatives.

Food Sovereignty and Security: Earth Democracy

"Earth Democracy is both an ancient worldview and an emergent political movement for peace, justice, and sustainability. Earth Democracy connects the particular to the universal, the diverse to the common, and the local to the global."[39]

With these words, the international human rights activist Vandana Shiva adopts the ancient worldview and promotes the emergent Earth Democracy movement. Shiva holds a doctorate in physics with an emphasis on quantum mechanics, but her career focuses more on India-grounded global social mobilization. Still, Shiva never forgets basic physical realities underpinning natural productivity. Food democracy, with a special focus on cultural rights and genetics especially through seed saving, are at the core of her work, including an emphasis on Earth Democracy and a related partnership with the Slow Food movement called Terra Madre.

All of Shiva's work and especially Earth Democracy reflects a deep understanding of the complex web of life and planetary potential, but much of it grows from concern for inalienable rights of farmers to the products of their cultural knowledge, especially as expressed in seed saving. Earth Democracy is a formidable opponent of corporatization of seed and knowledge with a special emphasis on local food production capability. Shiva explains both the problems and the needed response as follows:

> The globalized food system . . . is creating a fourfold crisis. The first is the crisis of non-sustainability because of overexploitation of soil and water, destruction of biodiversity, and the spread of toxic pollution from pesticides and chemical fertilizers. The second is the crisis faced by small farmers and producers. The third is the crisis of hunger, with a billion people denied their rightful share of the earth's produce. The fourth is the obesity crisis, of which one billion people are victims. This crisis is simultaneously ecological, economic, cultural, and political.[40]

Her recommendation in response to the crisis is democracy.

> Food safety and food security are a democratic challenge for North and South, for rich and poor, for producers and consumers. The right to safe, good, and adequate food is a universal human right and the basis of food democracy. No society can call itself free if it operates in violation of food democracy. . . .[41]
>
> By taking back control over our food systems, we can produce more food while using fewer resources, improve farmers' incomes and strengthen their livelihoods, while solving the problem of hunger and obesity. The future is not certain, but this much is, a better agriculture is possible than the one corporations offer.[42]

Earth Democracy and Terra Madre link ancient wisdoms, resistance to corporate domination grounded in analytical comparisons with the historic enclosure processes that privatized collective resources, and contemporary physics-grounded problems. According to Philpott, "Shiva pines for a 'carbon-rich' future—one in which agriculture systematically builds organic matter into the soil, capturing it from the atmosphere."[43] That future would enrich individual, cultural, and ecosystem productivity, especially regarding access to food, and democracy at every level.

Alternative Food Networks

Alternative food networks (AFNs) are webs of activity, including community gardens, urban agriculture, food cooperatives, farmers markets, community-supported agriculture (CSA), activist restaurants, and artisan agriculturalists and related activities with many labels.[44] Space allows for only limited discussion of a few such activities, all of which seek to shorten food supply chains and personalize food interactions in full accord with the three food-democracy prerequisites identified above and in direct contrast to industrial agriculture's impersonal, opaque, and often deceptive food system.[45]

A profound metaphor for AFNs is the 1960s Japanese housewives' slogan *Teikei* usually translated as "food with a farmer's face," which, in conjunction with older holistic European influences,[46] spawned CSA.[47] AFNs promote short, personalized, information-rich food supply chains. Like certain CSAs that contribute surpluses to food banks or encourage members to subsidize "shares" for low-income members, some AFNs champion effective food policy and food security as a fundamental human right.[48]

By facilitating collaboration among ordinary people in the production or supply chain of their own food, grassroots food activists enact the ultimate manifestation and the historically oldest version of food democracy. For example, collaborative gardening is surely a primary root of both agriculture and cities. Also, direct provisioning, including food service and the sharing of information and awareness that comes with it, must have accompanied trade routes throughout history. Furthermore, as is symbolized by both the Great Depression's unemployed apple peddlers and contemporary street food vendors everywhere, when other economic options fade, people still need to eat, and nearly anyone can earn at least something by helping to feed them.

Community gardens and urban agriculture are obvious roots of urban population aggregation. Immediate local food production was essential to precommodity, transport-based, urban food systems, and it remains significant today, especially to the urban poor and for food diversity. In many places significant shares of often unique foods are produced within or in proximity to cities.[49] Milwaukee community gardener and inner-city activist Will Allen just won a prestigious MacArthur Fellowship for his exceptional urban agriculture and inner-city cultural transformation program called Growing Power.[50]

Community gardens exist in nearly every city. A recent study of New York community gardens—the U.S. city with the most community gardens (nearly 2,000 in 1996, although it is tied for seventh place on a per capita basis)[51]—finds that they increase neighboring property values.[52] Another study confirms that community gardeners consume more fresh fruits and vegetables.[53] And recent and rapidly growing scholarship documents the nutritional superiority of fresh, diverse, naturally grown produce compared with homogeneous industrial alternatives.[54]

But scholarship on community gardening is thin. Laura Lawson's 2005 *City Bountiful: A Century of Community Gardening in America* provides a welcome academic perspective; however, as she acknowledges, it cannot fully make up for limited credible primary sources.[55] Although Lawson recognizes the possibility of a deeper history to community gardening,[56] she mentions only postcontact North American experience and focuses on policy experience since 1890 and thus fails to consider the full roots of collective gardening that not only predate but, quite literally, fed urbanization itself.

The thesis of this chapter is that food and democracy share deep, common, and widely shared roots, grounded in the garden, hearth, and food culture. Perhaps consideration of deeper roots could resolve the question of why interest in community gardens, though ever present and multifaceted, never gained the traction granted other public land uses like parks and playgrounds during the last century.

At least since fossil-fueled hauling replaced animal-powered cartage it has been common to think of agriculture, beyond gardening, as something that happens, or should happen, in "the country." But, in fact, much food is produced in or near most cities. Estimates of urban and peri-urban agriculture's (UPA) share of food consumed in the same city range from around 10 percent or so to upward of 50 percent. For reasons similar to those offered to explain urban gardening's lack of staying power during the last century in America, urban leaders have been uncomfortable embracing in-city agriculture. Thus, while UPA is important for food, employment, and learning, especially for the poor, as well as for enhancing public support for both UPA and sustainable communities generally, scholarship to analyze it and policy to develop it have been sporadic, even in the global south (except in isolated contexts like Cuba).[57]

Moreover, human-animal disease exchange and coevolution, recently associated with the bird flu, increase policy concerns about promoting some historically important forms of urban agriculture. These concerns are raised despite the growing awareness of the widespread, long-standing, and continuing significance of those activities for food security, diet quality, and employment for the poor.[58]

A recent analysis of the decline in UPA as Japan urbanized and struggled with associated planning and zoning conflicts, and of its current efforts to increase UPA activity, expresses the hope that Japan's experience may provide useful insights to other urbanizing areas.[59]

Thus, while many voices speak for the employment, food security, health, social cohesion, aesthetic, therapeutic, transport, and other virtues of UPA,[60] not even some of the most effectively planned cities are able to durably encourage it. Still, despite fundamental concerns like public health and safety and more superficial ones like "modern urban image," interest in UPA is growing and is increasingly fueled by concern for the global environmental consequences of historically conventional views of the "appropriate" division of economic activity between city and country in addition to food security, health, and other social concerns.[61]

Interest in UPA is at an all-time high among policy, philanthropic, and activist realms. The evolving concern for the global environmental consequences of the past century because of fossil fuel overindulgence,[62] now added to the health, food security, and broad social benefits of UPA, can only grow and perhaps bloom into a cornerstone of food democracy in the increasingly urban twenty-first century.

Activist Restaurants

Virtually every community of significant size enjoys one or often several activist restaurants. The activism may start from a cultural, including whole or wholesome food, or ethnic orientation but ever more frequently it also includes locally produced and often "organic" food. Perhaps the most famous such local-production-oriented restaurant is Alice Waters' *Chez Panisse* in Berkeley, California.[63] But in the spirit of the wide and rapid spread of this movement, let's focus on the White Dog Cafe in Philadelphia.

The White Dog Cafe started in 1983 as an informal coffee and muffin shop on the first floor of Judy Wicks's house. Dishes were washed in the corner of the dining room, and the restroom was upstairs in her home. The business took off, and Wicks added a kitchen in the basement and used space from the adjacent brownstone.

Today, the White Dog Cafe has a national reputation for its award-winning fare and leadership in the local-food movement, and Wicks has been named one of *Inc.* magazine's favorite businesswomen, because she put into place "more progressive business practices per square foot than any other entrepreneur." White Dog Cafe follows a four-part mission of serving customers, community, employees, and the natural environment; and uses humanely sourced meat and poultry, seafood from sustainable fisheries, and organic produce in season from local family farms.

The Cafe has created numerous educational and community-building programs focused on economic and social justice, environmental protection, peace and non-violence, drug policy reform, and community arts. Through "Table for Six Billion, Please!" the international "sister restaurant" project started in 1986, the Cafe has organized trips to Nicaragua, Cuba, Mexico, the Netherlands, Lithuania, Vietnam, Israel, and Palestine to understand the effects of U.S. agrifood and other policy. A local sister restaurant program promotes minority-owned restaurants in Philadelphia and Camden, Pennsylvania. The White Dog mentoring program began in 1992 to introduce inner-city high school students to the restaurant business through internships at the Cafe. An adjacent gift store, founded in 1989, features local and fair trade crafts. White Dog Enterprises employs more than 100 people and grosses approximately $5 million annually, demonstrating the concept of "doing well by doing good."[64]

Artisan Agriculture

As a cultural medium, from its roots agriculture frequently becomes a multidimensional art form in many realms. While some of these realms overlap with some of the collaboratively democratic modes discussed above, individual or family farms or food processors focused on producing distinctive high-quality foods, often with no explicit connection to any other cultural movement or phenomenon, abound. These food producers and processors often seek ways to distinguish their product and are symbolized by de Gaulle's quote that is the epigraph to this chapter. From rich dark-yolked eggs from genuinely free-range poultry; lean grass-fed meats from many specialty breeds and even species and sometimes overfed extravagances from goose livers to beer-fed beef; to every imaginable kind of cheese, beer, and wine; to specialty confections and pickled-everything, food artistry is everywhere. Outstanding forms of this expressive medium can provide enough market advantage to support hard-to-govern independent agriculturalists of the sort that Jefferson imagined would give a backbone to democracy and that de Gaulle laments.

Joel Salatin and his Polyface Farm, which was given a vast boost in public attention by Michael Pollan's bestselling *The Omnivore's Dilemma*, exemplify this yeoman agricultural art form.[65] Unlike industrial agriculture, whether organic or not, Salatin uses biology and multispecies interactions, rather than raw fossil-fueled power and industrial fertilizers, to achieve astounding productivity and profitability. Salatin considers himself a "grass farmer." His rotational grazing practices maximize the productivity and feed value of his pasture grass. He follows beef cattle with careful timing of chickens that scatter and enrich the cattle manure and break parasite cycles by, as Salatin puts it, "doing what chickens do," and eating grubs. In the winter, he raises rabbits in hoop houses with poultry under the rabbit cages to take advantage of waste feed and manure with worms under it all, and in the spring the area becomes garden. For Salatin, and many similarly creative farmers, farming is truly an art form and a never-ending process of creative improvement.[66] This kind of agriculture, and these kinds of farmers, are what Colin Tudge has in mind as he tells us *Feeding People Is Easy*, if only industrial agriculture and court rulings will stand aside in favor of a more democratic agrifood policy.[67]

Even without Pollan's bestselling boost, Salatin is a well-known public figure. He sponsors tours of his farm, writes extensively, especially in *Acres U.S.A.*, which calls itself "The Voice of Eco-Agriculture," and also contributes to books with titles like *Salad Bar Beef* and *Pastured Poultry Profit$*. In 2008, he was invited to testify on meat-processing standards before the House Committee on Oversight and Government Reform. His testimony grew out of his Polyface Farm transparency guiding principles, which are as follows:

1. Encourage a relationship among food, patron, farmer and processor . . .
2. Delivery limited to within four hours from the farm . . .
3. Diversified work stations . . . [with rotated workers to reduce physical and emotional stress and improve workers' ability to relate to visitors] . . .
4. Processing should be done on-farm or as close to the farm as possible.[68]

His testimony emphasized the need for transparent and culturally embedded food processing, including for slaughter and meat processing. He suggests establishing empirical thresholds for contamination enforced by random testing instead of rigid rules, which favor industrial-scale producers. Empirical thresholds with random testing would provide opportunities for real competition between industrially supplied and "serious entrepreneurial community-based food." Rules that make such community-based, culturally embedded agricultural processes competitively viable, Salatin argues, will "guarantee every American freedom of food choice." Among ten witnesses on the day he testified, Salatin was the only advocate of culturally and ethically grounded bottom-up, and hence inherently democratic, "regulatory" procedures. The other witnesses all were debating details of top-down regulation and enforcement.[69]

Salatin's summary states,

> The answer is more transparency through expanded market competition by freeing up community-based food systems to exist again . . . allow[ing] a community to at least try it. If people get sick, then it won't spread. But if in fact people begin eating better, the distribution carbon footprint is smaller, and area hospitals become vacant, then this system can be exonerated . . . and a self-directed community can choose *for itself* whether it wants government food or neighborhood food. . . . Food freedom can be allowed to proliferate organically and to make its own credentials within the culture.[70]

These recommendations, if generalized beyond meat processing, constitute a near manifesto for the future of food. The manifesto will be even more pertinent as time and contemporary human appetites continue, despite the current recession's dip, to press fossil fuel and thus industrially produced food prices upward. As this transpires, a broad transition to local food production and consumption will move ahead in rough parallel. As Pollan and Salatin make clear, locally appropriate farming is a learning process that, like any learning process, is furthered by collaboration and cooperation. Food giants that close their plants to the world's view and thereby to the openness of the democratic process must learn everything for themselves, however slowly, and their customers must pay for their learning in either prices or health consequences. Collaborating local farmers can learn from each other, their customers, and their suppliers as well as their advocates, like *Acres U.S.A.*, Rodale Press, and many authors in these two volumes. That these farmers are still out of the mainstream, and they are quite aware of this fact, means that they *must* learn together, trust each other, and develop the trust of their customers.

Such collective learning by those who are left out, in the spirit of Paulo Freire's *Pedagogy of the Oppressed*,[71] is the essence of democracy. This learning can be trusted to bring local food to the world's tables and democracy to its cultures despite practices and powers of corporate interests. In this regard, the continued leveling of the playing field, with increases in the price of fossil fuel, and associated incentives for carbon sequestration (at which low-input local food production is efficient) are all the policy support local agriculture and associated food democracy probably need. Indeed, "carbon farming" will likely dominate in the future, particularly as a policy to slow climate change matures with or without the currently corporate, "Big-Ag" and "big-food" dominated U.S. food policy.[72] Specific supports can help—for example, the land-grant agricultural college and extension systems, originated in the 1860s to promote food democracy, can be encouraged to attend at least as enthusiastically to local agricultural interests as they have historically to Big Ag interests.[73] Leveling the playing field in terms of what can be labeled "organic"—or better, carbon-friendly—also can help.

But even without explicit policy support, the sun's inherently democratic distribution of its immense energy—which was exactly why the physiocrats focused on the productivity of the land—ultimately will overwhelm the industrial food system that still seems incapable of reducing the mileage on, as well as the attendant fuel and carbon cost of, its products in the supermarkets.

CONCLUSION

The activities discussed in this chapter explicitly address the most fundamental of our modified version of Dahl's characteristics of democracy; they embody and reflect profound desire to infuse meaningful information into the food system. They also, at least implicitly but ever more openly, demonstrate a profound commitment to the ultimate sharing of information among eaters and to the foundation of the food system that is coming to be called "carbon farming." In the spirit of life's chemistry, perhaps it should be called "life farming."

Whatever we call it, food democracy is resilient and permanent. The mindlessness brought increasingly to eating by marketing in the last century is a temporary phenomenon. It will pass, and as it does, shared democratic consciousness regarding what and when to eat will return. The return of food consciousness will be greatly enhanced by the greatest social force on the twenty-first century horizon, carbon-conserving politics forced by climate change. We will soon, at least in historic context, embrace this consciousness and with it regionally democratic food practices. The more rapidly we move in this direction, the more comfortable humanity can be in its niche on Earth. As we move to embrace carbon consciousness, the sometimes-struggling activities reviewed in this chapter will provide useful perspective; and as the transition gains momentum, we will gradually begin to wonder, why were those pioneers so marginalized?

NOTES

1. Kenneth F. Kiple, *A Movable Feast: Ten Millennia of Food Globalization* (Cambridge, MA; New York: Cambridge University Press, 2007), 1–13; Marc D. Hauser, *Moral Minds* (New York: Harper Collins, 2006).

2. Ven. S. Dhammika, *The Edicts of King Ashoka* (1993), http://www.cs.colostate. edu/~malaiya/ashoka.html#INTRODUCTION (accessed September 12, 2008). "The contents of Asoka's edicts make it clear that all the legends about his wise and humane rule are more than justified. . . . State resources were used for useful public works like the importation and cultivation of medical herbs, the building of rest houses, the digging of wells at regular intervals along main roads and the planting of fruit and shade trees." Craig A. Lockard, *Societies, Networks, and Transitions: A Global History* (Boston: Houghton Mifflin, 2008), 309; Peter Linebaugh, *The Magna Carta Manifesto* (Berkeley: University of California Press, 2008); Ibn Khaldun, *The Muqaddimah, An Introduction to History*, trans. Franz Rosenthal (Princeton: Princeton University Press, 1967), vol. 3.

3. Henry William Spiegel, *The Growth of Economic Thought* (London; Durham, NC: Duke University Press, 1991), chapter 8.

4. Jack McIver Weatherford, *Indian Givers: How the Indians of the Americas Transformed the World* (New York: Fawcett Columbine, 1988) 117–50.

5. Smith, Adam, *An Inquiry into the Nature and Causes of the Wealth of Nations*, ed. Edwin Cannan (1776; repr., New York: Random House, 1937), 14.

6. James Gustave Speth, *The Bridge at the Edge of the World: Capitalism, the Environment, and Crossing from Crisis to Sustainability* (London; New Haven, CT: Yale University Press, 2008), chapter 8.

7. Ibid., 166. "In the 1886 Supreme Court case of Santa Clara County v. Southern Pacific Railroad, the chief justice merely said from the bench during oral argument that Southern Pacific was entitled to the protection of the Fourteenth Amendment. This comment, irrelevant to the Court's disposition of the case, made it into the clerk's notes on the case, not the decision itself, and the rest is history."

8. Ibid., 166–68.

9. Marion Nestle, *Food Politics: How the Food Industry Influences Nutrition and Health*, California Studies in Food and Culture, 3 (Berkeley: University of California Press, 2007).

10. Tim Lang and Michael Heasman, *Food Wars: The Global Battle for Mouths, Minds and Markets* (London; Sterling, VA: Earthscan, 2004), 16–20.

11. Millennium Ecosystem Assessment, http://www.millenniumassessment.org/en/ index.aspx (accessed November 8, 2008).

12. Amartya Sen, *Development as Freedom* (New York: Knopf, 1999), 51–52.

13. Garry Rodan, "The Internet and Political Control in Singapore," *Political Science Quarterly* 113, no. 1 (1998): 63.

14. Thomas F. Pawlick, *The End of Food: How the Food Industry Is Destroying Our Food Supply—and What You Can Do About It* (Fort Lee, NJ: Barricade, 2006); Paul Roberts, *The End of Food* (London: Bloomsbury, 2008).

15. Nestle, *Food Politics*.

16. Kiple, *A Movable Feast*, 293–94.

17. Michael Pollan, "You Are What You Grow," *New York Times Magazine*, April 22, 2007; Nicole Darmon and Adam Drewnowski, "Does Social Class Predict Diet Quality?" *American Journal of Clinical Nutrition* 87, no. 5 (May 2008): 1107–117.

18. Such appetites and associated abilities to follow the scent of burning meat, arrive first, gorge, and flee, sometimes with the need for great endurance that would have been enhanced by rapidly digestible energy-boosting foods like honey, when

available, would have been advantageous in times of scarcity or stress and thus concentrated in the evolving gene pool.

19. Tim Lang, "Food Security or Food Democracy?" *Pesticides News* 78 (December 2007): 12. Of course, our present system already edits choice, for example, toward foods high in inexpensive ingredients like fat, salt, and high fructose corn syrup; and, the editing is not all about cost fundamentals because production of certain ingredients like corn and sugar and practices like confined animal feeding are favored by policy.

20. Abraham Lincoln, *Gettysburg Address*, 1863, http://showcase.netins.net/web/creative/lincoln/speeches/gettysburg.htm (accessed April 16, 2009).

21. Said What?, "Government and Politics in Quotes" http://www.saidwhat.co.uk/articles/government.php (accessed April 16, 2009).

22. This statement is often attributed to Thomas Jefferson. However, it has not been found anywhere in Jefferson's recorded writings or speeches. http://www.geocities.com/peterroberts.geo/Relig-Politics/TJefferson.html (accessed April 17, 2009).

23. Robert Dahl, *On Democracy* (New Haven, CT: Yale University Press, 1998), 37–45.

24. Kiple, *A Movable Feast*, 292–94. Higher risk of hypertension among people of African heritage is probably just one of many genetic roots of dietary risk resulting from broad cultural and food processing practices, in this case overabundant salt in the U.S. diet.

25. Lucy Jarosz, "The City in the Country: Growing Alternative Food Networks in Metropolitan Areas," *Journal of Rural Studies* 24, no. 3 (2008): 231–44.

26. Anonymous, *Food Policy Councils*, http://www.worldhungeryear.org/fslc/faqs/ria_090.asp?section=8&click=1 (accessed December 28, 2008).

27. Toronto Food Policy Council, http://www.toronto.ca/health/tfpc_index.htm (accessed October 15, 2008).

28. Neva Hassanein, "Practicing Food Democracy: A Pragmatic Politics of Transformation," *Journal of Rural Studies* 19, no. 1 (2003): 79–80.

29. Ibid.; Wesley Mitchel, "The Backward Art of Spending Money," *The American Economic Review* 2, no. 2 (June 1912): 269–81.

30. Lynn Peemoeller, "Building Chicago's Community Food Systems: A Report by the Chicago Food Policy Advisory Council," Monograph (Chicago: Chicago Food Policy Advisory Council, 2008), http://www.chicagofoodpolicy.org (accessed December 28, 2008).

31. Ibid., 9.

32. Anonymous, "Terms of Reference for the London Food Board," http://www.lda.gov.uk/server.php?show=ConWebDoc.2877 (accessed December 28, 2008).

33. Ibid.

34. The Strategy Unit, *Food Matters: Towards a Strategy for the 21st Century* (Cabinet Office, U.K. Government, July 2008), http://www.cabinetoffice.gov.uk/media/cabinetoffice/strategy/assets/food/food_matters1.pdf.

35. Defra (Department for Environment, Food, and Rural Affairs), "Council of Food Policy Advisors," http://www.defra.gov.uk/foodrin/policy/council/index.htm. Links to three late-2008 press releases regarding formation of the Food Council Board, announcement of its chair, and announcement of appointments to the Food Council Board are available here. To date, 14 Council members have been announced with more to come. Four of these also sit on the London Food Board. The impressive slate of board members are "appointed . . . in a personal capacity, not as representatives of any sector, company, or organization." They come with critically appropriate food chain experience, including conventional and cooperative food industry interests, activist restaurant entrepreneurship, childhood and other at-risk food interests, insurance, and agriculture, including farming, public health, and academia. Four of the 14 are academics, including Professor Tim Lang, who is an outspoken critic of conventional corporate-dominated food policy. It will be

fascinating to see the minutes of their deliberations, which *must* be made transparently public to enhance the effort's credibility.

36. Lang and Heasman, *Food Wars*, 42–46.

37. Defra, "Council of Food."

38. Al Gore, *An Inconvenient Truth: The Planetary Emergency of Global Warming and What We Can Do About It* (New York: Rodale Press, 2006); Anonymous, *Food Policy Councils.*

39. Vandana Shiva, *Earth Democracy: Justice, Sustainability, and Peace* (Cambridge, MA: South End Press, 2005), 1.

40. Ibid., 151–52.

41. Vandana Shiva, "Food Democracy v. Food Dictatorship: The Politics of Genetically Modified Food," *Z Magazine*, April 2003, http://www.zmag.org/zmag/viewArticle/14050 (accessed December 31, 2008).

42. Shiva, *Earth Democracy*, 152.

43. Tom Philpott, "Terra Madre Notes: Vandana Shiva Rocks the House, A Food/Climate Manifesto Presents New Visions for Responding to Climate Change," http://gristmill.grist.org/story/2008/10/25/904/94558 (accessed November 18, 2008).

44. Jarosz, "The City in the Country."

45. Nestle, *Food Politics.*

46. Anonymous, "History of Community Supported Agriculture, Lecture Outline," http://casfs.ucsc.edu/education/instruction/tdm/download/4.1_CSA_History.pdf (accessed May 12, 2008). Despite limited documentation, this lecture outline is the most comprehensive single overview of the history of CSA.

47. Steven M. Schnell, "Food with a Farmer's Face: Community-Supported Agriculture in the United States," *Geographical Review* 97, no. 4 (2007): 550–64; Katherine L. Adam, "Community Supported Agriculture" (2006), http://attra.ncat.org/attra-pub/PDF/csa.pdf (accessed December 27, 2008).

48. The United Nations Universal Declaration of Human Rights, Article 25 no. 1, http://www.un.org/Overview/rights.html (accessed August 14, 2008), is the most universally cited authority naming food as a core element of an adequate standard of living, a basic human right.

49. Fred Pearce and Orjan Furubjelke, "Cultivating the Urban Scene," in *AAAS Atlas of Population & Environment*, ed. Paul Harrison and Fred Pearce (Berkeley: University of California Press, 2000), http://atlas.aaas.org/index.php?part=4&sec=urban (accessed December 26, 2008); Wendy Mendes et al., "Using Land Inventories to Plan for Urban Agriculture: Experiences from Portland and Vancouver," *Journal of the American Planning Association* 74, no. 4 (2008): 435–49.

50. 2008 MacArthur Fellows, "Will Allen," http://www.macfound.org/site/c.lkLXJ8MQKrH/b.4537249/ (accessed December 27, 2008).

51. American Community Gardening Association, "National Community Garden Survey" (ACGA Monograph 1998), http://7d8ca58ce9d1641c9251f63b606b91782998fa39.gripelements.com/docs/CGsurvey96part1.pdf (accessed November 18, 2008).

52. Ioan Voicu and Vicki Been, "The Effect of Community Gardens on Neighboring Property Values," *Real Estate Economics* 36, no. 2 (2008): 241–83.

53. Katherine Alaimo et al., "Fruit and Vegetable Intake among Urban Community Gardeners," *Journal of Nutrition Education and Behavior* 40, no. 2 (2008): 94–101.

54. See chapter 12 by Debra Pearson in volume 1, *Environment, Agriculture, and Health Concerns.*

55. Laura J. Lawson, *City Bountiful: A Century of Community Gardening in America* (Berkeley: University of California Press, 2005) 292–93.

56. Ibid., 2.

57. Alexandra Spieldoch, "The Food Crisis and Global Institutions" (Global Policy Forum, August 5, 2008), http://www.globalpolicy.org/socecon/hunger/general/2008/0805globalinstitutions.htm (accessed December 31, 2008); Sinan Koont, "Food Security in Cuba." *Monthly Review* 55, no. 8 (2004): 11–20, http://www.monthlyreview.org/0104koont.htm; Bill McKibben, *Deep Economy: The Wealth of Communities and the Durable Future* (New York: Times Books, 2007), 71–77.

58. Anonymous, *Urban and Peri-Urban Agriculture (UPA) in the Asian and Pacific Region* (Taipei: Food and Fertilizer Technology Center, 2007); London Food Link, *Edible Cities—A Report of a Visit to Urban Agriculture Projects in the U.S.A.* (London: Sustain, 2008).

59. Kunio Tsubota, *Urban Agriculture in Asia: Lessons from Japanese Experience* (Taipei: Food and Fertilizer Technology Center, 2007), 2–3.

60. Anne C. Bellows, Katherine Brown, and Jac Smit, "Health Benefits of Urban Agriculture" (Venice, CA: Community Food Security Coalition, 2005), http://www.foodsecurity.org/UAHealthArticle.pdf (accessed July 4, 2008).

61. Katherine H. Brown and Anne Carter, *Urban Agriculture and Community Food Security: Farming from the City Center to the Urban Fringe*, Monograph (Venice, CA: Community Food Security Coalition. 2003), http://www.foodsecurity.org/PrimerCFSCUAC.pdf (accessed July 4, 2008).

62. See chapter 5 by David Pimentel in volume 1, *Environment, Agriculture, and Health Concerns*.

63. Renee Montagne, "The Food Revolution of Alice Waters' Chez Panisse," *Morning Edition of National Public Radio*, April 27, 2007, http://www.npr.org/templates/story/story.php?storyId=9848900 (accessed December 1, 2008).

64. White Dog Café, http://www.whitedog.com (accessed December 1, 2008); David Kuppfer, "Judy Wicks on Her Plan to Change the World, One Restaurant at a Time," *The Sun*, August 2008, 5–13.

65. Michael Pollan, *The Omnivore's Dilemma: A Natural History of Four Meals* (New York: Penguin, 2006) 185–273.

66. Ibid., 208–25.

67. Colin Tudge, *Feeding People Is Easy* (Pari, Italy: Pari, 2007).

68. Joel Salatin, "After the Beef Recall: Exploring Greater Transparency in the Meat Industry," *Acres U.S.A.* 38, no. 6 (2008): 40–41.

69. Ibid., 42–45.

70. Ibid., 45.

71. Paulo Freire, *Pedagogy of the Oppressed*, trans. Myrna Bergman Ramos (New York: Continuum, 1970).

72. Tiziano Gomiero, Maurizio G. Paoletti, and David Pimentel, "Energy and Environmental Issues in Organic and Conventional Agriculture," *Critical Reviews in Plant Sciences* 27, no. 4 (2008): 239–54.

73. Daniel S. Greenberg, *Science for Sale: The Perils, Rewards and Delusions of Campus Capitalism* (Chicago: University of Chicago Press, 2007).

RESOURCE GUIDE

Suggested Reading

Berry, Wendell. *The Unsettling of America: Culture & Agriculture*. Berkeley: University of California Press, 1996 (1977).

Hawken, Paul. *Blessed Unrest: How the Largest Movement in the World Came into Being and Why No One Saw It Coming.* New York: Penguin, 2007.

Kiple, Kenneth F. *A Movable Feast: Ten Millennia of Food Globalization.* Cambridge and New York: Cambridge University Press, 2007.

Lang, Tim, and Michael Heasman. *Food Wars: The Global Battle for Mouths, Minds and Markets.* London and Sterling, VA: Earthscan, 2004.

Lawson, Laura J. *City Bountiful: A Century of Community Gardening in America.* Berkeley: University of California Press, 2005.

McKibben, Bill. *Deep Economy: The Wealth of Communities and the Durable Future.* New York: Times Books, 2007.

Nestle, Marion. *Food Politics: How the Food Industry Influences Nutrition and Health.* Berkeley: University of California Press, 2007.

Pollan, Michael. *The Omnivore's Dilemma: A Natural History of Four Meals.* New York: Penguin Press, 2006.

Speth, James Gustave. *The Bridge at the Edge of the World: Capitalism, the Environment, and Crossing from Crisis to Sustainability.* New Haven and London: Yale University Press, 2008.

Tudge, Colin. *Feeding People Is Easy.* Pari, Italy: Pari, 2007.

Web Sites

Community Food Security Coalition, http://www.foodsecurity.org/.

Department for Environment, Food, and Rural Affairs, Council of Food Policy Advisors, http://www.defra.gov.uk/foodrin/policy/council/index.htm.

Global Policy Forum, http://www.globalpolicy.org/visitctr/about.htm.

Growing Power, http://www.growingpower.org/Index.htm.

Millennium Ecosystem Assessment, http://www.millenniumassessment.org/en/index.aspx.

Navdanya, http://www.navdanya.org/.

Resource Centres on Urban Agriculture & Food Security, http://www.ruaf.org/.

Wiser Earth, http://www.wiserearth.org/.

World Hunger Year, http://www.worldhungeryear.org/about_why/why_programs.asp.

6

Consumers as Political Actors

Michele Micheletti and Dietlind Stolle

FOOD FOR POLITICAL THOUGHT

Globalized agricultural production offers consumers a steady supply of affordable fresh food all year long. It livens up meals with a good selection of produce and provides meat, poultry, and fish for the family dinner. Supermarket ads and food displays in grocery store aisles encourage consumers to indulge in seasonal food off-season. Thanks to the global food trade, consumers can purchase a wide variety of eatable goods on a daily basis. The list of global food constantly available on supermarket shelves grows longer and longer each year. Consumers can now plan meals around fresh berries, vegetables and fruit, inexpensive meat, poultry and fish, and plenty of good coffee, tea, and chocolates. Yet behind this enticing smorgasbord of affordable abundance is a series of problems directly related to global food supply and demand. Intensified agribusiness has led to global environmental problems with groundwater supply depletion, soil degradation, fresh water and air pollution, biodiversity loss, deforestation, and animal waste. It perpetuates the transmission of Bovine Spongiform Encephalopathy ("mad cow disease"), salmonella, and avian (bird) flu. Farming for the global supermarket also diverts land in poor countries from more local food crops and tends to treat farmworkers badly. The World Summit on Sustainable Development declared in 2007 that "fundamental changes in the way societies produce and consume are indispensable for achieving global sustainable development."[1]

The United Nations, World Resource Institute, European Union, national governments, corporate business, and civil society have problems associated with globalized food production on their agenda. The United Nations Convention on Biological Diversity identifies agriculture for its 2008 international day as "a major driver of biodiversity loss," and its agencies—the International Labour Organization (ILO) and the Food and Agriculture Organization of the United Nations (FAO)—work together because "the problems facing workers in agriculture need to be highlighted concerning social exclusion, poverty alleviation, fundamental rights, sustainable agriculture and sustainable development, food security and decent work in agriculture."[2] Local-to-global civil society campaigns mobilize grassroots consumer support to protect nature and humans from the negative effects of global agribusiness and to protest child labor in agricultural work and farm animal cruelty. This chapter focuses on why these groups believe that consumers must take responsibility for the food they eat, how they convince them to do so, and how successful they in campaigning.

THREE FORMS OF FOOD ACTIVISM

Civic groups use colorful language to draw consumers' attention to how their food choices and eating habits affect the world. They call farmworkers who help stock global supermarket shelves with fresh produce and candy "fruit slaves" and "chocolate slaves" to drive home problems with the lack of decent working conditions and wages in globalized food production. Their campaigns also identify large-scale agriculture as an industry—a "factory farm" system—that produces "Franken[stein] foods" from genetically modified seed and fodder and treats cows, pigs, and chickens like "animal machines" that only live to produce a steady high supply of milk, eggs, and meat. These groups urge consumers to think more broadly about agricultural products, protest against corporate practice, make different food choices, adopt new eating habits, and, in so doing, help change global food production.

Their mission is political consumerism. The consumer market, particularly the global supermarkets and fast-food chains in affluent nations, is their arena for politics. The groups inform shoppers about the "politics of products"—the social justice, health, and environmental aspects of food commodity production. Many of them target national and supranational governments. However, current free trade doctrines, the character of global problems, difficulties in legislating forceful national approaches, national protectionism, and the slow-moving consensual nature of international governmental organizations make public policy solutions less attractive.

Instead, these civic groups focus on the growing power of individual and even institutional consumers to influence the politics behind supermarket food. They support the three forms of political consumerism: boycotts, "buycotts," and discursive actions. Consumers are asked to support their cause by boycotting (refusing) to buy certain designated food brands and products. Examples include the 1960s grape boycott to protect grape pickers in California from deadly pesticides and give them better working and living conditions, the tuna boycotts of the 1980s to save dolphins caught in tuna fishing nets, and the Monsanto boycotts of the 1990s to oppose genetically modified organisms (GMOs).[3] In the ongoing Killer Coke Campaign, consumers pressure Coca-Cola to allow unions to represent workers in its bottling plants in Colombia, stop its overuse and pollution of fresh water in India, and protest its procuring of sugar harvested by child labor in El Salvador. The campaign criticizes the company's marketing of sweetened beverages to children globally. The boycott of Nestlé is well-known and long in duration. It charges Nestlé with responsibility "for more violations of the World Health Assembly marketing requirements for baby foods than any other company."[4]

Conversely, "buycotts" ask shoppers to buy (i.e., BUYcott) goods for ethical, political, and environmental reasons. Shopping guides and labeling schemes are the main forms of food buycotts today. Both types of guidelines, which have increased in number and importance, give consumers information about choosing among brands responsibly, replacing certain food choices with others, and a general understanding about how they can eat and promote sustainable food consumption in one easy bite. One of the first shopping guides, *The Green Consumer Supermarket Shopping Guide. Shelf-by-Shelf Recommendations for Products Which Don't Cost the Earth* (1984), is called a publishing phenomenon. It appeared in some 20 foreign editions, sold about 1 million copies globally, was updated in 1991 and functions as a role model for similar efforts.

Discursive actions, the third form of political consumerism, spread ideas rather than directly guiding consumers' choice. Although supportive of boycott causes and labeling schemes, they play an independent role by providing consumers with additional ways to speak out about how they view the connection between the food they eat and the way it is produced. At times, they are the only option open for consumers. Some examples include nongovernmental organization (NGO) "urgent alerts" that trigger consumers immediately to send corporations e-mails and faxes, animated films, culture jamming,[5] and efforts in "taste education" to teach food appreciation that discourages more globalized fast food. Food political consumerism even brings commercial culture and popular brands into activism. Interesting efforts include Free Range Studios' flash films, which successfully catch the public's eye by adapting blockbuster movie themes and music. *The Meatrix* award-winning films piggyback on *The Matrix*. They include interactive technology for consumers to learn more about factory farming and farm animal treatment and have been seen by more than twenty-five million people globally. The *Star Wars* theme is recognizable in *Grocery Store Wars*, a campaign film for organic food dubbed as a sci-fi supermarket saga by its sponsor, the Organic Trade Association. These films, which are easily found on YouTube and appeal to young people, hit hard at agribusiness and fast-food restaurants, and direct consumers into political consumerist activism.[6]

Food activism also employs culture jamming in its campaigns when it sponges off commercial advertising and corporate imagery in consumer society. After consumer pressure, celebrity support, and more than 800 protest actions worldwide, People for the Ethical Treatment of Animals (PETA) called off its 2001 "Murder King" campaign when Burger King, in an industry-leading commitment, began to source cage-free eggs.[7] Ongoing culture jamming is used to pressure Wendy's and Kentucky Fried Chicken to do the same.[8] Interestingly, the Kentucky Fried Cruelty campaign lets supporters devise their own activism. The Killer Coke Campaign also uses cultural resonance in the form of Coca-Cola's well-known marketing imagery, that is, its logotype and slogans. Previously McDonald's was an important target, but consumer activism led it to change its corporate practices. Nevertheless, its golden arches and the term "McDonaldization" still call attention to the negative effects of a fast-food lifestyle.[9] Discursive actions can even include friendly goal-oriented talks with the local grocer and restaurants about better procurement policy and with friends and neighbors about why food activism is important.

CERTIFICATION SCHEMES AND LIFESTYLE FOOD ACTIVISM

Certifying food has become an important vehicle in the struggle for sustainable food production and consumption. Certification and labeling schemes offer consumers concrete ways to change their purchasing choices and dietary habits. Most labeling schemes started as small activist campaigns that ran counter to established corporate policy and practice. Today, they successfully bring NGOs, farmers, consumers, and global food corporations together in constructive efforts to solve problems with global food production. They direct food activism away from contentious boycotts and reveal to businesses that consumer demand and a market exist for sustainable food. Labeling schemes are, therefore, an important innovation in food activism. Three global schemes for organic, fair trade, and sustainable fish are in operation today. Others are on the way. This section discusses what is called the "certification revolution" in global food production.[10] But first it is important to distinguish political consumerist labeling and certification schemes from those run by business. Both appear on common food goods. Political consumerist schemes are "type one" (third-party) in character. Business-driven ones (one-party schemes) are not. Type-one schemes are multistakeholder regulatory frameworks characterized by procedural and operational transparency. They bring together the major stakeholders—civil society associations, scientists, business, and government—to formulate certification criteria and use independent professional bodies to evaluate food for accreditation. Food production is then monitored to ensure that the accreditation standards are followed. If not, food producers are warned and, when necessary, certification is rescinded.

Organic Labeling for Ecological Food and Farming

Certification as organically grown is the oldest political consumerist food label. Concern for soil life and food for human health are the roots of today's global organic labeling industry. The first label (the Demeter biodynamic label) is from 1928. Broader consumer interest for organic food came after the publication of *Silent Spring* (1962), which addressed the problem of pesticide use in agriculture. In the early 1970s, alternative farmers and particularly a French farmers' association mobilized worldwide support for the creation of the International Federation of Organic Agriculture Movements (IFOAM). The British Soil Association (an important food activist group) established its organic label in 1973. IFOAM has grown from a small operation with member organizations from five countries (Great Britain, France, Sweden, South Africa, and the United States) to one with 739 affiliates from 106 countries (more than half of all countries in the world today). Many countries have more than one member. Canada has 11, China 33, Japan 17, Germany 69, India 48, Mexico 11, the Netherlands 25, the United Kingdom 16, and the United States 45. In the beginning, organic certification focused solely on the ecological aspect of farming (food produced from renewable resources, without antibiotics and growth hormones and that conserved the soil and water and enhanced biodiversity). As factory farming expanded and campaigns for pure or true non-GMO food, interest in fair trade, and consumer demand for community-supported local agriculture grew in importance, IFOAM expanded its standards to include the four principles of health, ecology, fairness, and care in its certification process. Health equates human and ecosystem well-being, ecology is biodiversity, fairness is fair treatment of farmworkers and farm animals, and care is the personal responsibility of farmers and consumers to safeguard the health and well-being of current and future generations and the environment.

Labeling schemes certify both organic food produced by "counterculture" green small farmers and food corporations, which shows the strength of the food "certification revolution." Some groups, like the Organic Consumer Association (OCA), view corporate activism as a threat to organic standards and ask consumers to boycott some U.S. Department of Agriculture (USDA) organic-labeled products. But in general, political consumerist food activists support it and use enticing, colorful, appealing, and even guilt-creating efforts to get shoppers to do so as well. Environmental, humanitarian, humane societies, and consumer-oriented associations as well as Global Exchange and special associations just for organic food even follow the lead of corporate commercial culture and prey on consumer vulnerabilities at holiday time. Like food and other retailers, they play up holiday generosity and gift-giving in special offers for Mother's Day, Father's Day, Valentine's Day, Thanksgiving, and Christmas. OCA plays off the classic hit "Unchain My Heart" to get North American consumers to unchain their hearts and open their wallets at Valentine's Day. Why? Because "by purchasing organic and Fair Trade chocolate and flowers . . . your consumer dollars will no longer be going towards toxic pesticides, child slavery, and farm worker exploitation."[11] Along with buying organic gifts, it suggests that consumers download a special Valentine's card and send prewritten e-mail messages to "anti-Valentines" businesses. In 2008, they included Nestlé, Dole, Wal-Mart, M&M-Mars Inc., and Hershey. It also gets animated in a simple and silly one-minute flash film that names, shames, and blames these businesses.[12]

Fair Trade Labels for Global Social Justice

The first fair trade label, Max Havellar, appeared on coffee in the Netherlands in 1988 after a plea from Mexican coffee farmers for help in stabilizing coffee prices and then expanded to other countries and products. Today the key institution is Fairtrade Labelling Organizations International (FLO-I from 1997) with twenty European and North American national fair trade certification marks operating in twenty-one countries that accredit eighteen different agricultural product categories and some processed food from the developing world. Fair trade certification is a global standard that ensures that food is traded under better conditions for producers and workers in developing countries. Its criteria include ILO core conventions, guarantee a minimum price considered as fair to producers, and require producers to invest in projects to enhance the local social, economic, and environmental development. Fair trade is also part of the certification revolution. A growing number of large-scale corporations—including up- and down-market coffee shops and large supermarket chains in Europe and North America—sell fair trade food, and corporate brand names seek to certify these products.[13]

Religious groups and churches as well as international humanitarian, human rights, developing world, environmental, and labor organizations conduct grassroots campaigns for fair trade. Again, holidays are a favorite opportunity. For example, British Oxfam, the oldest, largest, and leading fair trade actor, runs the campaign "Unwrap Oxfam Easter Gifts—100% of profits go to help fight poverty." Global Exchange, which aggressively opposes free trade and corporate globalization, appeals to kids in its Fair Trade Chocolate Easter Campaign message: "Every bunny loves fair trade." This campaign also asks adults to "make Easter sweeter for cocoa farmers by buying Fair Trade chocolate" and by faxing Nestlé USA about its use of child labor on cocoa farms.[14] Campaigners exert strength to mobilize entire geographic units as fair trade towns, now existing in Austria, Belgium, Canada, Finland, France, Ireland, Italy, Norway, Spain, Sweden, the Netherlands, and the United States. Even fair trade churches, islands, countries, and universities have emerged. In the United Kingdom, where the idea originated, three hundred towns have been certified and more than two hundred areas are currently campaigning toward this status. Fair trade certification is given to institutions or areas when they work toward five goals that show a political, retail, media, and activist commitment to promoting fair trade products.[15]

From Boycotts to Certified Sustainable Seafood

Supermarket activism has weight. Wide consumer support for the tuna boycott mentioned above forced the fishing industry to change its nets and led to national and multilateral government guarantees of dolphin safety and several dolphin safety seals of approval. A certification scheme can, thus, develop quickly when contentious grassroots consumer clout is harnessed. The case of the Marine Stewardship Council (MSC), the most comprehensive, ambitious, and only global eco-labeling scheme for seafood, shows that the driver can also be a partnership between green food activists and food corporations. MSC was cofounded in 1997 by the World Wildlife Fund for Nature (WWF, a large market-oriented global environmental organization) and the British-Dutch food conglomerated global corporation Unilever PLC. Finding a way to protect the oceans from overfishing caused by increased consumer demand for seafood globally and the limited capacity of ongoing regulatory programs explains WWF involvement. For Unilever, MSC is a risk management strategy that helps to ensure a continued future supply of seafood for its consumer products and a way of keeping consumer boycotts at bay.[16] Thus, unlike organic and fair trade labeling, this "sandals and suits" partnership[17] did not result from a long historical ideological commitment to small producers and does not include a raging social dilemma over the advantages and disadvantages of catering to global supermarkets and certifying food from global agribusiness. What it does, instead, is certify seafood on the basis of three principles—no overfishing, ecosystem maintenance, and compliance with local, national, and international fishery regulation—and harness "consumer purchasing power to generate change and promote environmentally responsible stewardship of the world's most important renewable food source."[18] Its focus on mainstream consumption is clearly shown on its "Where to buy" Web site, which offers information on MSC foods and where they can be found in more than thirty countries. Many environmental organizations, including Greenpeace and the Sierra Club, support it actively.[19]

Campaigning for New Eating Habits and Lifestyles

Getting a global labeling scheme in place can be difficult—even with consumer support, considerable civil society activism, government interest, and an attentive media. Finding mechanisms to improve farm animal treatment is a case in point. Environmental, agricultural, religious, and animal rights groups; humane societies and societies for the prohibition of cruelty against animals; and consumer-oriented associations support the better treatment of farm animals.[20] They maintain that farm animal treatment "is a marker for the entire industrial system's attitude toward farmers, communities, consumers and the environment"[21] and call on consumers to "end factory farming before it ends us," because it "causes environmental destruction, damages human health, contributes to global hunger and inflicts immense suffering on billions of animals across the world."[22] Both animal welfare organizations and the more adamant animal rights groups campaign for consumer supermarket activism. They emphasize farm animal sentience, complexity, and uniqueness—in other words, that farm animals should not be viewed or treated as "animal machines" for human consumption purposes—and supply consumers with statistics, reports, and video clips on meat consumption and animal treatment. With vivid titles like "Cruelty to Animals: Mechanized Madness," and "Living a Nightmare: Animal Factories in Michigan," activist reports urge consumers, producers, and governments to take action to solve the problems of industrial and global food production.

The more moderate animal welfare groups campaign for farm animals' "five freedoms"—that is, protection from hunger, thirst, and malnutrition; pain, injury, and disease; physical and thermal discomfort; fear and distress; and discomfort— and for animals' ability to express normal behaviors. They do what they can to promote existing animal welfare labeling (including organic food labeling) and better general farm animal treatment. So far, their efforts have not led to a global labeling scheme or widespread use of the ones in place. The European Union is slowly developing one such scheme. Examples of national and subnational schemes include Certified Humane Raised & Handled (United States, formerly entitled Free Farmed Certified), American Humane Certified, Freedom Food (United Kingdom, supported by celebrity cook Jamie Oliver), and the Canadian British Columbian Society for the Prevention of Cruelty to Animals (SPCA) certification, as well as special schemes for free-range eggs. Because animal rights groups do not think that these schemes go far enough, they openly criticize them for failing to ensure good farm animal treatment and promote their own smaller non-third-party vegan labels.

Without a trustworthy global food label, farm animal activism mobilizes consumers into a larger register of responsibility. In particular, it attempts to convince consumers to play a direct role by becoming vegetarians. PETA and other animal rights' groups argue that "the best way to stop the destruction and the cruelty is to stop eating animals now" and advocate veganism (a complete plant-based diet and lifestyle).[23] Both animal rights and animal welfare groups support vegetarianism (a plant-based diet that may include milk, cheese, and eggs) and know that vegetarianism does not come easy. It is often viewed as time-consuming, dull, and outside most social conventions. So they strive to create positive social pressure by offering scientific evidence about the positive personal health effects of a vegetarian diet and by showing that growing numbers of ordinary consumers make easy everyday dietary changes. Their long lists of famous and even "sexy" vegetarians from different age and pop culture backgrounds makes vegetarianism look cool and socially acceptable. "You're not alone" announces the Free Farmed™ Consumer Action Center of the Humane Society of the United States and cites polling data to back this up. Animal welfare groups give advice about gradual lifestyle change in their "three R's program—Reduce (eat fewer animal products), Refine (choose organic or cage- and crate-free animal products), and Replace (become vegetarian). PETA provides its 1.6 million members and others with a "Go Veg" Web site and a free vegetarian starters' kit to try a plant-based diet for 30 days. Dating sites and blogs for vegetarians and vegans illustrate that both are acceptable lifestyles, easy food recipes for family meals and pot luck encourage dietary change, and campaign apparel and buttons reinforce the sense of a shared lifestyle identity.

Letting food-related changes play a central role in how consumers take everyday, hands-on responsibility for their lifestyles, their communities, and global affairs is the goal of the Slow Food® movement. It pushes for "ecogastronomy" (traditional local food culture) to strengthen the connections between "plate and planet." Slow Food began in the mid-1980s as a protest against a McDonald's restaurant near Piazza di Spagna in Rome. Now it has more than 85,000 members in 132 countries. Like all food political consumerism, it continues to broaden its scope and, thus, gives weight to the centrality of food in contemporary global political activism. Ideas about organic farming, fair trade, and animal welfare are part of its philosophy of good, clean, and fair food. Its taste education (mentioned above) aims to lessen the distance between the farm and fork by informing consumers about food production, actively supporting labeling schemes, and considering consumers as coproducers of food. Its mission of maintaining food cultures and the love of well-cooked food have now spiraled into another effort, Cittaslow International, which, reminiscent of Fair Trade Towns' certification initiative, uses the politics of food to bring people sharing the same food goals together in local food communities.[24]

FOOD SHOPPING AS RESPONSIBILITY FOR GLOBAL FOOD PRODUCTION

How successful is political consumerist activism in creating awareness about the problems of consumption in the world today? In answer to the question whether people had participated in a consumer boycott, comparable data available for eight Western democracies from 2002 show a clear rise from 4.7 percent in 1974 to an average of 15.2 percent in 1999. Buycotts are even more popular. Overall, when asked whether they purchased products for ethical, environmental, or political reasons, about 24 percent of Europeans in 20 countries said they had done so in a 12-month period.[25] Northern Europeans are often the most active. In Sweden, for example, buycotting has become somewhat of a mainstream form of shopping. About 55 percent said they have buycotted in the last year, and 95 percent claimed that they understood organic labeling and 63 percent understood the fair trade labeling scheme.[26] Political consumerism has not taken off this way throughout Europe: among Southern Europeans and Eastern Europeans only 7 to 12 percent are political food activists. Americans—with 23 percent buycotting and 18 percent boycotting—take a middle position between the high and low political consumerist regions of Europe. Yet when asked specifically about organic labels, more than half (52 percent) of Americans indicated that they bought organic foods in 2006; 26 percent bought organic beverages, and nearly one-third reported purchasing organic products "as often as possible." This shows a rise when compared with the one-third who said they bought either organic food or beverage products in 2002.[27] The conclusion is that consumers clearly feel increasingly drawn into political consumerism and, more specifically, toward food boycotts and labeled food.

But what do consumers think about when shopping for food? Available data are sparse. Findings from a Swedish national mail survey from 2003 as well as ethnological studies provide some insight.[28] These studies show that consumers who say they frequently buycott are much more likely to think about the working conditions, environmental consequences, and farm animal treatment when they decide what to eat. What is interesting is that at least Swedish buycotters do not differ from other consumers when it comes to concerns about personal health and food price as well as quality and taste. Thus, political consumers express a heightened awareness of the political, environmental, and ethical significance of their purchasing choices but, otherwise, are just like other consumers when it comes to valuing personal health and other aspects of food consumption.

Some consumers do more and adapt their personal lifestyles to their political and moral values. Vegetarians are a good case in point. They "boycott" meat, poultry, and fish. Many strive to purchase the labeled farm products discussed above. Together with others, they engage in the boycotts of fast-food chains and lobby businesses to change their values and codes of practice. Some go further and "boycott" the use of animals for all forms of human consumption—food, leather, cosmetics, and so on. Vegetarianism and veganism are, therefore, an interesting form of lifestyle food activism. How widespread is vegetarianism in Western democracies? In seven European countries, researchers estimated about 4.6 percent are vegetarians, with a high of about 8 percent in the United Kingdom, and a low of about 1 percent in France.[29] The Vegetarian Resource Group (a nonprofit organization that educates the public on vegetarianism and the interrelated issues of health, nutrition, ecology, ethics, and world hunger; see more at www.vrg.org) estimates that about 2.3 percent of adult Americans consider themselves vegetarian because they indicate that they never eat meat, poultry, and fish. Another 6 to 10 percent said they were "almost vegetarian," and another 20 percent to 25 percent are "vegetarian inclined" and intentionally reduce meat in their diet. Over the last 10 years, the number of Americans rejecting or "boycotting" red meat has been steady at around 6 percent. But what is interesting is that those "boycotting" fish have climbed from 4 to 15 percent; and those "boycotting" eggs changed from 4 to 9 percent. There seems, therefore, to be a growing category of specialized vegetarians who reject certain animal products but not others. Even the number of occasional (nonrigid) vegetarians is increasing as they try to follow a vegetarian lifestyle whenever possible. It seems that the "three R's" concept is catching on. In general, overall interest in a vegetarian lifestyle and diet is on the rise, a development also reflected in the increase of U.S.-based vegetarian food sales, which doubled since 1998, hitting $1.6 billion in 2003, and with steady increases since then. Similar trends are noticeable in Europe as well.

Increasingly specialized and fluctuating interest in vegetarianism suggests a variety of reasons for choosing a more plant-based diet. A 2002 Time/CNN poll shows that health concerns lead the American list with 47 percent, whereas about 21 percent are vegetarians because they are concerned about animals and animal rights. Five percent mentioned a more global concern for our planet and world poverty. Another 22 percent expressed other private reasons for their vegetarianism.[30] Thus, it seems that campaigns based on personal health are most successful so far, but we can expect that once active, vegetarians become increasingly aware and interested in other reasons for a plant-based diet like farm animal treatment, environmental pollution, and climate change.

Similar general sociodemographic characteristics are behind all forms of political consumerist food activism. More women, people between 25 and 40 years of age, the highly educated, those with higher incomes, urban residents, and even pet owners are more involved in various political consumerist food activities. Particularly women stand out as an increasingly important group, especially in countries where political consumerism is high. Survey research shows that women, more than men, are more knowledgeable about health issues and care more about the consequences of consumption for animal rights and child labor.[31]

Consumers' attitudes about food are, obviously, changing, and this change is leading them to purchase alternative food in supermarkets. The overall sale of major fair trade food products was nearly eight times higher in 2005 than in 1997.[32] The sale of organically grown labeled products is also on the rise, and consumers spend more of their money on these products.[33] Global sales of organic food quadrupled to $40 billion within the last 10 years. The demand for organic food products is concentrated, with the big consuming G7 countries[34] alone accounting for more than 80 percent of the total sales. However, whereas actual behavioral change is visible and citizens appear to be more open to choosing labeled over conventionally produced food, their market share remains relatively low. So, for example, the market shares of organic food consumption compared with the entire food market is highest for Switzerland at 4.5 percent, followed by Germany, and Austria and Denmark with around 3 percent, but hovers around 1 to 2 percent in other countries of the Western Hemisphere.[35] In sum, whereas the sale of labeled food products is clearly on the rise, they have not penetrated major markets and remain at small though increasing market shares overall.

Yet, regardless of small market share, agribusiness has taken notice. Several mainstream global supermarkets—Wal-Mart, Safeway, Tesco, and others—now carry organically labeled, fair traded, and MSC goods. Multinational food corporations—Nestlé, Dole, Del Monte, and others—certify some of their products. But as with other market share data, certified goods do not dominate their assortments. Interestingly and perhaps because of its founding as a partnership between a market-friendly environmental organization and a global food corporation, MSC-labeled products are more widely distributed. As of late 2006, 467 MSC labeled products were available in the food market. It labels 6 percent of the world's total edible wild capture or about 3.5 million tons of fish and shellfish, and about 25 large supermarket retailers (including big names like Wal-Mart, Safeway, Marks & Spencer, Tesco, and Sainsbury) purchase MSC-certified marine food.[36] This is a higher market penetration compared with most other food labeling schemes.

The certification revolution does not only affect consumers and global agribusiness. International governmental organizations (e.g., the World Bank), the European Union, and different national governments are following suit and changing their procurement policies to include fair trade, by supporting fair trade and organic production directly, and even by insisting on selling fair trade coffee in cafeterias in government buildings. The conclusion is that political consumerist campaigns are paying off.

But do these changes have the desired effect? In other words, is food activism aiding the struggle against child labor in agriculture, improving working conditions in agriculture, and protecting the environment? Again, fair trade production will be used to answer this question. Studies show that farmers benefit materially and socially from fair trade.[37] Its guaranteed fair price gives, for instance, fair trade coffee farmers a significantly higher income than other ones. The fair trade price "social premium," which FLO-I encourages coffee co-ops to use for local development investments, has gone to economic diversification, community infrastructure, social community development, and education scholarships, or has been distributed evenly among co-op members. Fair trade—like all political consumerism—is not flawless, and improvements are necessary. Demand in industrial countries is still limited, not all farmers wanting to certify their products can do so, the FLO model is criticized as a top-down affair, and farmers in the global south (i.e., the developing world) do not have enough say and decision-making power. But most important, fair trade (and this goes for all food activism) cannot—and is not intended to—solve the structural problems of global food production. Yet even with these limitations and flaws, political consumerist food activism has put sustainable consumption on the global food agenda and has developed innovative mechanisms that help solve complex problems in the global food system.

CONSUMERS, SUSTAINABLE CITIZENSHIP, AND FOOD DEMOCRACY

Multinational agribusiness and globalized food production have turned consumer choice about what to eat into a decision-making effort. Consumers from industrialized nations, in particular, now shoulder responsibility for global developments and problems. This responsibility may sound daunting, but the food activism discussed in this chapter shows how each and every consumer can contribute by making small, good, clean, and fair quality food choices. For Slow Food, these small contributions are an "act of civilization and a tool to improve the food system."[38] Surveys show that in growing numbers consumers in the industrialized world agree. They engage in boycotts and buycotts, change their lifestyles, and voice their concerns about the politics of food publically. They are questioning the steady supply of affordable and abundant global food. Supermarkets have become an arena for these consumers to vent concern and motivate others to act.

Political consumerist food activism is contagious. More people engage in it, more labeling schemes are in operation in more countries today, and the market share of labeled food is small but rising. Governments are also participating more actively. Some observers are skeptical. They maintain that agribusiness' interest is a form of corporate takeover that slows down and even impedes the march toward sustainable food production and consumption. For others, this warming of transnational agribusiness is a sign that they too have begun to understand the responsibility that they must take to solve the human rights, animal welfare, and environmental problems tied to the globalization and industrialization of food production. Their small steps in addressing these problems are given as evidence of the "certification revolution."

But the consumer, corporate, and government trend toward sustainable food is more than that. It is part of broad-based global efforts now under way to solve the dual problems of overconsumption in the global north and underconsumption in the global south and to apply the fundamental right of all humans to have an adequate, safe, and nutritious supply of food. Private food consumption has been directly linked to climate change and environmental problems. The year 2008 is marked with increased food scarcities, food riots in developing nations, and producer protests in the industrialized nations. Today, it is hard to get around the centrality of this fundamental right to food globally. The new terms "food democracy" and "food citizenship" mark this centrality. Civic projects, such as the Food Democracy Network Society in British Columbia, Canada, take on this challenge. In the Western nations, they imply that consumers should demand better quality food, not more choices of food from globalized and industrialized agriculture. These civic groups encourage consumers to help change multinational agribusiness operations and turn around bad government agricultural policy through labeling schemes and other market-based mechanisms. Attention is, therefore, cast on the role that consumers can and must play in better "farm to the fork" policy globally.

This chapter discusses how concern over food stretches the spatial, temporal, and material bounds of the private lives of consumers. Food shopping and eating habits have become part of what is now called "sustainable citizenship," another new idea that stresses the personal responsibility of each individual for the total relationship between their political, social, economic, and natural environment.[39] This responsibility knows no political, territorial, or economic bounds and signifies that the wealthier nations must think about how their food consumption not only affects their own health and well-being but that of families and communities around the globe. Food shopping and other consumer choices have become a junction filled with opportunities to decide about which path to take for taste, convenience, affordability, and global responsibility. Political food consumerist campaigns and labeling schemes call on consumers to make the link between themselves and others.

NOTES

1. World Summit on Sustainable Development, *Plan of Implementation 2002* (adopted on September 4, 2002, Paragraph 14), http://www.environment.gov.za/Documents/Documents/Summit_ImplementationPlan/wssd_pi_12-22.htm (accessed July 29, 2008).

2. United Nations Convention on Biological Diversity, "Biodiversity and Agriculture" in *The International Day for Biological Diversity* (May 22, 2008), http://www.cbd.int/ibd/2008/?tab=1 (accessed July 17, 2008); ILO (International Labor Organization), *Symposium on Decent Work in Agriculture September 15–18, 2003*, http://www.ilo.org/public/english/dialogue/actrav/new/agsymp03/index.htm (accessed July 18, 2008). See also FAO (Food and Agriculture Organization of the United Nations), *Food, Agriculture & Decent Work. ILO & FAO Working Together*, http://www.fao-ilo.org/ (accessed July 29, 2008).

3. Monroe Friedman, *Consumer Boycotts: Effecting Change through the Marketplace and the Media* (New York; London: Taylor & Francis, 1999).

4. Baby Milk Action, "Nestlé-Free Zone," http://www.babymilkaction.org/resources/boycott/nestlefree.html (accessed June 30, 2008); Killer Coke Campaign, "Campaign to Stop Killer Coke," http://www.killercoke.org/ (accessed May 17, 2008); Human Rights Watch, "Following the Supply Chain: The Link between Child Labor and the Coca-Cola Company," in *The Complicity of Sugar Mills and the Responsibility of Multinational Corporations* (2004), http://www.hrw.org/en/node/12067/section/6 (accessed January 4, 2009).

5. Culture jamming (also called ad-busting) uses corporate imagery in consumer society to alert consumers about the environmental, ethical, and social justice problems of production and consumption. It criticizes corporations in humorous ways and changes their logotypes and marketing slogans to reveal the politics behind products.

6. Free Range Studios, http://www.freerangestudios.com/ (accessed June 5, 2008).

7. PETA (People for the Ethical Treatment of Animals), "Murder King Campaign," http://www.goveg.com/corp_murderk.asp (accessed July 10, 2008).

8. PETA, "Kentucky Fried Cruelty Campaign," http://www.kentuckyfriedcruelty. com/ (accessed July 29, 2008); Humane Society of the United States, Factory Farming Campaign, "Wendy's Attitude toward Animal Welfare: Frosty," http://www.hsus.org/ farm/news/ournews/wendys_frosty.html (accessed July 17, 2008); Stop Killer Coke Campaign, http://www.killercoke.org/newflyers.htm (accessed July 29, 2008).

9. George Ritzer, *The McDonaldization of Society* (Thousand Oaks, CA: Pine Forge Press, 1993).

10. Michael E. Conroy, *Branded! How the "Certification Revolution" Is Transforming Global Corporations* (Gabriola Island, BC: New Society Publishers, 2007).

11. OCA (Organic Consumers Association), "Unchain Your Heart," http://www. organicconsumers.org/valentines/index.cfm (accessed July 8, 2008).

12. Ibid.

13. Marie-Christine Renard, "Fair trade: Quality, Market and Conventions," *Journal of Rural Studies* 19 (2003): 87–96.

14. For general information on Oxfam's gifts see Oxfam International, "Oxfam Unwrapped," http://www.oxfam.org/en/getinvolved/unwrapped (accessed July 29, 2008); Global Exchange, *Every-bunny Loves Fair Trade!!*, http://www.globalexchange. org/campaigns/fairtrade/cocoa/easter2006.html (accessed July 7, 2008).

15. Fair Trade Foundation, "Fair Trade Towns," http://www.fairtrade.org.uk/get_ involved/campaigns/fairtrade_towns/default.aspx (accessed July 1, 2008).

16. Cathy Roheim and Jon G. Sutinen, *Trade and Marketplace Measures to Promote Sustainable Fishing Practices* (Issue Paper No. 3, International Center for Trade and Sustainable Development, Geneva, Switzerland, 2006).

17. Sebastian Matthew, "When Sandals Meet Suit: Letter from Sebastian Matthew, Executive Secretary of ICSF to Michael Sutton, Director, Endangered Seas Campaign, WWF International, August 7, 1997," *Samudra* January (1998): 31–35.

18. MSC (Marine Stewardship Council), *MSC Environmental Standard for Sustainable Fishing*, http://www.msc.org/about-us/standards/msc-environmental-standard (accessed August 7, 2008).

19. Bruce Philips, Trevor Ward, and Chet Chaffee, eds. *Eco-labelling in Fisheries: What Is It All About?* (Oxford: Blackwell Publishing, 2003).

20. Ronald T. Libby, *Eco-Wars: Political Campaigns and Social Movements* (New York: Columbia University Press, 1991).

21. Sierra Club, "Clean Water and Factory Farms: Inhumane Treatment of Farm Animals," http://www.sierraclub.org/factoryfarms/factsheets/inhumane.asp (accessed June 6, 2008).

22. Viva (Vegetarians International Voice for Animals), "Welcome to Viva," http:// www.viva.org.uk/ (accessed July 16, 2008).

23. Ibid.

24. Carlo Petrini, *Slow Food: The Case for Taste* (Irvington: Columbia University Press, 2006); Cittaslow, http://www.cittaslow.net/sezioni/Rete%20Internazionale/ (accessed July 29, 2008).

25. European Social Survey, "Cross-National Social Scientific Survey in 20 European Countries" (2003), http://www.europeansocialsurvey.org/ (accessed July 29, 2008).

26. Michele Micheletti and Dietlind Stolle, "Politiska Konsumenter: Marknaden Som Arena För Politiska Val," in *Ju Mer Vi Är Tillsammans. Tjugosju Kapitel om Politik, Medier Och Samhälle*, ed. Sören Holmberg and Lennart Weibull, Report No. 34 (Gothenburg, Sweden: SOM Institute, 2004), 103–16; Michele Micheletti and Dietlind Stolle, "Swedish Political Consumers: Who They Are and Why They Use the Market as an Arena for Politics," in *Political Consumerism: Its Motivations, Power, and Conditions in the Nordic Countries and Elsewhere* (TemaNord 517, 2005): 145–65.

27. Business Wire, "Eating it Up: Organic Market Booms as Consumers Seek Healthier, More Natural Food and Drink" (November 12, 2007), http://findarticles.com/p/articles/mi_m0EIN/is_2007_Nov_12/ai_n21095138 (accessed July 29, 2008).

28. Dietlind Stolle and Michele Micheletti, "Warum Werden Käufer zu 'Politischen Verbrauchern?'" *Forschungsjournal Neue Soziale Bewegungen* 18, no. 4 (2005): 41–52; Daniel Miller, *The Dialectics of Shopping* (Chicago: University of Chicago Press, 2001).

29. "Animal Welfare Survey, 2005," http://ec.europa.eu/food/animal/welfare/euro_barometer25_en.pdf (accessed July 29, 2008).

30. "Do You Consider Yourself a Vegetarian?" Time/CNN Poll (July 7, 2002), http://www.time.com/time/covers/1101020715/poll/ (accessed July 29, 2008).

31. Dietlind Stolle and Michele Micheletti, "The Gender Gap Reversed," in *Gender and Social Capital*, ed. Brenda O'Neill and Elisabeth Gidengil (London: Routledge, 2005), 45–72.

32. Jean-Marie Krier, *Fair Trade in Europe 2005*, http://www.european-fair-trade-association.org/efta/Doc/FT-E-2006.pdf (accessed in July 2008).

33. Helga Willer and Minou Yussefi, *The World of Organic Agriculture: Statistics and Emerging Trends 2007* (Germany: IFOAM, 2007).

34. The G7 countries are Canada, France, Germany, Italy, Japan, the United Kingdom, and the United States.

35. Ibid.; For organic production, see Ulrich Hamm, Friederike Gronefeld, and Darren Halpin, *Analysis of the European Market for Organic Food* (Aberystwyth: University of Wales, 2002).

36. MSC, *Annual Report 2005/6*, http://www.msc.org/documents/annual-report-archive/MSC_annual_report_05_06.pdf/view (accessed June 12, 2008).

37. Sarah Lyon, "Fair Trade Coffee and Human Rights in Guatemala," *Journal of Consumer Policy* 30, no. 3 (2007): 241–61; Douglas Murray, Laura T. Raynolds, and Peter Leigh Taylor, "One Cup at a Time: Poverty Alleviation and Fair Trade Coffee in Latin America" (Colorado State University, Fort Collins, 2003), http://www.colostate.edu/Depts/Sociology/FairTradeResearchGroup (accessed June 12, 2008).

38. Slow Food," "Manifesto for Quality" in *Slow Food: Welcome to Our World Companion*," http://www.slowfood.com/about_us/img_sito/pdf/Companion08_ENG.pdf (accessed June 30, 2008).

39. Ruth Lister, "Inclusive Citizenship: Realizing the Potential," *Citizenship Studies* 11, no. 1 (2007): 49–61.

RESOURCE GUIDE

Suggested Reading

Conroy, Michael E. *Branded! How the 'Certification Revolution' Is Transforming Global Corporations*. Gabriola Island, British Columbia: New Society Publishers, 2007.

Friedman, Monroe. *Consumer Boycotts: Effecting Change Through the Marketplace and the Media.* New York; London: Taylor & Francis, 1999.

Libby, Ronald T. *Eco-Wars: Political Campaigns and Social Movements.* New York: Columbia University Press, 1991.

Micheletti, Michele. *Political Virtue and Shopping: Individuals, Consumerism, and Collective Action.* New York: Palgrave, 2003.

Princen, Thomas, Michael Maniates, and Ken Conco. *Confronting Consumption.* London: The MIT Press, 2002.

Ritzer, George. *The McDonaldization of Society.* Thousand Oaks, CA: Pine Forge Press, 1993.

Shopping for Human Rights. Special issue of *Journal of Consumer Policy* 31, no. 3 (2007).

Stolle, Dietlind, Marc Hooghe, and Michele Micheletti. "Politics in the Super-Market—Political Consumerism as a Form of Political Participation." *International Review of Political Science* 26, no. 3 (2005): 245–69.

Web Sites

Baby Milk Action, http://www.babymilkaction.org/.

Consumers' International, Coffee Campaign, http://www.consumersinternational.org/Templates/Internal.asp?NodeID=95754&int1stParentNodeID=89650&int2ndParentNodeID=94997?NodeID=94997.

Fairtrade Labelling Organizations International, http://www.fairtrade.net/; http://www.european-fair-trade-association.org/efta/Doc/FT-E-2006.pdf.

Free Range Studios, http://www.freerangestudios.com/.

IFOAM, http://www.ifoam.org/.

Killer Coke Campaign, http://www.killercoke.org/.

Marine Stewardship Council, http://www.msc.org/.

McSPOTLIGHT, http://www.mcspotlight.org/.

People for the Ethical Treatment of Animals, http://www.peta.org/.

Sierra Club, http://www.sierraclub.org/factoryfarms/.

Soil Association, http://www.soilassociation.org/.

Vegetarian Resource Group, http://www.vrg.org/index.htm.

Welfare Quality Science and Society Improving Animal Welfare, http://www.welfarequality.net/everyone.

7

Choosing Quality: The Knowledge-Intensification Shift

JoAnn Jaffe

The following commentary on baking by a forty-eight-year-old supermarket baker expresses the ambiguous status of knowledge in the commercial-industrial food system today:

> People coming in the [bakery] shop [to work] now won't be able to learn what I was able to learn and I didn't get to learn what the guys before me knew. It's getting really difficult to find somebody who knows what they're doing . . . it's a balancing act. You still need a feel, [but] we use the mixes and the bases and who knows how those work and how to fix them when they go wrong. We do a few basic things. [He pulls out a 100 lb. batch of French White bread dough]. It will be turned into white bread, kaiser rolls, baguettes, could be crusty rolls and many others, depending on the shape and whether it's baked on a bare pan or paper . . . it's the same thing with the Canadian Grain mix. The trend is for bakeries to move to frozen breads that you proof and bake, or that are partially pre-baked. We do some of that, particularly the breads we can't get mixes for like multigrain or the specialty breads that sell maybe a dozen in two weeks.[1]

From one perspective, each successive generation seems to know less about their craft and to depend more on manufactured products to produce what they formerly made relying mostly on their own expertise. From another perspective, the market seems to be filled with more variety than ever—implying a broadening of knowledge even though the plethora of choices may be more apparent than real. Contemporary consumers seem to know more about food, health, and the environment, and to demand more quality characteristics based on that knowledge. These demands present opportunities for those who recognize in consumer concerns an opening to remake a piece of the food system.

After 25 years of relatively slow growth, the agrifood sector is now experiencing a new round of intensified accumulation based on selective responses to public concerns about health, food safety, environmental impacts, animal welfare, and rural decline.[2] These quality-focused projects take place in the context of rapid technological change, new product introductions, and the creation of new product subsectors—all intended to improve competitive positions, increase market share, and achieve greater flexibility and control through the rationalization of every phase of the production process. Food manufacturing and preparation processes are standardized so that they can be carried out by minimally skilled, low-wage workers. The knowledge that is deployed is a technical, abstract knowledge, mostly controlled by the designers of ingredients, machines, and production lines. The shifting of the terrain of competition toward knowledge-intensive, patentable technologies accelerates the incorporation of results of strategically targeted, technoscientific research and development.

This turn to knowledge-intensity, and to particular attributes and claims of quality, intersects with a dual strategy of creating and exploiting niche markets, while also selling in mass markets that persist for certain staple commodities. Standardized and predictable prepared foodstuffs are produced for all market segments, while new market niches or segments are constantly being created. To make space for novel products, existing tastes, preferences, and traditions have been overthrown or reworked.[3] As more foods are manufactured rather than being made from scratch, they are modified with an eye toward using standardized and interchangeable basic inputs (starches, sweeteners, extenders, fiber sources, and so on) in manufacturing processes.[4] The result is a homogenization of diets despite surface appearances to the contrary. In much of the world, many people now consume substantially similar diets. Regional and ethnic specialties are diluted and made palatable to mouths now accustomed to the tastes and textures of fat, sugar, and salt.[5] Moreover, diets are subject to a class bifurcation, in which the majority consumes processed, high fructose, bulk-commodity foods with large quantities of genetically modified and pesticide-treated ingredients, and the relatively well-to-do eat higher quality specialty and specially prepared products.[6]

Some people have been unwilling to accept the "deskilled," passive relations of consumption and constrained choices imposed by these practices.[7] One result of this resistance by certain consumers and producers has been a shift toward more knowledgeable production and consumption as exemplified in the movement toward artisanal foods, such as breads and cheeses, and specialty varieties of fruits, vegetables, and grains. Artisanship in this context represents an engagement with the sensory attributes of foods, craftsmanship, hands-on work, variable products, and high standards. It often involves creation with older techniques, machines, or varieties.

In raising and responding to questions of quality, however, the contemporary development of artisan production has proceeded through a double movement. In some cases, specific social conditions make artisanship a strategy that has the potential to build alternatives to the present system. In other cases, it provides new spaces for profit-making by agri-industry by turning this production into another niche market—and, in the process, it blurs the boundaries of artisan production. Which face of artisanship has the upper hand in any particular instance may have everything to do with the relations of agrifood knowledge and intellectual property undergirding these options.

DYNAMICS OF AGRIFOOD KNOWLEDGE

The feelings of this 60-year-old woman of mixed Aboriginal and non-Aboriginal ancestry tell us something about the role of early experience in developing tastes:

> I love saskatoon berries [*Amelanchier alnifolia*, also known as service berries], which I ate as a kid, but the flavor of blueberries is just too strong. Especially the wild berries from up north. I really prefer the big industrial blueberries that are more bland. I had to throw out a bag of wild blueberries that was stinking up my freezer, because the smell was just too strong. It made me sick every time I opened my freezer.

Her ancestors would have depended on the wild blueberry to add to meat from hunting and trapping to make pemmican, a winter staple. She, however, grew up eating the food of urban Canada. Ingested from our earliest moments, the blander salty, sweet, and fatty flavors of industrial food conditions us to prefer a mild palate and to reject the stronger flavors of wild or nonengineered foods.

Much of what we understand about the world, and our place in it, is rooted in the experience of our bodies. The nature of our embodiment is that substantial learning happens through interactions with the world outside ourselves, becoming our "second nature" without our specifically trying to acquire knowledge or skill.[8] The resulting capacities are not those that lend themselves to verbal explanation and likely they will escape conscious awareness until we make a mistake or find ourselves doing something we are unable to explain, such as riding a bike.

While embodied knowledge may be characterized as discovery of self and nature, practical knowledge can be thought of as apprenticeship.[9] It is through watching and imitation that we learn practical knowledge and skills, including complex combinations of motor skills and judgment, such as those that are displayed when baking bread from scratch (particularly without a recipe), and social skills that are needed when moving from one social context to another. Along with embodied knowledge on which it depends, it is often described as "knowing how" in opposition to the "knowing what" of discursive knowledge.

Discursive knowledge is developed through language and meaning created through talking, listening, and, especially, writing and reading. It has the potential to allow knowledge to be divorced from context and experience. Cookbooks are good examples of discursive knowledge—the extension of technical rationality is shown in the transformation of recipes from listed collections of ingredients to their measurement expressed in exact quantities. The development of science and technology, as well as technological rationality embedded in industrial capitalism, both depend on the development and transmission of discursive knowledge. In practice, science and technology often depend on the embodied and practical knowledge of scientists, engineers, and technicians.

People's agrifood knowledge and skill develop in the context of particular social sites and relationships, and in this way, they are intrinsically local as well as social. Agrifood knowledge thus is highly relational and reflects the culture from which it arises. Early experiences develop tastes. While later years can modify them, family plays an important role in constructing tastes by exposing children to particular diets, which themselves are produced by different socioeconomic and cultural constraints, conditions, and possibilities.[10] These then become expressed as preferences.

Tastes are strongly influenced by culture, wealth, region, and gender, and they also play a strong role in reproducing social differences. People develop strong aversions to particular flavors, foods, cuisines, appearances, and food combinations that are not local to their social group, which serves to develop social boundaries. This drive for social distinction complements a drive for conformity as people use consumption to show that they belong to particular groups or have certain identities, but also try to distinguish themselves from those in groups whose social position is closest.[11] People in lower social positions may imitate those in positions above them, however, leading those in the higher positions to abandon some foods and move on to new options in their own quest for distinction.

Corporate agribusiness contributes to this dynamic process of distinction with the constant development of new or pseudo-novel foods. Agribusiness recognizes the wealth-stratified nature of consumption and targets its products accordingly, with some novel products aimed at wealthier consumers and others directed at those not so wealthy.[12] In parallel, many alternative practices are structured by class. Specialty products and special experiences such as farmers markets, which are aimed at increasing returns to farmers and shortening supply chains, tend to be targeted at privileged or relatively high-income consumers. Strategies focused on low-income consumers concentrate on lessening consumers' dependence on prepared and packaged foods and developing the skills to transform commodity foods into quality meals.

The more one is distanced from necessity, the more one is free to enjoy food without being concerned about the balance between money spent and belly filled. The rich, thus, pursue and refine a taste for luxury. Those with cultural sophistication (or "high cultural capital"), but with relatively moderate incomes—in distinction from the truly wealthy—are more likely to consider a wide variety of objects as being deserving of aesthetic appreciation and to hold an abstract aesthetic sense in which many things theoretically could be considered worthy of appreciation. Particularly for younger people, education does not so much mean that one will cook daily or eat well as it does that one will be willing to eat foods in styles that are considered foreign, high status, and not typically "comfort foods."[13] Conversely, the consumption of foods that carry symbolic status or display particular quality characteristics can be a way for individuals to signify new identities or to "social climb."

Low-income consumers tend to rely on the complex of foods that are subsidized and cheap, which are apt to be made from bulk commodities and provide a high calorie count per dollar spent.[14] Economic necessity encourages people to eat prepared foods. This is a risk-avoidance strategy in that flavors are predictable and engineered to be satisfying to a palate conditioned to like industrial food. It is a reliable way to vary one's diet and try novel foods, whereas preparing new foods may require new knowledge and demand an investment that may not be recouped if one does not like the novel food.[15]

Broadly speaking, food production practices are structured by the logics and justifications of two different settings. The first is the setting of conviviality, in which production and consumption are oriented toward the provisioning and eating activities of families and households. It is structured by the logics of status and identity, comfort and care, familiarity and traditions. Many current alternatives to the dominant industrial system emerge from this setting, with activists anxious to reclaim the social and cultural roles of food and agriculture.

The second is the setting of commercial-industrial food production, structured primarily by the business rationality of capitalist production and marketing. This setting is dominated by logics of efficiency and productivity, with standardization, flexibilization, rationalization, calculability, and predictability important design criteria for products and processes. It is characterized by a disembedding of knowledge in which embodied and practical knowledge of food producers across the food system is replaced by discursive knowledge allied with the products of science and technology. Industrial bread bakers today, for example, find that their hands punch buttons of control panels rather than dough, which itself has been created using precisely calculated recipes of components of partially unknown composition.[16] Many chefs and cooks warm the frozen products of food service companies or have been replaced by unskilled machine-minders in fast-food restaurants.[17] Many agrifood workers experience a gap between what they know and what is necessary to know to be autonomous and in control of their labor process. Fewer people are able to create legitimate knowledge, and fewer people are able to gain access to it.

This centralization of knowledge comes at a cost. All knowledge is embedded in social contexts, but one can distinguish between that which is locally embedded (also referred to as "situational" or "local" knowledge) and that which is more abstract, procedural, and applicable to a wide variety of contexts and which emerges in more technical or scientific contexts. The latter knowledge, however, may not contribute to the proficiency, autonomy, or creativity of the knower in particular local contexts. Knowledge and its products often confront food producers as "black boxes" all across the food system.[18]

THE TURN TO QUALITY AS KNOWLEDGE-INTENSIVE PRACTICE

Quality is multidimensional; what is considered "quality" depends on the goals and standpoint of the evaluator. Conventional approaches divide quality into three components: objective elements, subjective aspects, and perceived quality. Objective elements are those that would be the same to anyone who measured them, such as nutritional content, bacterial load, and pesticide residues. Their measurement is normally accomplished through scientific analysis, and they are often the target of regulation and standards. Subjective elements, which also could be the object of standards, are those evaluations that differ based on individual consumer preferences, such as appearance, texture, and flavor. They take into account few factors and are evaluated as simple taste attributes—does the food have the right amount of saltiness, fattiness, or sugariness? They include some superficial exterior properties—is the food nonblemished, a good shape, and the right color? Perceived quality is based on opinion or image of the good and is often the subject of branding and advertising.[19] The commercial-industrial agrifood system combines these approaches with the macro-quality orientations of low cost, convenience, consistency, reliability, and predictability to guide food development. This focus is consistent with the "food-as-fuel perspective,"[20] which views food as routine consumption leading to short-term satisfaction.[21]

Conventional approaches treat qualities as intrinsic to the good itself. Through another lens, complex socioeconomic processes can shape those goods that come to be described as having particular qualities and others not. These are contested, discursive processes in which interests and goods come together to create rankings that, by favoring some values over others, redistribute power and advantage across the agrifood chain. Quality is a lens through which products, processes, and people are judged—a good apple implies a good grower with good practices.[22] Being the result of contestable processes, these quality assignments are always provisional and open to change.[23]

Conventional approaches correspondingly regard consumers as if they all had the same pregiven preferences[24] and as if their interests were satisfied at the moment of consumption. They view the capability of consumers to consume as competent, the acquisition of knowledge and information about quality as untroubled, and the communication between consumers and producers as unproblematic. Agrifood corporations, however, tend to see consumers as malleable—the focus of tremendous effort—from product and marketing research, to branding, advertising, and packaging.[25] Agrifood corporations seek to solidify old preferences into brand loyalties and to incorporate the already-developed tastes of consumers into new allegiances. Brand loyalty reduces competitive pressures for the brand and thereby allows corporations to charge more. Corporations use symbols, metaphors, and stories to help consumers place themselves in relation to these products, to imagine who they would be by buying a particular product.[26] Corporations draw on these already-constituted understandings of consumers and reformulate and repackage them to get them to buy and to consent—to the product in particular and consumerism in general.

People use consumption to accomplish many things, from signifying status, confirming identity, conveying love, remembering parents, and showing self-control to providing nutritious and healthy food. Consumption is structured by the interpenetrating logics of conviviality and the commercial-industrial system and its strategies, technologies, and products.[27] The result is socially constructed consumers, who may lack the information, knowledge, and analytical frameworks needed to make informed decisions, and whose attention to quality is shaped by the latest concerns of the commercial-industrial system—although not always in the desired ways.[28]

Different consumer judgments of quality are supported by different kinds of knowledge. Some knowledge is immediately available to consumers through the experience of consumption. One knows, for example, that the bread is white, soft, and tasty. One may lack the ability to judge whether these characteristics are good or bad, but the act of seeing and eating will give consumers access to information, including whether they like it or not.[29] Other quality judgments are supported by knowledge not immediately accessible through direct experience. In these cases, quality refers to credence attributes that derive from scientific, social, ethical, and environmental commitments. It takes knowledge on the part of the producer to produce a product that satisfies the quality demand and on the part of the consumer to know to make that demand. Where these kinds of quality judgments are not part of the deep culture in which agriculture and food are embedded, they may require third-party involvement to bridge the knowledge gap between field or factory and fork, both in terms of setting standards and of verifying that the standards have been met.

Quality concerns provide a link between producers and consumers. The supply of quality, and information about it, logically precedes demand because in a marketplace, consumers cannot express preferences for nonexistent things. The best that consumers can do is to recombine preexisting elements.[30] Furthermore, the messages consumers can send regarding quality via the medium of purchasing decisions are blunt, at best. How do sellers know which of many potential messages buyers are trying to convey through purchase or nonpurchase?

In the last 25 years, civil society has acted as a vehicle whereby collective consumer concerns can be expressed in public arenas.[31] Activists have expanded notions of quality into extrinsic categories of the social, ethical, political, and environmental, providing discursive foundations for consumer demands beyond the narrow basis of quality judgments presently at play in mass markets. In some cases, they have refocused attention on intrinsic characteristics, such as flavor, texture, and nutrition. Attention to quality has provided openings for alternative value chains to operate alongside or beyond conventional systems.[32] In relation to agrifood systems, reembedding is about putting into play principles of conviviality and reducing the degree to which purely economic considerations are determinate. Reembedding must address how food networks and chains are qualitatively linked to social, economic, and political issues and how values beyond profit can assert claims in agrifood systems. Reembedding does not necessarily imply a more just agrifood system, however. What is required is that the agrifood economy be embedded in more equitable social relations and subordinated to democracy and ecosocial justice.

Maria Fonte[33] offers a framework that helps explain why particular quality concerns and conventions are adopted within different agrifood knowledge contexts based on research on local food networks in the European Union.[34] She identifies two general approaches to the development of local foods and relates them to the social and cultural importance of agriculture and food in the area. The reconnection perspective, typical of Northern Europe, emphasizes deriving quality from rebuilding links between producers and consumers and reembedding agriculture into the interpersonal world. In places where export agriculture and perhaps specialization are long-standing practices, with an absence or loss of food culture and knowledge and no outlet for local agricultural production, the task is to revive locally oriented agriculture and rebuild people's social and cultural connections to agriculture and food. This approach is characterized by explicit documentation of quality characteristics of foods and the processes that produce them. This is necessary because some of the new characteristics being produced are credence qualities and because, in these contexts, people tend not to know enough to ascertain quality on their own. Activities that bring local food to local people, such as farmers markets and organic food boxes, exemplify the reconnection perspective.

The origin of food perspective, typical of Southern Europe, is a territorially based strategy of local development meant to revitalize socially and economically marginal areas. In this case, local has been expanded to include tradition and history; what is local, and thus of quality, is that which shares the "raw materials, taste, and dishes" of food traditions that form a robust part of the embodied and practical knowledge of cultures. This view of local goes beyond the view of food as essential to sociality to regard it as the rudiments of deep identity and patrimony. In local markets with knowledgeable producers and consumers, trust and communication provide the assurance of quality. According to Fonte,[35] in these regions, multidimensional commitments to the quality of food and of the processes that produce it are implicitly part of a knowledgeable agrifood culture in which food consumption and agricultural production grow up together, as part of the cultural fabric of place. Acquaintance with foodways, culture, practical knowledge, and tradition take the place of certification that guarantees quality at a distance.

Although some local products are produced and remain in local regions, many enter global value chains and are consumed as elements of diets and social life far removed from their origins.[36] This shift, in which product and process remain linked to the local area and tradition but local evaluation is not possible, requires a shift in knowledge relations. At a distance, the product is no longer embedded in the practical knowledge of consumers, and possibilities of trust, shared culture, and communication are eroded. Long value chains require movement to discursive knowledge, with the simultaneous introduction of scientific experts and technicians to establish and measure relevant quality characteristics.[37] Many of these products enter the market with labels of origin, which connect qualities presumed inherent in regional cultures and environments with labels only available to those products from the region.[38] These products may be subject to certification—private and public—guaranteeing that products or production processes meet culinary, environmental, or social quality standards. These efforts depend on a knowledgeable and skilled consumerate base to support the different kinds of quality produced.

These approaches draw on strategies linking quality to distinguishing characteristics that command premiums in the marketplace—a focus of innovations across the agrifood sector. Quality certification, however, has an ambivalent character. Certification that reduces quality to a set of technical characteristics, as seen in organic production, permits capital to subject quality to processes of standardization and rationalization. Certification has the potential to flatten existing diversities in products, processes, and crop and animal varieties that are sources of creative variation in local foods by regulating their production and content. Certification may favor some producers over others because of the relative advantage of some in meeting the additional capabilities or costs associated with meeting quality standards. Conversely, being able to carve out spaces where the establishment of quality monopolies is possible may allow local producers a bulwark against their appropriation by commercial-industrial interests.

Changing the agrifood system requires constructing new quality through an engagement with a different kind of politics—one that links quality to the more broadly conceived multifunctionality of agriculture and food.[39] Building alternative approaches involves creating new meanings—and thus, one might presume, new possibilities for action—in five interrelated dimensions of the politics of quality. These fields include information (what we know), science and technology (how we know), knowledge (the context and focus of concern), communication (how we represent what we know), and standards and innovation (appropriate judgments and values).[40] In each dimension, the questions of who decides and who controls the process are of utmost importance. The process of negotiating over and consolidating meanings around quality characteristics gradually endows them with an objective character.[41]

One might argue that commercial-industrial systems—in league with dominant conventions in science and technology—have usurped processes of qualification and made them essentially one-sided. However, "the questioning of the legitimacy of the 'institutions' which provide knowledge about food: mothers as the experts, public agencies and even 'science,' which together functioned in a way that guaranteed the productivist model of industrialization and the safety of food during the so-called modern period,"[42] has reopened questions of quality and brought them back into the political arena. Alternative approaches to agrifood systems have the potential to democratize and broaden notions of quality beyond that which is possible in conventional commercial-industrial systems. This points to the importance of movements reopening questions about the meaning and significance of food and agriculture, and of knowledgeable consumers and producers supporting a transition to deep-quality politics.

RED FIFE WHEAT: A COMMON PROPERTY RESOURCE

The rediscovery of Red Fife, the original commercial variety of wheat grown in Canada, provides an interesting case from which to view issues of knowledge and quality. Wheat is the most important cultivated crop in Canada by area and by contribution to gross domestic product.[43] It is the single most important source of plant protein in the world and the second highest volume of cereal grain produced after corn.[44] The importance of wheat is due to its use in cereal, bread, pasta, pastries, beer, animal feed, and now as feedstock for biofuel production. One of the earliest domesticated plants, wheat has been the most important staple crop in modern history, having been key to the establishment of the world food economy as well as to the formation of many settler nations.[45]

Saskatchewan is the source of 60 percent of wheat grown in Canada. Much of that is hard red spring wheat, planted in May or June, harvested in early fall, and destined for flourmills and bread factories at home or (especially) abroad. The few varieties that are most important crystallize a complex mix of quality considerations that combine the interests of growers, processors, and, presumably, eaters within a commercial-industrial economy. To be acceptable to all of these interests, a good bread wheat variety must combine yield, milling quality, baking quality, and appropriate alpha-amylase content, which affects the conversion of starch to sugars in dough.[46] Wheat yields are a complex mix of multigenetic factors, agronomic practices (especially timing at planting), weather, and soil type. Milling quality is a balance between flour yield and lightness of color. Lightness is important because quality is determined by white bread being the largest use of bread wheat. Baking quality combines measures of elasticity (strength) of gluten, volume and crust of the loaf, and quantity of water able to be absorbed by the dough.[47] Varieties considered to be of highest baking quality are those suited "to production of the conventional light and fluffy breads of the conventional marketplace."[48] Few wheat varieties have the genetic potential to combine all of these qualities, and genetic expression depends on environmental conditions and agronomic practices.[49]

A small percentage of wheat produced will end up at artisan bakeries. Although there is no agreed-on or regulated definition of artisan, which allows this term to be appropriated by industrial bakeries, according to most artisan bakers, bread can only be called "artisan" if it is weighed, rounded, shaped, and slashed by hand, and then baked on the hearth.[50] In these bakeries, the concern for craft and complex flavor shape the baker's assessment of quality. Artisan bakers often favor wheat varieties with different qualities than those preferred by commercial industry. For example, artisan bakers generally prefer lower-protein wheats, as high-gluten flours may not support the use of preferments and the long fermentation associated with artisan breads.[51] High-gluten flours are particularly good for producing high-volume breads that rise quickly in a pan[52] and for withstanding the rigors of industrial mixing.[53]

Artisan breads gained some limited popularity in the early 1970s with the rise of social movements that rejected industrial approaches to agriculture and nutrition and that favored "whole, natural" foods. In recent years, artisan breads—either real or so-called—have become widely popular along with other quality foods such as extra-virgin olive oil and premium dark coffees. Today, the fastest growing segment of the bread sector is the supermarket and industrial "artisan" category.[54] Many artisan bakeries that were once small and local have been acquired by the commercial agrifood industry. A notable example is LaBrea Bakery, credited with helping to reintroduce artisan bread to the North American public and which was purchased by the Irish agribusiness conglomerate IAWS in 2002.[55] Its products are now produced as prebakes that can be finished in-store and offered as fresh artisan products from scratch. They are now sold in more than 2,500 supermarkets in the United States.[56]

Saskatchewan has few strong food traditions. Its rural sector is dominated by family-based export agriculture—primarily wheat, but also other grains and livestock—and has experienced rural depopulation and farm concentration at accelerating rates since the mid-1970s. Here, alternative quality implies the reconnection perspective: organic, sold in local farmers markets or food co-ops, relatively small scale, and presumably healthy and nutritious. It may also imply few preprepared foods; vegetarian diets or, at least, nonindustrial livestock; and a core population of somewhat knowledgeable consumers and producers willing to try nontraditional products. Heritage varieties of foods (meaning before 1950) are becoming fashionable, especially in a few products, such as tomatoes, that are considered to be the most degraded in taste or for visual appeal. The culinary basis to support a widespread transition to quality, however, is arguably limited.

Red Fife wheat is rooted in local value chains,[57] but distinguished as a quality product and traded—albeit in extremely limited quantities—in national and global value chains. The first common bread wheats in Canada were grown from seed that individual farmers saved and reproduced on their own. Although the origin of Red Fife is shrouded in mythology, some say that in 1842 David and Jane Fife of Ontario planted wheat seeds they received from a friend in Scotland.[58] They noticed that one plant in a plot of what they had thought was winter wheat was actually hard red spring wheat. They reproduced this wheat from one plant, which gave rise to a hardy, disease-resistant, high-yielding variety possessing excellent milling and baking qualities and exceptional flavor according to the requirements of the period.[59] It was introduced into western Canada in 1882, where it remained the leading variety until 1908 when its progeny, Marquis wheat, replaced it, primarily due to its earlier ripening.[60] Red Fife is an ancestor of many improved British, French, and U.S. wheat varieties.[61]

Limited amounts of Red Fife once again became available to Saskatchewan farmers when a wheat breeder planted one pound of seed in 1988 as part of the Heritage Wheat Project, a preservation trust of seven early Canadian wheat strains. About 13 years later, the main Saskatchewan grower organized a group of

26 small and medium-size producers into the Prairie Red Fife Wheat Organic Growers Co-operative.[62] These are, in essence, artisan farmers who produce small amounts of special quality products that will be used by alternative and quality-seeking consumers and artisan food producers. Red Fife's profile was raised when the Vancouver Island Slow Food® Chapter succeeded in its campaign to place the wheat in Slow Food's 2003 Ark of Taste. It is furthermore Canada's first and only Slow Food Presidium.[63] With foods that are designated as presidia, Slow Food replaces official certification with their guarantee that these products will meet process and product quality requirements, but do so in ways that contribute to the social and ecological diversity and knowledge that created the presidia food.[64] Saskatchewan farmers produced more than 500 tons of Red Fife wheat in 2007, up from 70 tons in 2004.[65] Although negligible compared with total spring wheat production of almost 6 million tons, producers of Red Fife received a price of more than 50 percent more per bushel compared with hard red spring wheat in 2007.[66] Furthermore, studies show Red Fife producing comparable or better yields to widely planted modern cultivars such as 5602HR or ACBarrie under organic management.[67]

People disagree in their assessment of Red Fife's quality characteristics. Some artisanal bakers consider Red Fife to be "a fantastic baking wheat because it is low in gluten and it has a crumbing effect when ground into flour—meaning that it makes a hay yellow crumb—with a scent of herbs like anise and fennel. In the mouth, it has an herby, spicy flavour to it."[68] Other artisanal bakers report not liking the taste of Red Fife and finding it difficult to work with. They talk about having trouble getting it to rise properly if it is the only variety in use or without the addition of white flour or dough conditioners.[69] A study comparing Red Fife to wheats used in industrial baking rates it as having the poorest baking quality because of its low protein content and low flour yield—meaning that too much material has to be removed to make white flour.[70]

Variety registration is the gatekeeper for the grain system in Canada. The Canadian Wheat Board is the federal orderly marketing agency that sells all western Canadian wheat and barley destined for human consumption. The Wheat Board sells only registered grain. This translates into approximately 20 percent of the world's wheat trade, with annual revenues above $4 billion.[71] Red Fife, however, is not on the list of varieties of Canadian Red Spring Wheat registered with the Canadian Grain Commission, so it cannot be sold through conventional channels.[72] Heritage varieties appear to be ineligible for registration because of a combination of factors. Although Red Fife has a common core of subjective qualities, as a landrace,[73] its desirable characteristics appear to be due to interactions and redundancies of multiple genes. Together, these genes express particular traits (known as horizontal resistance) as opposed to one gene being responsible for one trait (vertical resistance) that can be easily identified through testing, as is the case with contemporary breeding.[74] Moreover, neither the process nor the outcome of traditional cross-breeding can be patented. They are considered by the courts of Canada "neither new nor an invention, but rather a natural biological process which occurs according to the laws of nature."[75] In effect, Red Fife is an open-source wheat with genetics that make it difficult to monopolize by commercial interests.

Red Fife growers use the producer direct-sale system set up by the Wheat Board for organic farmers. This system keeps grain out of the conventional elevator system and avoids cross-contamination with nonorganic products. Farmers then sell their Red Fife wheat by declaring it to be (animal) feed wheat, which acknowledges that it is not registered. Although this puts limitations on how Red Fife can be marketed, it also may be a strength, as this is what keeps it from being easily appropriated.

It is not clear whether present efforts by some Red Fife advocates to extend the patenting system to encompass traditional, farmer-bred varieties will succeed, but their conservation as common property represents a partial movement away from commodification and is likely key to providing a bulwark against conventionalization, or their co-optation by the commercial-industrial system.[76] Some artisan producers treat quality as a property that can be made proprietary and from which rents can be derived. This strategy turns these distinguishing characteristics into things, something to be regulated and controlled, encouraging standardization where previously the product had diversity. Ironically, efforts to control and standardize efface the very artisanship—the embodied and practical expertise—that through the interaction with diverse conditions, applications, and responses builds deep quality knowledge. This has the effect of creating "frozen commodities" that reflect static notions of the real conditions and culture that originally produced the product.

At present, producers can command a premium for Red Fife because it is a fashionable specialty product that allows artisan bakers to gain a competitive market position. In the words of one baker, "Red Fife is a nostalgia product, a peasant flour that today produces an expensive bread. Having Red Fife on the label guarantees you'll sell your bread, even if it's just 20%."[77] Ideas of quality and local tend to imply a "small is beautiful" approach. But nothing prevents that value added from being captured equally by large centralized producers. Indeed, the additional costs associated with quality may favor the large producer who has enough volume to spread those costs across the enterprise or who might have the specialized connections necessary to provide an outlet for the quality product. The legal and intellectual property issues related to Red Fife make it unlikely that industry will appropriate this product, but in the quest for something new to offer the public emulating the privileged consumer, the industry could just as easily promote another named "quality" variety.

REFLECTIONS ON QUALITY AND KNOWLEDGE

Constructing successful agrifood alternatives to the current system involves creating new knowledge contexts for agrifood practices. In some cases, this will mean developing new relationships to food in which attention to the multiple dimensions of quality is broadly supported by embodied and practical knowledge. In other cases, this means reinforcing or recreating traditions in ways that do not allow them to become frozen or open to monopolization by rent-seekers. The success of Red Fife as an alternative, for example, depends on its uptake by artisanal and home bakers who have a deeper appreciation of the multidimensional aspects of quality than that offered by conventional supermarket breads, including its relation to preserving the livelihoods of artisanal farmers. At present, industrial producers have been able to take advantage of the shift to quality bread to realize large margins as they appropriate the meanings of artisanship in the face of indeterminate definitions and unaware consumers.

By highlighting the fact that all varieties are not the same, the move to Red Fife has made consumers and producers more aware of the role of wheat varieties in constructing bread quality. Many quality-stream products are based on proprietary knowledge and on branding that mixes liberal quantities of image and imaginary with some characteristics that have substantive importance. Because the impetus is fundamentally commercial, the efforts are focused on privatizing the benefits of knowledge rather than on sharing information that might help all participants make more savvy choices. In the end, consumers wind up purchasing so-called quality products that may be lacking in certain important dimensions of quality that impinge on human and animal welfare, as well as other spheres of environmental and social concern. Similarly, producers end up foreclosing the potential for knowledge about quality to become a vehicle for wider social enrichment. Consumers may have more quality consciousness, but may not be aware of how to best carry out their concerns. By being unwilling or unable to truly share information with their customers and patrons, producers lose an opportunity to get informed feedback and form a partnership in developing products and processes.

A real transition to quality will require consumers as well as producers who have deep knowledge across the issues. Expanded conceptualizations of quality will need to be developed and supported with knowledgeable and skillful partners in the food system, including a publicly oriented range of researchers who will use common intellectual property as a basis for building the public good.

NOTES

1. All quotes are from a research project, "Thought for Food: Essential Skills and Food System Performance," funded by the Social Sciences and Humanities Research Council (SSHRC, Canada). Participant's identities have been disguised to protect anonymity and confidentiality.

2. Harriet Friedmann, "From Colonialism to Green Capitalism: Social Movements and Emergence of Food Regimes," in *New Directions in the Sociology of Global Development*, ed. Frederick H. Buttel and Philip McMichael (Oxford: Elsevier, 2005), 227–64.

3. JoAnn Jaffe and Michael Gertler, "Victual Vicissitudes: Consumer Deskilling and the (Gendered) Transformation of Food Systems," *Agriculture and Human Values* 23, no. 2 (2006): 143–62.

4. Harriet Friedmann, "Distance and Durability: Shakey Foundations of the World Food Economy," *Third World Quarterly* 13, no. 2 (1992): 371–83.

5. Donna R. Gabaccia, *We Are What We Eat: Ethnic Food and the Making of Americans* (Cambridge, MA: Harvard University Press, 1998).

6. Jaffe and Gertler, "Victual Vicissitudes."

7. Ibid.

8. Margaret Archer, *Being Human: The Problem of Agency* (Cambridge: Cambridge University Press, 2000).

9. Ibid.

10. Pierre Bourdieu, *Distinction: A Social Critique of the Judgement of Taste* (Cambridge, MA: Harvard University Press, 1984).

11. Ibid.

12. Jaffe and Gertler, "Victual Vicissitudes."

13. Omar Lizardo and Sara Skiles, *Beyond the Distinction Myth: Rethinking the Relevance of Bourdieu's Class Theory for the Sociology of Taste* (University of Notre Dame, 2007).

14. Adam Drewnowski and Anne Barratt-Fornell, "Do Healthier Diets Cost More? (Policy Update)," *Nutrition Today* 39, no. 4 (2004): 161–68.

15. JoAnn Jaffe, "Understanding Food Knowledge and Domestic Skills: Three Generations in the Family Kitchen" (paper presented at the annual meeting of Agriculture and Human Values, New Orleans, June 4–7, 2008).

16. Richard Sennett, *The Corrosion of Character: The Personal Consequences of Work in the New Capitalism* (New York: W.W. Norton & Company Inc, 1998); Anonymous, personal communication, 2007.

17. Ester Reiter, *Making Fast Food* (Montreal, Kingston: McGill-Queens's University Press, 1991).

18. Harry P. Diaz and Bob Stirling, "Degradation of Farm Work on the Canadian Prairies," in *Farm Communities at the Crossroads: The Challenge and the Resistance*, ed. Harry P. Diaz, JoAnn Jaffe, and Bob Stirling (Regina, SK: CPRC Press, 2003), 31–44.

19. Vickie Vaclavik and Elizabeth Christian, *Essentials of Food Science* (New York: Kluwer Academic/Plenum Publishers, 2003).

20. Jaffe, "Understanding Food Knowledge."

21. Gianluca Brunori, "Local Food and Alternative Food Networks: A Communication Perspective," *Anthropology of Food* S2 (2007), http://aof.revues.org/document430.html.

22. After Elizabeth Ransom, "Defining a Good Steak: Global Constructions of What Is Considered Good Meat," in *Agricultural Standards: The Shape of the Global Food and Fiber System*, ed. Jim Bingen and Lawrence Busch (Dordrecht, Netherlands: Kluwer Press, 2006) 159–76.

23. Mark Harvey, Andrew McMeekin, and Alan Warde, "Quality and Processes of Qualification," in *Qualities of Food,* ed. Mark Harvey, Andrew McMeekin, and Alan Warde (Manchester, UK: Manchester University Press, 2005), pp. 192–208.

24. Gilles Allaire, "Quality in Economics: A Cognitive Perspective," in *Qualities of Food,* ed. Mark Harvey, Andrew McMeekin, and Alan Warde (Manchester, UK: Manchester University Press, 2005), pp. 61–93.

25. Tim Lang and Michael Heasman, *Food Wars: The Global Battle for Mouths, Minds, and Markets* (London: Earthscan, 2004).

26. Stuart Ewen, *Captains of Consciousness: Advertising and the Social Roots of the Consumer Culture* (New York: McGraw-Hill, 1974).

27. Jaffe, "Understanding Food Knowledge."

28. Jaffe and Gertler, "Victual Vicissitudes."

29. Their attention still may have been directed to particular features and not others.

30. Allaire, "Quality in Economics."

31. Lang and Heasman, *Food Wars.*

32. At present, the most important movement for extrinsic quality is the one for fair trade; however, for the moment, it appears to be feasible in only a narrow range of specialty value chains.

33. Maria Fonte, "Knowledge, Food and Place: A Way of Producing, a Way of Knowing," *Sociologia Ruralis* 48, no. 3 (2008): 200–222.

34. See Corazon Project, http://www.corason.hu (accessed August 29, 2008).

35. Fonte, "Knowledge, Food and Place."

36. These products are called "locality" foods by Brunori, "Local Food."

37. See Maria Fonte, "Local Food Production and Knowledge Dynamics in the Rural Sustainable Development" (local food production input paper for the Working Package 6, CORASON Project, 2006), www.corason.hu, for a similar argument.

38. Elizabeth Barham, "Towards a Theory of Values-based Labeling," *Agriculture and Human Values* 19, no. 4 (2002): 349–60.

39. Michael Gertler and JoAnn Jaffe, "Agri-Food System Performance: Competing Frameworks and Development Alternatives" (paper presented at the meeting of the Rural Sociological Society, Manchester, NH, July 27–31, 2008).

40. Brunori, "Local Food."

41. Ibid.

42. Allaire, "Quality in Economics," 61.

43. Statistics Canada, "Farm Cash Receipts, 2008," http://www40.statcan.ca/l01/cst01/agri03a.htm; Statistics Canada, "Field and Specialty Crops, 2008," http://www40.statcan.ca/l01/cst01/prim11a.htm.

44. USDA (United States Department of Agriculture), "World Agricultural Production, 2007)," www.pecad.fas.usda.gov/wap_current.cfm.

45. Harriet Friedmann, "The Political Economy of Food: The Rise and Fall of the Postwar International Food Order," *The American Journal of Sociology* 88 (1982): S248–S286.

46. F. Lupton, "Advances in Work on Breeding Wheat with Improved Grain Quality in the Twentieth Century," *Journal of Agricultural Science* 143 (2005): 113–16.

47. Stephan Symko, "From a Single Seed: The Quality of Wheat, Flour and Bread" (Agriculture and Agri-Food Canada, 1999), http://www4.agr.gc.ca/AAFC-AAC/display-afficher.do?id=1181313724319.

48. Brenda Frick, "Going with the Grains" (January 2007), http://www.organicagcentre.ca/NewspaperArticles/na_cog_grains_bf.asp (accessed August 26, 2008).

49. H. Mason, A. Navabi, B. Frick, J. O'Donovan, D. Niziol, and D. Spaner, "Does Growing Canadian Western Hard Red Spring Wheat under Organic Management Alter Its Breadmaking Quality?" *Renewable Agriculture and Food Systems* 22 (2007): 157–67.

50. Maggie Glezer, *Artisan Baking* (New York: Workman/Artisan, 2000).

51. Jeffrey Hamelman, *Bread: A Baker's Book of Techniques and Recipes* (Hoboken, NJ: Wiley, 2004); Anonymous, personal communication, 2008.

52. Hamelman, *Bread*; Anonymous, personal communication, 2007.

53. Anonymous, personal communication, 2008.

54. Katherine Bryant, "Modern Art," *Restaurant Business* 103, no. 7 (2004): 60–61.

55. This process is reminiscent of earlier processes of labor and workshop centralization. IAWS merged with Zurich-based Heistand Holding AG in August 2008. Together they form the Arytza Group, the global leader in value-added baked goods, http://www.labreabakery.com/affiliates.aspx (accessed September 12, 2008).

56. Julia Moskin, "Taking the Artisan out of Artisanal: Good Bread Goes Commercial," *New York Times*, March 10, 2004.

57. This point is somewhat ironic because many local foods in Saskatchewan are either imports or diasporic foods adapted into local socioecological contexts.

58. Sharon Rempel, "Red Fife Wheat" (*Canadian Encyclopedia Online*, 2008), http://www.thecanadianencyclopedia.com/index.cfm?PgNm=TCE&Params=A1ARTA0010468.

59. Red Fife is apparently a descendent of (Ukrainian) Halychanka wheat.

60. Marquis has since been replaced by other varieties.

61. Bob Belderok, "Developments in Bread-Making Processes," *Plant Foods for Human Nutrition* 55 (2000): 1–14.

62. Sharon Rempel, "The Heritage Wheat and 'Red Fife' Projects: Developing Community Wheat Projects Linking Consumers, Artisan Bakers, Pastry Chefs and Organic Farmers to Heritage Varieties of Wheat" (2007), www.grassrootssolutions.com.

63. Slow Food is a nonprofit, member-supported organization founded in Italy in 1989. Primary activities of Slow Food are to rediscover and catalogue heritage foods threatened with extinction by placing them in the Ark of Taste and to develop projects around these foods, called presidia, with local artisan producers. The theory behind presidia is that foods with economic importance should be given the means to be preserved.

64. Fondazione Slow Food per la Biodeversità, http://www.fondazioneslowfood.it/eng/arca/dettaglio.lasso?cod=547&prs=PR_1192.

65. Rempel, "The Heritage Wheat and 'Red Fife' Projects."

66. Saskatchewan Agriculture and Food, "Spring Wheat Production and Value" (2008), http://www.agr.gov.sk.ca/apps/agriculture_statistics/HBV5_Result.asp; Heliotrust, "Red Fife: The Grandmother of Wheat," http://heliotrust.squarespace.com/storage/Red%20Fife%20article.pdf.

67. J. C. Pridham, M. H. Entz, R. C. Martin, and P. J. Hucl, "Weed, Disease and Grain Yield Effects of Cultivar Mixtures in Organically Managed Spring Wheat," *Canadian Journal of Plant Science* 87 (2007): 855–59.

68. Jack Klassen, "Return of Red Fife Wheat Bodes Well for Organic Producers" (quoted in Action Committee on the Rural Economy, 2005), http://www.ei.gov.sk.ca/acre/Stories/RedFifeWheat.asp.

69. Personal communication, artisan bakers (2007, 2008).

70. Brenda Frick, "Going with the Grains," Organic Agriculture Centre of Canada, http://www.organicagcentre.ca/NewspaperArticles/na_cog_grains_bf.asp (accessed April 24, 2009.

71. Canadian Wheat Board, www.cwb.ca.

72. Rules governing the sale of heritage varieties in other countries, such as France, also limit the commercialization of Red Fife.

73. Landraces are domesticated varieties of plants and animals adapted to local climate, culture, disease, and pests. They have been developed by communities and farmers through traditional breeding methods.

74. Raoul Robinson, *Return to Resistance* (Ottawa, ON: International Development Research Centre, 1995), http://www.idrc.org.sg/en/ev-9339-201-1-DO_TOPIC.html.

75. James Mallett, "Patentability of Seed Varieties" (2003), http://www.grassrootsolutions.com/heritage-wheat/patents.html.

76. Julie Guthman, *Agrarian Dreams: The Paradox of Organic Farming in California* (Berkeley: University of California Press, 2004).

77. Personal communication, artisan baker (2008).

RESOURCE GUIDE

Suggested Reading

Fonte, Maria. "Knowledge, Food and Place: A Way of Producing, A Way of Knowing." *Sociologia Ruralis* 48, no. 3 (2008): 200–222.

Glezer, Maggie. *Artisan Baking.* New York: Workman/Artisan, 2000.

Harvey, Mark, Andrew McMeekin, and Alan Warde. *Qualities of Food.* Manchester: Manchester University Press, 2005.

Jaffe, JoAnn, and Michael Gertler. "Victual Vicissitudes: Consumer Deskilling and the (Gendered) Transformation of Food Systems." *Agriculture and Human Values* 23, no. 2 (2006): 143–62.

Lang, Tim, and Michael Heasman. *Food Wars: The Global Battle for Mouths, Minds, and Markets*. London: Earthscan, 2004.

Nestle, Marion. *Food Politics. How the Food Industry Influences Nutrition And Health*. Berkeley: University of California Press, 2002.

Vileisis, Ann. *Kitchen Literacy: How We Lost the Knowledge of Where Food Comes from and Why We Need to Get It Back*. Washington, DC: Island Press, 2007.

Web Sites

Grassroots Solutions, www.grassrootssolutions.com.
Slow Food International, www.slowfood.com.

PART II

Culture

8

Sustaining Regional Food Systems and Healthy Rural Livelihoods

Gail Feenstra and Jennifer Wilkins

The past century has seen a dramatic change in how our food is produced, processed, and distributed. Industrialization, globalization, and concentration have shaped agricultural production, food processing, and retailing. Tens of thousands of food products developed from a diminishing set of commodities compete for shelf space in supermarkets where a year-round supply of fresh and processed foods from around the world is the norm.

Interrelated trends are intensifying within the food system: obesity and diet-related diseases, food-borne illness, inequity and social injustice, economic imbalances, increasing food costs, and energy and other natural resource limits. As public concern about the food system and its impacts escalates, communities across the United States are creating alternatives to how food is grown, distributed, and consumed. These new food systems explicitly incorporate sustainability as a priority.

The manifestations of sustainable food systems are varied; however, their values are consistent: health (environmental, personal), equity (working conditions to community food security), and regional identity. These characteristics are woven throughout the "new generation" food systems emerging from rural towns to urban centers. Although vulnerable in some ways, these food systems are restructuring in ways that sustain public health, the natural resource base, economic vitality, and the social fabric of communities.

The food system, then, is at an interesting and critical juncture. While it has become globalized and concentrated, the emergence of local community-based food systems suggests a counterforce. Whether these emerging food systems flourish will depend in large part on community engagement, consumer demand, and public policy.

THE BACKDROP

Sustainable, regional food systems exist in the shadow of a dominant food system that has been shaped by at least three interrelated trends: (1) industrialization, (2) globalization, and (3) economic concentration.

Industrialization

For the last century, agriculture has become more mechanized, technological, and larger in scale.[1] Average farm size more than tripled from 1900 to 1997 from 146 acres to 487 acres, and the total number of farms decreased from more than 5.7 million to 1.9 million in the same period.[2] The percentage of the U.S. population living on farms dropped from 39 percent in 1900 to less than 2 percent in 1990.[3]

From the narrow perspective of yield per acre, agriculture has become more productive. However, not all farms have shared equally in terms of profitability. Midsize family farms, in particular, are disappearing from the landscape.[4] Kirschenmann and colleagues suggest that the midsize farm enterprises—those generating between $100,000 and $250,000 annually—are too small to compete in the vertically integrated commodity markets and too big and specialized to take advantage of direct markets. As data from coast to coast indicate, these farms are fast becoming "endangered."[5]

As these farms are either lost to development or consolidated with other holdings, along with them goes the infrastructure—that is, the local processing facilities, input suppliers, and small businesses that accompany family farming enterprises. In addition, regions lose diversified farmland, crops, and soils that provide ecosystem services, such as wildlife, carbon sinks, and the ability to hold water and reduce erosion. To the extent that these small and midsize family farms are associated with sales within their geographic regions, when they fail, communities lose access to foods with the place-based values increasing numbers of consumers are demanding.[6]

Globalization

Lyson linked the emergence of a global food system beginning about the mid-twentieth century to the growth of nationally organized food corporations. He describes, "A wave of mergers among food processors, input suppliers, and marketers resulted in a tremendous consolidation of power in the food sector."[7] These mergers resulted in large, multinational food corporations, functioning in a global food economy and sourcing and transporting foods coast to coast and country to country. The typical morsel of food we eat has traveled 1,500 to 2,500 miles from farm to fork.[8] For the most part, the dominant food system is no longer based on regional production, processing, and distribution, but rather on global markets that depend on efficiency and least-cost suppliers to remain viable.

Economic Concentration in the Food System

Today, a relative few multinational corporations control the majority of the agrifood markets from seed to table. Since the mid-1980s, Heffernan and Hendrickson have been collecting data on the market share of the four largest processing firms for many of the major commodities produced in the U.S. Midwest, as well as dairy and food retailing.[9]

According to economists, when four or fewer firms control 40 percent or more of an industry's market, that sector loses characteristics of a competitive market. This holds true in a number of food commodities, including beef packing (81 percent), soybean crushing (80 percent), flour milling (61 percent), pork packers (59 percent), and broilers (50 percent).[10] Heffernan and Hendrickson maintain that the consolidation of the food system is organized around five or six "global food chain clusters," occurring as a result of horizontal and vertical integration and global expansion. Examples of these clusters include Cargill/Monsanto/Kroger, DuPont/ConAgra, and Novartis (Syngenta)/ADM.[11] Kroger, once the largest U.S. retailer, is now second only to Wal-Mart, which claimed $98.7 billion in U.S. sales in 2006, compared with Kroger's $58.5 billion. In 2005, the top five food retailers controlled 48 percent of supermarket sales.[12]

FOOD SYSTEM IMPACTS: HEALTH, JUSTICE, AND THE ENVIRONMENT

The implications of industrialization, globalization, and economic concentration have been profound. The oft-touted consumer benefits—particularly an abundant, cheap, and consistent food supply—have come at a cost. Key drivers inspiring food system change emanate from its detrimental impacts, particularly on public health, equity and social justice, and natural resource conservation and renewal.

Crisis in Public Health

As a result of the integrated, industrial global food system, many U.S. consumers have easy access to too much food or the wrong kind of food, and have become, as Michael Pollan describes in *The Omnivore's Dilemma*, "industrial eaters."[13] Per capita daily servings of added fats and oils in the U.S. food supply have more than doubled from 1909 to 2000. Total per capita consumption of added caloric sweeteners— 150 pounds of sugar annually—increased 20 percent between 1970–1974 and 2000. One particular sweetener, high fructose corn syrup (HFCS), has risen dramatically in that time period to almost 63 pounds per capita per year.[14]

Although our diet is not solely to blame for our health problems, long-term health impacts of eating habits are increasingly clear. Diet-related diseases along with physical inactivity constitute leading causes of preventable death (15 percent of total deaths), just below smoking (18 percent of total deaths).[15] Nearly two-thirds of American adults are overweight or obese.[16] Since the 1970s, the rate of childhood overweight or obesity tripled to almost 20 percent for some age-groups.[17] Obese children are more likely to become obese adults, threatening Americans' long-term health profile. Direct and indirect health care costs of obesity are estimated at $117 billion.[18]

Agricultural practices can also negatively impact public health. According to the American Public Health Association (APHA), "there is clear evidence of the human health consequences due to resistant organisms resulting from nonhuman usage of antimicrobials."[19] APHA also issued a policy statement warning about negative public health impacts stemming from the source of most U.S. beef, pork, and chicken: Confined Animal Feeding Operations (CAFOs). CAFOs have been associated with declines in community economic and social well-being, which undermine the foundations of community health.[20] CAFOs annually require city-scale sewage treatment, impose a nitrogen burden on the environment, and contain by-products, including heavy metals, antibiotics, pathogenic bacteria, nitrogen and phosphorus, as well as dust, mold, bacterial endotoxins, and volatile gases. APHA has urged federal, state, and local governments "to impose a moratorium on new CAFOs until additional scientific data on the attendant risks to public health have been collected and uncertainties resolved."[21]

While small- and large-scale food production and processing systems are both vulnerable to accidental (or intentional) contamination with bacteria and other toxic substances, the centralized nature of the dominant food system aggravates the consequences of such problems when they do occur. Every year 5,000 deaths, 325,000 hospitalizations, and 76 million illnesses are caused by food-borne illnesses within the United States. The recent rash of food recalls provides tangible evidence of weaknesses in the U.S. food safety system and ample cause for an erosion of public confidence in the government's ability to keep food safe.

Concerns about Social Justice

From living and working conditions of farm and food system laborers to food security for low-income inner-city residents, the impacts of the food system on health and livelihoods are increasingly problematic. Recent studies in California show that many farmworkers suffer from poor health even though they are young and physically active. They have high rates of serum cholesterol, high blood pressure, anemia, obesity, and dental problems. They are exposed to high levels of agricultural chemicals and suffer from pesticide poisonings. Many lack health insurance.[22]

The general situation for urban residents in low-income communities is depressingly similar. Obesity, diabetes, and other diet-related diseases are more common than in the general population, and poverty exacerbates these conditions. Inner-city and rural residents often find themselves in "food deserts," areas that lack grocery stores that carry wholesome food. As Winne carefully outlines in Closing the Food Gap,[23] the poor in both urban and rural areas pay more for food and have less access to quality products. Both factors lessen their ability to use government food assistance dollars effectively.

One common thread running through both urban and rural populations is that for the poor, often ethnic minorities, the food system is not meeting their basic needs. Many communities are not "food secure," a condition at the household level in which "all members have access at all times to enough food for an active, healthy life."[24]

Natural Resource Limits

Prime farmland continues to disappear across the landscape in the United States, replaced by houses, shopping malls, and other nonfarm uses. The American Farmland Trust's studies show that farmland is disappearing at an alarming rate—two acres per minute from 1992 to 1997. If trends of the 1990s continue and estimates are accurate, the Central Valley of California can expect to lose another 882,000 acres of farmland to urbanization and "ranchettes." Productive capacity will be reduced by about $814 million per year with a total cumulative loss of $17.7 billion in farm gate sales.[25]

One of the most limited natural resources, particularly in the arid west, is water. In California, population increases, drought, decline in the Sierra snowpack, and court orders to limit water transfers in order to protect endangered fish species all contribute to restricted water for food production.[26]

Crisis in Energy and Carbon Emissions

Energy is one of the most critical resources associated with food production in this century. In the United States, approximately 10 percent of the energy used annually is consumed by the food system. Most of transportation, food processing, storage, and tillage, not to mention our reliance on petroleum-based agricultural chemicals, are dependent on fossil fuel. According to Heinberg, "over 400 gallons of oil equivalent are expended to feed each American each year."[27]

When we add up the energy costs of food production, processing, and transport, the current food system consumes approximately seven calories of fossil-fuel energy for every calorie of food energy produced.[28] So, what allows this to happen? To maintain our current food system "standard of living," we are using up the world's energy and other natural resource reserves as well as our human communities.

EMERGING SUSTAINABLE, REGIONAL FOOD SYSTEMS

It is possible to grow and eat food in ways that protect the environment, conserve energy, preserve family farms, support our farm and food system workers and rural communities, and promote healthful eating and community food security. One option is for citizens, policymakers, and others to begin to plan for healthy, livable communities by thinking about their food supply in terms of a local or regional, sustainable food system. Communities from coast to coast are already engaged in this challenge in a variety of ways.

Consumer Interest in Local Food

Interest in local food has increased so dramatically in recent years that a new word was coined to describe someone who strives to dine on foods grown within a one hundred-mile radius of where they live: "locavore." Survey research suggests that consumers believe local fruits and vegetables are fresher, look better, and taste better than produce imported from other regions or countries.[29] The Hartman Group, a consumer research firm, found that for 55 percent of consumers, whether the food to be purchased is "locally grown" was more important than whether it is "organically grown."[30] Responding to demand, supermarkets are increasing sales of foods produced within their states and regions.[31]

What Does a Sustainable, Regional Food System Look Like?

According to a definition by the University of California Sustainable Agriculture Research and Education Program, a sustainable food system is based on values and practices that simultaneously achieve the following:

- Ensure agriculture systems that are both productive and ecologically sound.
- Provide access to an adequate, affordable, nutritious, and culturally appropriate diet.
- Provide all those working within the food system with equitable economic rewards and safe and dignified working and living conditions within healthy communities.

- Promote food and agricultural businesses and organizations that strengthen local and regional economies and communities.
- Engage and empower citizens in becoming actively involved in the food system and policy decisions affecting it.

In this context, we define a sustainable food system as one that is environmentally sound, economically viable, socially just, and geographically bounded.

Communities, nonprofits, researchers, city planners, and businesses nationwide are beginning to support the values of stewardship and sustainability by putting their energies into designing and implementing sustainable food systems. Strategies include farmers markets, community-supported agriculture, regional marketing and place-based labeling, farm-to-school and farm-to-institution programs, community gardens and urban farms, and food policy councils (FPCs), as well as innovative combinations of the above. Most of these strategies create direct marketing opportunities for regional growers to sell products to the public, institutions, or retail outlets and simultaneously encourage social and cultural connections that contribute to more sustainable communities. The term "civic agriculture," coined by Lyson, encompasses many of the multiple benefits these direct marketing strategies provide.[32]

Farmers Markets

Farmers markets, one of the most common and widely available venues for linking local farmers directly with consumers, have been growing in number and popularity over the past decade, providing valuable opportunities for thousands of full- and part-time farmers. In 2007, the U.S. Department of Agriculture (USDA) counted more than 4,680 farmers markets nationwide, benefiting more than 19,000 small and midsize family farmers, thousands of consumers, and hundreds of communities. In addition to the direct economic benefits to growers, farmers markets also bring healthful food directly to consumers, create tourism destinations, allow money to be recirculated in a local economy, and provide a setting for community celebrations and gatherings.[33]

An important way in which farmers markets connect urban and rural people is by bringing healthful food to low-income communities (community food security). The USDA funds two subsidy programs—one for pregnant and lactating women and their children (Women, Infant and Children Farmers Market Nutrition Program—FMNP) and the other for seniors (the Senior Farmers Market Nutrition Program—SFMNP), providing coupons to low-income people to purchase fresh produce at farmers markets. Food stamps also may be used at farmers markets and, in some markets, bring in a sizable portion of the revenues. Case studies in California highlight how some of these programs work in ethnic neighborhoods. According to one study of the Stockton, California, farmers market, low-income Southeast Asian residents have easy access to fresh, seasonal, locally produced produce, fish, chicken, and other food products at reasonable prices.[34]

Community-Supported Agriculture

Another strategy for creating an even more committed connection between consumers and growers is through community-supported agriculture (CSA). This strategy relies on consumers paying in advance for a "share," or portion of the year's harvest, which they receive in weekly installments throughout the season. In the early models, a farmer would add up all the costs of production and agree on a division among customer-shareholders. In many instances today, the arrangement is more akin to a "subscription," where members pay a particular fee for a month, a quarter of a year, or a season in exchange for weekly shares from the farm. The CSA movement has picked up momentum since it was introduced in the northeastern United States from Japan and Europe in the mid-1980s. An estimated 1,200 CSA farms nationwide now participate in this unique alliance between farmers and consumers.

The original goals of CSA included saving family farms and the environment; increasing fresh, local produce in members' diets; and providing a consumer-based option for resistance to the dominant agrifood paradigm; however, a number of researchers have questioned whether these goals have been fully realized.[35] Whatever the economic and political changes that have resulted from the CSA movement, thousands of committed consumers have emerged and begun to change the way they think about the food system. Perhaps even more important, as Ostrum suggests, is the "transformative potential" of the CSA movement and its ability to work toward "democratizing" the agrifood system in local settings.[36]

Regional Marketing Programs

Across the country, programs are emerging to identify for consumers where foods are produced and simultaneously to provide a price premium for growers, with product differentiation based on a sense of place. These regional brands can be as local as a valley within a county or as large as a region encompassing several states. They all, however, offer farmers a way to add value to their products and meet a growing demand for "place-based" foods. Barham suggests these "values-based labeling" programs are motivated by a growing need to re-embed the agrifood economy in the larger social economy.[37]

A study of 13 programs that exist throughout California was conducted in 2005 and 2006.[38] Each program has a distinctive label describing where the products are from. In addition to the label, programs have several common goals, including (1) increased production of local products, (2) increased consumer awareness of local agriculture, (3) improved local infrastructure for marketing and distribution, and (4) technical expertise for growers who want to explore this marketing dimension.

All of the programs studied were voluntary, membership-based associations, some of which were nonprofit organizations. Although core members were farmers and ranchers, program organizers recognized the benefit of having a diverse membership base, including retailers, restaurants, consumers, nonprofits, university partners (particularly Cooperative Extension), and other local organizations. Marketing and education activities varied and included many creative ideas, such as an "agro-art" festival, locally sourced dinners for the public, farm and range tours, and local tastings. Funding also varied; however, all agreed that a part-time staff person coordinating these programs was important. The biggest challenges faced for expanding these initiatives were time, resources, and local politics. It requires persistence to work through challenges and see positive results—at least five years, according to some program organizers. For most of the programs studied, however, participants generally felt the efforts were worth it. Among the biggest benefits cited were new opportunities for networking within and outside of the agricultural community. More research is needed to measure long-term impacts of these organizations and their contributions to communities.

In addition to the local labels developed in California and around the country, most states have marketing programs that promote their food and agricultural products.[39] A 2006 study found that of the 44 states with an agricultural identity branding program, the main objectives were to promote the state's products, increase consumer consumption of these products, and develop new markets and businesses. The challenges were similar to county-level programs—dealing with funding constraints for staffing and activities, and building consensus among participants with diverse points of view. The advantages were also similar—most programs were viewed positively as contributing to statewide agriculture and developing a higher market share for growers.

Some local labeling programs have pursued a hybrid between a local and state program, by adopting state-recognized labels of origin. As Barham describes in the case of the producers of Charlevoix in Quebec, this new label is actually a form of intellectual property recognizable at the global level. This "place-making" label can integrate the social, economic, and environmental goals of a location as its products enter a global marketplace.[40]

Farm-to-School Programs

The last decade has seen rapid growth in kindergarten through twelfth-grade (K–12) school districts in North America that are interested in serving farm fresh food in their cafeterias to provide healthy food to children in school meal programs, while simultaneously providing a market for small and midsize family farmers. These programs are improving their school food environments by sourcing locally grown farm fresh ingredients for school meals, starting school gardens, recycling and composting, including nutrition and food education in classrooms or cafeterias, and conducting farm tours for school children.

As of July 2008, the National Farm to School Network had identified more than 2,000 farm-to-school programs in 39 states. More than 8,700 schools and 1,900 school districts are involved.[41] Resources abound documenting the benefits, challenges, and impacts of farm-to-school programs in many states.[42] A recent review of farm-to-school evaluation studies suggests that these programs contribute to more healthful eating patterns among children, as well as to more diversified income streams for regional growers. Successful farm-to-school programs tend to have three key ingredients: (1) active leadership, (2) complementary partnerships among diverse community stakeholders, and (3) creative, resourceful use of assets.[43] Additionally, regionally based mid-tier food distributors can play an important role in making procurement options more economically viable for schools.[44] As the cost of initiating and maintaining such programs is often still more than many school districts can afford on their own, supplementary income in the form of grants or donations is necessary. The future of these programs will be determined by whether public and private funds, leadership, and local, state, and federal policies support ongoing farm-to-school development.

Farm-to-Institution Programs

The farm-to-school movement has fueled a broader movement to purchase locally grown, sustainable foods for cafeterias at other institutions, including colleges, universities, hospitals, corporate cafeterias, and prisons. There has been a big growth in this arena in the last five years; as with farm-to-school programs, initial work began in other institutions at least two decades ago. The advantage for institutions other than K–12 schools is that they are often less restricted financially, because they often do not depend on government subsidies like the School Meals Program or the Commodities Program to purchase foods.

The Economic Research Service estimates that Americans spent $556 billion on food away from home in 2007 and at least 14 percent of that is captured by institutions (about $77 billion).[45] Farm-to-institution programs can create win-win situations for farmers and consumers. As with schools, customers have access to fresher foods, while farmers benefit from new market niches. So far, these markets have been largely untapped by small and midsize farms. New research results from a California study that interviewed college students, food service managers, farmers, and distributors show farm-to-institution programs hold potential as long as farmers, distributors, and food service buyers address transaction costs and distribution issues.[46] The surveys show that college students and food service managers are interested in local and sustainably produced foods. Twenty-eight percent of colleges surveyed in California have local produce buying programs and another 22 percent are developing them. In-depth case studies of food service directors showed that, on average, food service buyers purchased about 26 percent of their produce from local growers in 2006 (about $226,000 per institution per year). Research from this study showed that smaller colleges currently buy the most produce (as a percentage of total produce purchases) from local growers, and they tend to use smaller "nonprofit allied" distributors and direct purchases from growers to accomplish this.

Significant challenges have surfaced in the logistics, timeliness, and consistency of the delivery system, as well as the seasonality, bidding regulations, liability insurance, and understanding and valuing of local food, but new solutions are emerging.[47] Case study interviews[48] showed that nearly 70 percent of food service buyers considered "quality" to be an advantage of working with local growers, and more than 60 percent mentioned "supporting the local economy" as an advantage. It is interesting that the California study and a similar Colorado study found that price is not the most important criterion in purchasing decisions; quality is.[49] Many feel that the advantages are worth the time it takes to establish new working relationships and new purchasing protocols for a portion of their business.

Values-based Supply Chains

New models for "values-based supply chains" are emerging across the country. Values-based supply chains are institutional purchasing arrangements whereby an agreed-on set of environmental, social, and economic values drive the provision— from production to marketing—of a given product or service. In value chains, partnering businesses form long-term networks and work together to maximize these values for the partners and customers.[50]

Examples of value chains include the New Seasons Market, a regional grocery chain in Portland, Oregon, that is committed to a Northwest regional food economy; Country Natural Beef in the Pacific Northwest; Ozark Mountain Pork in Missouri; and the Organic Valley of Farms headquartered in Wisconsin. In a study of these and other value chain models, Stevenson and Pirog identified several "best practices." The most successful value chains include high levels of performance and trust, a shared vision, transparency with respect to information and decision-making, and ample recognition of the contributions made by strategic partners.

To see values-based supply chains succeed in the future, the authors suggest that attention should be paid to achieving the following: (1) differentiation and pricing structure; (2) a sufficient volume and supply of high-quality products; (3) adequate capitalization and competent management; (4) technical, research, and development support; and (5) meaningful standards and consistent certification.

Community Gardens and Urban Farms

Many of the strategies outlined thus far have involved rural farms producing food and selling it to urban dwellers through various marketing venues. Food production can also happen much closer to urban centers and can involve urban consumers in producing their own food. In the first instance, "urban farms" are enterprises in which food production within the city limits is organized to provide food for many families. These farms range from independent sites on the urban edge that derive their main source of income from local consumer sales such as Fairview Gardens[51] in Goleta, California, to those such as the Food Project in Boston, Massachusetts,[52] or Red Hook Community Farm in Brooklyn, New York,[53] that involve youths or low-income residents in growing their own food. Since these urban farms are so close to their constituents, many include an education and experiential component that often is funded by an associated nonprofit organization. Through these programs participants learn how food is grown using sustainable production practices and how it can be marketed directly to consumers or shared with local food banks.

Community gardens provide benefits similar to urban farms. Community gardens have proliferated throughout urban centers nationwide and have served many different functions, from providing food security, neighborhood development, and strengthening ethnic or cultural connections, to forming a connection with the environment and enhancing public spaces.[54] Most importantly, they provide fresh, wholesome food to community residents and opportunities for positive, healing interactions among people. In a study of the association between household participation in a community garden and fruit and vegetable consumption among urban adults, "adults with a household member who participated in a community garden consumed fruits and vegetables 1.4 more times per day than those who did not participate, and they were 3.5 times more likely to consume fruits and vegetables at least 5 times daily."[55]

In many urban neighborhoods, community gardens are located on a separate lot near housing. However, in some developments, edible landscaping and gardening have become a central feature of the community. In such communities, gardening is part of a larger sustainable community design that is consistent with the Ahwahnee community design guidelines, which are considered a positive alternative to urban sprawl. Village Homes in Davis, California,[56] is considered part of the New

Urbanism that focuses on creating human-scale neighborhoods better able to meet residents' social needs.[57] Along with a new vision for pedestrian-friendly urban design, accessible and beautiful public spaces, community gathering places, and landscapes that celebrate local history, these new developments also encourage the production, processing, and consumption of local food.

All of these alternative approaches to food marketing and acquisition are considered key elements of local and sustainable food systems. Whether they exist in communities often depends on how engaged stakeholders are in assessing assets, identifying needs in the current food system, and developing concrete steps or plans to meet those needs.

CONNECTING SUSTAINABLE REGIONAL FOOD SYSTEMS TO COMMUNITY DEVELOPMENT

Food System Analysis and Planning

In the last decade, professional planners have begun to view the food system as an important component to community design.[58] Planners use tools such as GIS (geographic information system) mapping and zoning to plan for infrastructure and transportation systems that support a more sustainable community food system. Some strategies also detail how low-income residents can better access food in their communities. Additionally, the planning community has adopted a set of decision-making guidelines that include food systems in community plans.[59] These guidelines will contribute to a built environment that supports a more sustainable food system.

Meeting Consumer Food Needs: Adequacy of Local Supplies

Efforts to make food systems local or regional often raise the question of food self-reliance. How much of the food needs of the people living in a defined area can be provided by local agriculture? The exercise of analyzing food needs and agricultural capacity can often enlighten food system planning and lead to additional questions worthy of exploration.

One study of food self-reliance was conducted for the Canadian province of British Columbia.[60] The 2006 report concluded that "B.C. farmers produce 48 percent of *all* foods consumed in B.C. and produce 56 percent of foods consumed that can be economically grown in B.C." This might be considered a measure of the province's food self-reliance. When researchers considered what consumers *should* eat, based on Canada's *Food Guide to Healthy Eating,* however, food self-reliance dropped to 34 percent largely because fruit and vegetable is currently below recommended levels.

A similar conclusion was reached in comparisons of New York State fruit and vegetable production with New Yorkers' food consumption, and how much is recommended in the Food Guide Pyramid.[61] New York vegetable farmers produce enough vegetables to provide 38 percent of total demand. In a similar analysis for fruit, researchers found that New York fruit production could meet only 18 percent of the fruit New Yorkers demand, plus 256 million pounds of "surplus" of a few crops—namely, apples and cherries—that were produced in excess of consumption. Both of these analyses suggest opportunities for increasing food self-reliance by orienting current and future agricultural production toward local consumer food preferences as well as dietary guidelines. The studies highlight the need to protect land from development and to bring available land into production of high-value, high-nutrition specialty crops.

Economic Development Impact of Local Food Self-Reliance

One of the potential benefits often ascribed to local or regional food systems is the contribution they make to community economic development. In the past decade, research has begun to document and measure this economic benefit.

Several recent studies have looked at potential income and job growth from a shift in food consumption toward local sources. An 18-month study was conducted by the Michigan Land Use Institute and the C. S. Mott Group at Michigan State University to assess the impact of efforts to increase sales of fresh, local foods in Michigan on employment and personal income across the state. The study found that such a shift in marketing would generate 1,889 new jobs across the state and result in $187 million in new personal income.[62]

Another study assessed the potential net economic impacts that could accrue to Iowa from each of four scenarios of fruit and vegetable production and direct and grocery sales to consumers.[63] For each scenario the economic impact was calculated. In one scenario in which Iowans ate five servings of fruits and vegetables per day and ate solely local produce for three of the five servings, the total economic output came to $331.2 million, including $123.3 million in total labor income, which generated 4,484 total jobs in Iowa.[64]

This report shows that "by substituting in-state production for out-of-state purchases, money that otherwise would have left the state remains in the state. Keeping money in the state is desirable because money that leaves the state rarely returns. Money that remains in the state has an economic multiplier effect on the whole economy."[65] This strategy of "import substitution" and capturing the economic benefits is at the core of many efforts to rebuild local and regional food systems.

Building a Policy Framework for Local Sustainable Food Systems

Should public schools serve food produced by local farmers? Should farmland near communities be protected from development? Should good food be more affordable than calorie-rich products in local food stores? What incentives exist in communities to establish food markets in areas with limited access to wholesome food? These and other food system related questions are ideal for local and state Food Policy Councils (FPCs) to entertain.

Federal law sets a framework for action, but it cannot provide a local response to the needs and interests of consumers and farmers or respond to the natural, economic, and cultural conditions of a particular place. Hence the need for, and value of, state and local FPCs.

Because FPCs are generated locally or at the state level, they reflect place-specific participation and process. For example, an FPC may be an official advisory body on food system issues to a city, county, or state government, or it may be a grassroots network focused on educating the public, coordinating nonprofit efforts, and influencing government, commercial, and institutional practices and policies on food systems. However, all FPCs "bring together stakeholders from diverse food-related areas to examine how the food system is working and propose ways to improve it."[66]

The first city-level FPC was founded in Knoxville, Tennessee, in 1982 to address food system problems experienced by community members. Soon after, FPCs began in St. Paul, Kansas City, Charlotte, Philadelphia, Hartford, Austin, Los Angeles, Syracuse, Portland, Seattle, and Toronto. A number of state-level FPCs have also formed—Connecticut, Iowa, Utah, New Mexico, and North Carolina. New York now has several FPCs, and a number are emerging in California, Oregon, Oklahoma, Michigan, Maine, and Colorado.

The issues FPCs address and the decisions they reach are as diverse as the constituents they represent. As an example, in December 2005, the City Council of Oakland authorized the Mayor's Office of Sustainability to develop an Oakland food policy and plan enabling the city to get 30 percent of its food from local area food production. Its goal is to establish a sustainable food system in Oakland, thereby addressing food security, public health, local agriculture, energy efficiency, environmental resource preservation, zero waste, and community and economic development, and to increase food literacy through education, outreach, and advocacy.

Are Regional Food Systems the Only Answer?

While strategies to "relocalize" food supplies can provide multiple benefits, this framework is only a partial answer to making food systems more sustainable. If we examine the definition of sustainability, the alternative production, marketing, analysis, education, and policy options suggested here may not lead to achieving all the goals. As Allen has pointed out, broader policy reforms, especially targeting social justice, are also needed.[67] "Localness" alone may, in fact, lead us astray unless we uncover and name the other dimensions of a sustainable food system that are important, for example, food democracy, control of decisions affecting our food system, social justice, and community empowerment.

Although we want to avoid what Born and Purcell call the "local trap,"[68] we agree with Hinrichs' rationale for pursuing regional food systems strategies:

> Remaking the food system then suggests neither a revolutionary break nor a radical transformation but rather deliberate, sometimes unglamorous multipronged efforts to do things differently. Seen together, these initially isolated efforts to remake the food system begin to form a platform from which people might continue to work.[69]

Such work provides encouraging signs of change that motivate us and provide a sense of hope as we come together to create a sustainable food system for ourselves and our children.

NOTES

1. Steven C. Blank, *The End of Agriculture in the American Portfolio* (Westport, CT: Quorum Books, 1998); Rick Welsh, "The Industrial Reorganization of U.S. Agriculture" (Policy Studies Report no. 6, Henry A. Wallace Institute for Alternative Agriculture, Greenbelt, MD, 1996).

2. USDA (U.S. Department of Agriculture), National Agriculture Statistics Service, "Trends in U.S. Agriculture," http://www.usda.gov/nass/pubs/trends/farmnumbers. htm (accessed January 3, 2009).

3. Ibid.

4. Fred Kirschenmann et al., "Why Worry about the Agriculture of the Middle?" in *Food and the Mid-Level Farm: Renewing an Agriculture of the Middle*, ed. Thomas A. Lyson, G. W. Stevenson, and Rick Welsh (Cambridge, MA: The MIT Press, 2008).

5. Kirschenmann et al., "Why Worry about Agriculture," 7.

6. Eileen Brady and Caitlin O'Brady, "Consumer Considerations and the Agriculture of the Middle," in *Food and the Mid-Level Farm: Renewing an Agriculture of the Middle*, ed. Thomas A. Lyson, G. W. Stevenson, and Rick Welsh (Cambridge, MA: The MIT Press, 2008); Robert Feagan, "The Place of Food: Mapping Out the 'Local' in Local Food Systems," *Progress in Human Geography* 31, no. 1 (2007): 23–42.

7. Thomas A. Lyson, "Civic Agriculture and the North American Food System," in *Remaking the North American Food System: Strategies for Sustainability*, ed. C. Clare Hinrichs and Thomas A. Lyson (Lincoln: University of Nebraska Press, 2007): 19–32.

8. Brian Halweil, "Home Grown: The Case for Local Food in a Global Marketplace" (paper no. 163, Worldwatch Institute, Washington, DC, 2002).

9. William Heffernan, Mary Hendrickson, and Robert Gronski, "Consolidation in the Food and Agriculture System" (Report to the National Farmers Union, 1999), http://home.hiwaay.net/~becraft/NFUFarmCrisis.htm; Mary Hendrickson et al., "Consolidation in Food Retailing and Dairy: Implications for Farmers and Consumers in a Global Food System" (report to the National Farmers Union, 2001).

10. Phil Howard, "Consolidation in Food and Agriculture: Implications for Farmers and Consumers," *The Natural Farmer* (Spring 2006).

11. Ibid., 18; Heffernan, Hendrickson, and Gronski, "Consolidation."

12. William Hendrickson and Mary Heffernan, "Concentration of Agricultural Markets" (report to the National Farmers Union, April 2007), http://www.nfu.org/wp-content/2007-heffernanreport.pdf.

13. Michael Pollan, *The Omnivore's Dilemma: A Natural History of Four Meals* (New York: Penguin Press, 2006): 90–99.

14. Judy Putnam, Jane Allshouse, and Linda Scott Kantor, "U.S. per Capita Food Supply Trends: More Calories, Refined Carbohydrates, and Fats," *FoodReview* 25, no. 3 (2002): 2–15, http://www.ers.usda.gov/publications/FoodReview/DEC2002/frvol25i3.pdf.

15. Ali H. Mokdad et al., "Actual Causes of Death in the United States 2000," *The Journal of the American Medical Association* 291 (2004): 1238–245, http://dying.about.com/causes/tp/actual_death.htm.

16. National Center for Health Statistics, "Prevalence of Overweight and Obesity among Adults: United States, 2003–2004" (*Health and Stats*, 2006), http://www.cdc.gov/nchs/products/pubs/pubd/hestats/overweight/overwght_adult_03.htm.

17. CDC (Centers for Disease Control and Prevention), "Overweight and Obesity: Overweight Prevalence," http://www.cdc.gov/nccdphp/dnpa/obesity/childhood/prevalence.htm.

18. Elizabeth Frazao, "High Costs of Poor Eating Patterns in the United States," in *America's Eating Habits: Changes and Consequences*, ed. Elizabeth Frazao, Agriculture Information Bulletin No. 750 (Washington, DC: USDA, Economic Research Service, 1999): 5–32, http://www.ers.usda.gov/publications/aib750/.

19. American Public Health Association, "Helping Preserve Antibiotic Effectiveness by Stimulating Demand for Meats Produced without Excessive Antibiotics" (Policy

Statement 2004–13, 2004), http://www.apha.org/advocacy/policy/policysearch/default. htm?id=1299.

20. Jan L. Flora et al., "Social and Community Impacts in Iowa State University and the University of Iowa Study Group," *Iowa Concentrated Animal Feeding Operations Air Quality Study* (Iowa City: University of Iowa Press, 2002), 147–63.

21. American Public Health Association, "Precautionary Moratorium on New Concentrated Animal Feed Operations" (Policy Statement 2003–7, 2003), http://www. apha.org/advocacy/policy/policysearch/default.htm?id=1243.

22. Don Villarejo, "Suffering in Silence: A Report on the Health of California's Agricultural Workers" (Davis, CA: CIRS, 2000) cited in Guzman et al., *A Workforce Action Plan for Farm Labor in California: Toward a More Sustainable Food System* (report to the Roots of Change Fund, 2007), http://www.cirsinc.org/Documents/Pub0707.1.pdf.

23. Mark Winne, *Closing the Food Gap: Resetting the Table in the Land of Plenty* (Boston: Beacon Press, 2008).

24. USDA, ERS (Economic Research Service), "Food Security in the United States: Measuring Household Food Security," http://www.ers.usda.gov/Briefing/FoodSecurity/ measurement.htm (accessed August 7, 2008); Sue Ann Andersen, ed., "Core Indicators of Nutritional State for Difficult to Sample Populations," *The Journal of Nutrition* 120 (1990): 1557S–1600S.

25. American Farmland Trust, "What's Happening to Our Farmland?" (*Farming on the Edge Report*, n.d.), http://www.farmland.org/resources/fote/default.asp; American Farmland Trust, "Where is the Central Valley Heading? Projection of Current Trends," *The Future Is Now: Central Valley Farmland at the Tipping Point?*, http://www.farmland. org/programs/states/futureisnow/projections.asp.

26. The Polaris Institute, "Water Stewardship: Ensuring a Secure Future for California Water" (California Agricultural Water Stewardship Initiative, 2008), http://www. agwaterstewards.org/Water_Stewardship.pdf.

27. Richard Heinberg, "Threats of Peak Oil to the Global Food Supply #159" (paper presented at the FEASTA Conference, "What Will We Eat as the Oil Runs Out?" Dublin, Ireland, June 23–25, 2005).

28. Martin C. Heller and Gregory A. Keoleian, "U.S. Food System Factsheet" (Ann Arbor: Center for Sustainable Systems, University of Michigan), http://css.snre.umich. edu/css_doc/CSS01-06.pdf.

29. Jennifer L. Wilkins, Jennifer C. Bokaer-Smith, and Duncan Hilchey, "Local Foods and Local Agriculture: A Survey of Attitudes among Northeastern Consumers: A Survey of Northeast Consumers" (Ithaca, NY: Division of Nutritional Sciences, Cornell University, 1996).

30. Hartman Group, Inc., "Organic Food & Beverage Trends 2004: Lifestyle, Language & Category Adoption," Pub ID: HAR1032427 (Bellevue, WA: The Hartman Group, Inc., 2004).

31. Packaged Facts, "Locally Grown Foods Niche Cooks Up at $5 Billion as America Chows Down on Fresh" (press release June 20, 2007), http://www.packagedfacts. com/about/release.asp?id=918.

32. Thomas A. Lyson, *Civic Agriculture: Reconnecting Farm, Food and Community* (Medford, MA: University Press of New England, 2004).

33. Agricultural Marketing Service, "Farmers Markets: Wholesale and Farmers Markets, United States Department of Agriculture," http://www.ams.usda.gov/AMSv1.0/ams. fetchTemplateData.do?template=TemplateC&navID=FarmersMarkets&rightNav1=Far mersMarkets&topNav=&leftNav=WholesaleandFarmersMarkets&page=WFMFarmers MarketsHome&description=Farmers%20Markets&acct=frmrdirmkt; Gail Feenstra,

"The Roles of Farmers' Markets in Fueling Local Economies," *Gastronomic Sciences* January, no. 2 (2007): 56–64.

34. Christopher C. Lewis, "The Saturday Stockton Certified Farmers Market: An Urban Community Market" (Direct Marketing, UC Sustainable Agriculture Research and Education Program, 2001), http://www.sarep.ucdavis.edu/cdpp/stockton.htm.

35. Patricia Allen et al., "Shifting Plates in the Agrifood Landscape: The Tectonics of Alternative Agrifood Initiatives in California," *Journal of Rural Studies* 19 (2003): 61–75; C. Clare Hinrichs, "Embeddedness and Local Food Systems: Notes on Two Types of Direct Agricultural Markets," *Journal of Rural Studies* 16 (2000): 295–303.

36. Marcia Ruth Ostrom, "Community Supported Agriculture as an Agent of Change," in *Remaking the North American Food System*, ed. C. Clare Hinrichs and Thomas A. Lyson (Lincoln: University of Nebraska Press, 2007), 99–120.

37. Elizabeth Barham, "Towards a Theory of Values-based Labeling," *Agriculture and Human Values* 19 (2002): 349–60.

38. Erin Derden-Little and Gail Feenstra, "Regional Agricultural Marketing: A Review of Programs in California" (Local Food Systems in a Global Environment, UC Sustainable Agriculture Research and Education Program, 2006), http://www.sarep. ucdavis.edu/cdpp/foodsystems/MarketingReportFinal_5_10.pdf.

39. C. Clare Hinrichs and Eric Jensen, "State Labeling of Food and Agricultural Products: Organization, Governance and Outcomes" (paper presented at the annual meeting of the Rural Sociological Society, Louisville, KY, August 10–13, 2006).

40. Elizabeth Barham, "The Lamb That Roared: Origin-labeled Products as Place-Making Strategy in Charlevoix, Quebec," in *Remaking the North American Food System*, ed. C. Clare Hinrichs and Thomas A. Lyson (Lincoln: University of Nebraska Press, 2007).

41. National Farm to School Network, "Welcome to National Farm to School Online," http://www.farmtoschool.org/ (accessed July 25, 2008).

42. Barbara C. Bellows, Rex Dufour, and Janet Bachman, "Bringing Local Food to Local Institutions: A Resource Guide for Farm-to-School and Farm-to-Institution Programs" (ATTRA), http://attra.ncat.org/attra-pub/PDF/farmtoschool.pdf.

43. Anupama Joshi, Andrea A. Azuma, and Gail Feenstra, "Do Farm to School Programs Make a Difference? Findings and Future Research Needs," *Journal of Hunger and Environmental Nutrition* 3, no. 2, 3 (2008): 229–46.

44. Betty Tomoko Izumi, "Farm to School Programs in Public K-12 Schools in the United States: Perspectives of Farmers, Food Service Professionals, and Food Distributors" (PhD dissertation, Michigan State University, 2008).

45. USDA, ERS, "Food Away from Home, Table 3: Food CPI, Prices and Expenditures," http://151.121.68.30/Briefing/CPIFoodAndExpenditures/Data/table3.htm.

46. Patricia Allen et al., "Bringing Students, Farmers and Food Service to the Table" (paper presented at the annual meeting of the Agriculture, Food and Human Values Society, New Orleans, LA, June 4–8, 2008).

47. Allen et al., "Bringing Students"; Mary B. Gregoire, et al., "Iowa Producers' Perceived Benefits and Obstacles in Marketing to Local Restaurants and Institutional Foodservice Operations," *Journal of Extension* 43, no. 1 (2005): article # 1RIB1, http://www.joe.org/joe/2005february/rb1.shtml; Harriet Friedmann, "Scaling Up: Bringing Public Institutions and Food Service Corporations into the Project for a Local, Sustainable Food System in Ontario," *Agriculture and Human Values* 24 (2007): 389–98.

48. Allen et al., "Bringing Students."

49. Amory Starr et al., "Sustaining Local Agriculture: Barriers and Opportunities to Direct Marketing between Farms and Restaurants in Colorado," *Agriculture and Human Values* 20 (2003): 301–21.

50. G. W. Stevenson and Rich Pirog, "Values-Based Supply Chains: Strategies for Agrifood Enterprises of the Middle," in *Food and the Mid-Level Farm: Renewing an Agriculture of the Middle*, ed. Thomas A. Lyson, G. W. Stevenson, and Rick Welsh (Cambridge, MA: The MIT Press, 2008): 119–43.

51. Fairview Gardens, http://www.fairviewgardens.org/.

52. The Food Project, http://www.thefoodproject.org/.

53. Lisa McLaughlin, "Inner City Farms," *The New York Times Magazine*, July 24, 2008, http://www.time.com/time/magazine/article/0,9171,1826271,00.html.

54. Laura Lawson, *City Bountiful: A Century of Community Gardening in America.* (Berkeley: University of California Press, 2005).

55. Katherine Alaimo et al., "Fruit and Vegetable Intake among Urban Community Gardeners," *Journal of Nutrition Education and Behavior* 40, no. 2 (2008): 121.

56. Mark Francis, *Village Homes: A Community by Design* (Washington, DC: Island Press, 2003).

57. Judy Corbett and Michael Corbett, *Designing Sustainable Communities: Learning from Village Homes* (Washington, DC: Island Press, 2000).

58. Kami Pothukuchi and Jerry Kaufman, "Placing Food Issues on the Community Agenda: The Role Of Municipal Institutions in Food Systems Planning," *Agriculture and Human Values* 16 (1999): 213–24.

59. Jerry Kaufman, Kami Pothukuchi, and Deanna Glosser (in consultation with American Planning Association members), "Community and Regional Planning: A Policy Guide of the American Planning Association" (adopted by APA Legislative, Policy Committee, and Chapter Delegates, APA National Conference, Philadelphia, PA, 2007), http://www.planning.org/policyguides/food.htm.

60. British Columbia Ministry of Agriculture and Lands, "B.C.'s Food Self-Reliance: Can B.C.'s Farmers Feed Our Growing Population?" (2006), http://www.southlandsin thealr.ca/b-c-s-food-self-reliance (accessed August 7, 2008).

61. USDA, Center for Nutrition Policy and Promotion, "Food Guide Pyramid: A Guide to Daily Food Choices" (1992), http://www.nal.usda.gov/fnic/Fpyr/pmap.htm (accessed July 28, 2008).

62. C. S. Mott Group, *Eat Fresh and Grow Jobs* (East Lansing: Michigan State University, 2006).

63. Dave Swenson, "The Economic Impacts of Increased Fruit and Vegetable Production and Consumption in Iowa: Phase II" (prepared for the Regional Food Systems Working Group Leopold Center for Sustainable Agriculture, 2006), http://www.leopold. iastate.edu/pubs/staff/health/health.htm (accessed August 18, 2008).

64. Ibid.

65. Ibid.

66. World Hunger Year, Food Security Learning Center, "Food Policy Councils, 2008," http://www.worldhungeryear.org/fslc/faqs/ria_090.asp?section=8&click=1 (accessed August 18, 2008).

67. Patricia Allen, *Together at the Table: Sustainability and Sustenance in the American Agrifood System* (University Park: The Pennsylvania State University Press, 2004).

68. Brandon Born and Mark Purcell, "Avoiding the Local Trap: Scale and Food Systems in Planning Research," *Journal of Planning Education and Research* 26 (2006): 195–207.

69. C. Clare Hinrichs, "Introduction: Practice and Place in Remaking the Food System," in *Remaking the North American Food System*, ed. C. Clare Hinrichs and Thomas A. Lyson (Lincoln: University of Nebraska Press, 2007), 1–15, 5–6.

RESOURCE GUIDE

Suggested Reading

Halweil, Brian. *Eat Here: Reclaiming Homegrown Pleasures in a Global Supermarket.* Washington, DC: Worldwatch Institute, 2004.

Hinrichs, Clare, and Thomas A. Lyson. *Remaking the North American Food System: Strategies for Sustainability.* Lincoln: University of Nebraska Press, 2008.

Kingsolver, Barbara. *Animal, Vegetable, Miracle: A Year of Food Life.* New York: Harper-Collins, 2007.

Patel, Raj. *Stuffed and Starved: Markets, Power, and the Hidden Battle for the World's Food System.* London: Portobello Books Ltd., 2007.

Pollan, Michael. *The Omnivore's Dilemma: A Natural History of Four Meals.* New York: Penguin Press, 2006.

Pollan, Michael. *In Defense of Food: An Eater's Manifesto.* New York: Penguin Press, 2008.

Roberts, Paul. *The End of Food.* Boston: Houghton Mifflin Co., 2008.

Smith, Alisa, and J. B. MacKinnon. *Plenty: One Man, One Woman, and a Raucous Year of Eating Locally.* New York: Harmony Books, 2007.

Weis, Anthony. *The Global Food Economy: The Battle for the Future of Farming.* London: Zed Books, 2007.

Web Sites

Community Food Security Coalition, http://www.foodsecurity.org/.

Food System Research Group, University of Wisconsin-Madison, http://www.aae.wisc.edu/fsrg/.

Local Harvest, http://www.localharvest.org.

World Hunger Year, Food Security Learning Center, http://www.worldhungeryear.org/fslc/.

9

Social Movements: Slow Places, Fast Movements, and the Making of Contemporary Rurality

Daniel Niles

In September 2004 the often sleepy grounds of Mexico City's Monument to the Revolution were briefly brought to life. A group of campesinos was using the monument's cement embankments as a staging ground for a protest and occupation of several government ministries concerned with rural development. Some had donned their best shirts and hats for the occasion, but many had arrived as if straight from their fields, in their rubber boots, patched pants and thin shirts open wide at the neck. Most came with only a few pesos in their pockets or tucked into their brassieres, yet prepared to stay for the duration. They slept on the monument grounds under a large canvas tarp that provided shelter from the cold fall rain, if not the wind, or on their buses until such time as the demonstration organizers were granted hearings with the appropriate government ministries. Then the group would discuss whether or not their objectives had been or would be realized, and whether they should return to their towns, villages, and hamlets, at least for the time being.

The presence of an unaffiliated *estadounidense* (U.S. citizen) wandering through the campesino crowd generated a fair amount of interest and commentary, and plenty of invitations to stop and talk for a while. Conversation often turned to the United States. Almost all of these rural people, especially the men, had been to the United States and knew it well. It is now rare to meet in the Mexican countryside a man of mature age who has not lived in and between Oregon, Idaho, California, and Colorado, or increasingly Illinois, North Carolina, New York, and even Maine, for 2, 8, 20 years, or more. Such men and women have passed half a lifetime as shadow labor in the United States. Rural women who have not been to the States themselves have husbands, sons, and daughters, sometimes all of their sons and daughters, absent for years on end often with little or no contact sometimes, gone forever to another life, or to a faraway death.

Fewer of the campesinos on the monument grounds had been to Mexico City. In the small groups standing around or squatting comfortably, varied commentary discussed the cross-dressed prostitutes now visible in the early night, general fear of crime, and the shadowed streets, and no confidence in the capital's food. Some resolved not to venture into the surrounding neighborhood at all: the Monument to the Revolution would be their island.

Before long, a small group of farmers from Michoacan struck out for a protest several blocks away, one of several occurring simultaneously at different buildings in the central city. The group stuck closely together as it moved quickly beneath the polished-glass high rises and across the ill-lit striated avenues, sometimes suspiciously devoid of traffic. As we crossed one median after another, someone joked that here I was the *coyote*—the cunning characters on whom most migrants depend to guide them across the U.S. border—and that even in Mexico's capital, the campesino is always on the run.

We arrived at the offices of SAGARPA (the Secretary of Agriculture, Cattle Ranching, Rural Development, Fisheries, and Food), where several hundred campesinos were cramped between the pulsing avenue and the glass ministry high-rise building. Most of the lights were turned off; the functionaries had long since slipped out the back. Only a few police guarded the front door and the brightly lit street-level showroom in which choice pieces of folk art and other items—some obviously updated to appeal to more urbane taste—were on display at top-dollar prices. The campesinos, whose home regions I could sometimes guess based on a particular style of hat or blouse, quickly made their initial point, calling out *Presente!—We're here!*—in response to a speaker who called off the names of the Mexican states. Even though most people had arrived earlier that day and were in good spirits, after a short while, there did not seem to be much to do—the office lights were mostly turned off, few other people passed on the sidewalk—and it appeared that the whole demonstration might dissipate at any moment in the chill air. Then, it seemed mostly to keep spirits up, a group of campesinos with dented horns and drums set into their instrument, mounting an impromptu *huapango* (or village *fête*) right there on the avenue.

Despite the "constant change" in Mexico's countryside, and the morbid predictions for the future of its people,[1] what Bonfil Batalla[2] called *México Profundo*, or deep Mexico, still exists and remains largely rural or indigenous. This Mexico is still the source, or at least the referent, of much Mexican popular art and culture, and often at the base of what is considered most quintessentially Mexican. Here, in the darkened streets of the strange capital, flickering in the glass of the ministry showroom and propelled by the band's ragged tunes, the shuffle-dance of a few bold couples, and the encouraging shouts and whistles from the crowd, the assembly took on a strangely un-protest-like feel: the deep contrast and irony between the well-lit "folk" culture managed, promoted, and updated at will by the state, and the folk themselves seemed lost on no one. Displacing the standard practical and political demands, at least for the moment, were country people unabashedly celebrating themselves in the political center of the nation that claims to represent them.

That rural people would have cause to protest the plans of an authoritarian, rapidly modernizing, and technocratic state should come as no surprise. Their reasons for doing so in different periods have been well described in various contexts.[3] One of the classic texts on rural rebellion and political economy is James Scott's *The Moral Economy of the Peasant: Rebellion and Subsistence in Southeast Asia.*[4] It describes the series of peasant rebellions against colonial powers in 1930s and 1940s Burma and Vietnam as fundamentally conservative: their objective was to reestablish the variety of social and economic arrangements that had ensured a minimum income to all. In such settings,

> [t]he appeal [of rural rebellion] was in almost every case to the past—to traditional practices—and the revolts I discuss are best seen as defensive reactions. Such backward-looking intentions are by now a commonplace in the analysis of peasant movements. As Moore, citing Tawney, put it, "the peasant radical would be astonished to hear that he is undermining the foundations of society; he is merely trying to get back what is rightfully his."[5]

In essence, Scott's thesis is that colonialism violated rural peoples' sense of themselves *as producers of their own livelihoods and patterns of social reproduction.* This thesis is still pertinent to rural social protest today. But the implication that such action is referenced to the past alone, to "closed and autonomous utopia,"[6] that it has no engaged or substantive interest in the wider political and economic conditions, and that it certainly offers no *proposal* for alternative political economies, is now plainly out of date.

On the contrary, contemporary agrarian politics look to the future, combining awareness of human-ecological interdependence with political-economic critique and a strong sense of cultural potential. For example, Via Campesina, an international alliance of small farmers and rural peoples, is a mass political movement. The food-centered Slow Food® organization is a kind of social network with goals beyond those of most social networks. Both Via Campesina and Slow Food emerged in response to the dominant course of twentieth-century agricultural development, a course that has—with few exceptions—seen the steady undermining of the structural conditions that would support small-scale producers, so that now the very idea of agrarian society is in jeopardy.[7] Rural places have come to be seen as little more than sources of raw materials and sinks for urban and industrial waste, or to be of value *in spite* of rural peoples themselves.[8] Via Campesina organizations experienced this devaluation of rural people and places at the point of production, as support for small farmers has declined along with the percentage of the food dollar that stays on-farm, and as local products have been displaced from local markets.

In contrast, Slow Food began its critique of industrial agriculture and food systems from the point of consumption: it rejected the very food produced in industrial food systems—the "rivers of grain"—as a false abundance that transformed the gastronomic and social experiences of cooking and eating into banal, pleasureless acts. Via Campesina and Slow Food attempt to change this course of development. In its place, they struggle to create circuits of small-scale agrobiodiverse agricultural production and rich food cultures, each of which supports the other. Both organizations blend place-based development projects with international networking and solidarity, and thus can operate consistently in local, national, and international contexts.

However critical are their practical actions and proposals, these organizations also attempt to reassess and reassign the meanings associated with food production and consumption, and of the role of rural peoples in these processes. In this sense, both are guided by a vision of rural places and peoples, and of the wider circuits of food production and consumption in which much of the planet is ultimately involved, which is simultaneously *preservationist* and *prefigurative*. Their great project is to discover what could be called "contemporary rurality."

NEW RURAL MOVEMENTS

Via Campesina

Via Campesina is a grassroots rural popular movement calling itself, and calling for, "the country people's way" to rural social and ecological change. Its roots stretch back to the early 1990s, when it was formed out of a series of exchanges and collaborations between farmer organizations in the Americas and Western Europe. These organizations had decades of experience in all kinds of rural development projects, and yet their participants—and rural peoples more generally—had seen steady declines in their living conditions in the previous decades of state-led agricultural development.[9]

The organizations that would form Via Campesina took an early interest in the conditions of farmers in different places and began to explore the similarities in their experience that might allow them to work together. For one, they noted that local development had become increasingly intertwined with, and subject to, policies and forces operating beyond national borders. They sensed their organizational weakness at this important transnational scale and also realized that influencing such highly fluid transnational authorities as the World Trade Organization (WTO) would require a whole new bag of movement tools. Via Campesina was formed to take up the task of organizing a coherent presence for farmers at the transnational scale, and especially to confront the ideology of neoliberalism[10] as it was applied to rural and agricultural development.[11]

Via Campesina quickly established itself as an authentic voice of rural peoples, and has become a point of reference at high-level forums, such as WTO Ministerials or meetings of the Food and Agriculture Organization of the United Nations (FAO) and the United Nations Committee on Trade and Development (UNCTAD). Its prominence is largely due to its first major campaign (dating to 1996) for "food sovereignty," a plan for farmer-centered agricultural production and rural development.[12] Food sovereignty addresses the micro and macro policies that could support relatively localized circuits of food production and consumption as a basis for rural economic development and cultural survival. It is therefore opposed to neoliberal development—that is, development based on narrow interpretation of international competitive advantage rather than directed to satisfy objectives that are debated through an accessible political process. In clear contrast to the kind of agricultural development designed within the WTO (which favors trade-based development, even requiring nations to import a certain percentage of their food), food sovereignty claims the rights of nations to determine the agricultural and food policies that best meet the needs of it citizens. On this level, Via Campesina clearly sees the nation-state as a useful buffer to undesirable advances in transnational governance, even as its organizations are often involved in entrenched negotiations with their national governments. Its stance against neoliberal development puts Via Campesina at odds with the most powerful interests in the food and agricultural industries, the landed elites of many developing countries, and the ubiquitous conventional wisdom regarding the inherent superiority of free markets.

Rather than streamlining international trade in the food products most easily produced in an industrial food system, and so smoothing the ground for further expansion of the empty landscapes of industrial agriculture, food sovereignty supports "busy" agrarian landscapes with production primarily corresponding to local, national, and regional patterns of food production. It involves a profound change in practical and conceptual orientation. According to Peter Rosset, a former director of the Institute for Food and Development Policy (better known as Food First),

> To me the most important thing about food sovereignty are local and national markets. Just totally rejecting the whole ideology of export production. Not that there shouldn't be any exports, but as that being the driving force behind agricultural policy, as if a farmer's be-all and end-all is to manage to export. Completely rejecting that because, looking at farmers in the third world, only a tiny minority of wealthy farmers benefited from policies that favored exports, while a huge majority of farmers would benefit if there were policies that supported production for domestic markets. And so [Via Campesina] finally said, look all this ideology sounds great but the bottom line is it's benefiting 3% and we're 97%. It's displacing us: the more that the 3% grows the more we get pushed off our land.
>
> Then U.S. and European farmers realized that in the export boom in the US and Europe from the early 1970s on, even if the volume exported from both areas went up dramatically, farmer incomes had actually declined. You hear American or European farmers saying "now we produce twice as much as we did before, and we earn half as much," and the figures actually support those kinds of ratios. That's when family farmers in the U.S. begin to reject this ideology of "feeding the world." First of all they're getting screwed in the process, as I said, and then they start to have conversations and dialogues with farmers in the third world and realize that [the same export-centered ideology is] screwing them too.
>
> So food sovereignty says, wait a minute, it's not access to other people's markets that we need, it's access to our own markets. This mania of exportation at cheap prices is driving us all out of our local markets. It's driving crop prices down, creating a global food market where the lowest price, whoever self-exploits the most, is the one who "gets ahead" (because even the one who gets ahead is going broke at the same time). So food sovereignty finally says "Enough! We can't take this anymore. This is complete bull. We've been sold hook, line and sinker into this ideology of export and it's just wrong."[13]

It is worth stressing that food sovereignty is a vision for *agrarian* societies. Put slightly differently by a Via Campesina organizer in Mexico:

> As distinct from other campesino movements, we [in Via Campesina] assert, shall we say, the campesino way of life, and the right to be campesino, to continue to be the producers and suppliers of our own foods. We are not searching for the best economic conditions in which to buy maize, but in which to continue producing maize.[14]

It is largely due to the sensibility and flexibility of the food sovereignty platform in the context of global economic liberalization that Via Campesina has expanded both within and beyond its initial core area of operations. In recent years the locus of Via Campesina activity has notably shifted to Asia. One of the innovations in Via Campesina organization is that the headquarters are designed to rotate, and they shifted from Honduras to Indonesia in early 2005. The move corresponded to an increase in Via Campesina activity in the region because of the affiliation of large, well-organized, and active farmer organizations in India, Indonesia, the Republic of Korea, and the Philippines in the early 2000s. The 2006 conference on food sovereignty in Nyeleni, Mali, demonstrated that African farmer organizations also increasingly view their national predicaments through an international lens and seek common counterproposals to conventional development.[15]

Beginning in 2004, Via Campesina mounted a second campaign in defense of public access to seeds, which are described as the common inheritance of humankind, and as critical to the cultural, ecological, and economic past and futures of rural peoples.[16] As distinct from the proposal for food sovereignty, which is in large part directed toward the policymaking world, the seeds campaign can be seen to be primarily oriented toward rural peoples themselves. The seeds campaign highlights the fact that rural peoples are de facto stakeholders—and so legitimate participants—in the debates surrounding privatizations and sensible use of natural resources. The campaign asserts the role of rural peoples in the generation and maintenance of biodiversity, and of rural communities as actual and potential stewards of rural natural resources.

According to the same Mexican Via Campesina organizer quoted above,

> I think that the seeds campaign has two ends. One, it has a real cultural importance, because it makes it clear that we are biodiverse, and that there is real wealth and real importance within campesino territories. Demonstrating this I think gives us strength and credibility because it shows that we are not just talking about any old thing; all of these plants are valued by and attractive to many food and pharmaceutical companies.
>
> On the other hand, the seeds campaign internationalizes the ownership of those genetic resources. Now a seed is no longer the exclusive patrimony of Mexico, no, but one that fellow producers in Brazil or Guatemala or Costa Rica can have as well. And they can have it as part of their patrimony. Between ourselves this sharing is no problem. With luck [one of our plants] will serve as a nice forage crop there, or has medicinal qualities, or is well adapted to a particular altitude in some other place. This wealth can be shared.[17]

Though the campaign is relevant to contemporary debates surrounding intellectual property rights and genetic engineering, its wider project is to develop the political potential within the idea of a peasant way of life. It attempts to mobilize cultural ties to seeds, food, social life, and landscapes, and to promote these as a kind of collective wealth that is of significance to the wider world, that is indeed the basis of worldwide food security. A goal of the seeds campaign is to insert rural communities into the contemporary world not as "backward," relentlessly "traditional," "underdeveloped . . . have-nots," but as active participants in, and contributors to, the circuits of life on which all humanity is dependent. The phrase "la Via campesina" (literally "the country peoples' path or road") in addition to being a metaphor for a kind of development, has something of the sense of a political journey as well.

The two campaigns describe the principal characteristics of Via Campesina. While it is deeply entrenched in the structural conditions—local, national, regional, and transnational—of rural development, it also attempts to expand the conceptual and practical space in which the place of rural peoples in contemporary development can be reconsidered. In both campaigns, Via Campesina is revealed as a place-based social movement of rural peoples with explicitly internationalist agenda. It is not against globalization per se, but rather against the kind of globalization that centers on urban and industrial development and leaves little opportunity for viable rural social life. It is not necessarily antimodern, but it is against the kind of modernity that is taken as the opposite of all that is traditional. It is against the (false) choice of "either modernist development or social and economic stagnation" and against the view of traditional cultures implicit in that problematic.

Via Campesina represents an evolution in the character of local and national rural popular movements.[18] Farmer organizations can no longer be assumed to be purely parochial, conservative, and averse to change or contact with the outside world.[19] Certainly one of the remarkable features of Via Campesina is that it has managed to extend the reach and influence of disparate local and national farmer organizations and to develop a coherent analysis of rural development that can be articulated at strategic points, without overextending its constituent organizations. In organizational skill, it has proven itself to be as fluent in the digital age as most nongovernmental organizations (NGOs), while its analysis of international trade dynamics and WTO negotiations is as detailed as that of any academic. At the same time, it is a popular movement: its influence within the WTO, FAO, or most other organizations is entirely related to its ability to mobilize people. To be taken seriously, it must literally *manifest* its legitimacy in the streets, and so mass mobilization is its primary strategy.[20] As a movement, it must deliver some real advantage to the people in the streets to remain credible with them. It therefore is involved in a whole field of activity beyond that necessary for the FAO or other smaller, specialized NGOs or think tanks—it must maintain a popular movement.

While Via Campesina has focused its energies on the international context, its constituent organizations have never left off the tasks of local and national organization. These organizations are willing to engage with the state but are more cautious than party-based peasant federations were about incorporation into state policies and projects. They are also cautious about incorporation in NGO-led projects, even as they have learned from close contact with NGOs.[21] Many contemporary farmer organizations now attempt to deal directly with the state almost as if they were agencies with development projects of their own. Even while engaged in bitter struggles with local landlords and local governments, farmer organizations sometimes tailor their proposals to suit federal mandates, for example, when they stress the foreign exchange benefits that will accrue to the state through their plans for export-production of coffee, or some other product.[22] Peasant organizations now present themselves not as poor peasants seeking handouts from the state, but as frustrated agricultural entrepreneurs and potential agents of agricultural modernization. They highlight the contrast between themselves, small farmers eager to increase production, and the large rural landholders who often prefer superexploitation of their workers to real productive investment in their grand estates.[23]

As mentioned above, local and national farmer movements increasingly recognized that what were formerly largely sectoral or national issues (such as land reform) have become increasingly exposed to influences from transnational entities. As part of Via Campesina, farmer organizations attempted to delegitimize new transnational governance, especially that led by the WTO, on the basis that in its neoliberal guise it is undemocratic, corporate-driven, and ecologically reckless.[24] Via Campesina charges that designs to privatize seeds, water, common lands, and plants amount to a commodification of the entire agrarian landscape, and thus deny and exclude the communal knowledge and practices involved in the creation of the very resources now declared private property. Via Campesina organizations have responded to such development by opposing it on the ground and at the international forums where it is discussed, advocated, or legitimized. As described in one Via Campesina document:

> Regarding WTO, World Bank and IMF, Via Campesina has a "confrontative strategy." The goal is to de-legitimize these institutions and decrease their influence. Via Campesina does not engage in dialogue or consultative processes with these institutions as these efforts do not bring any positive changes and would contribute to [these groups'] legitimation [*sic*].[25]

Via Campesina attempts to negotiate with organizations that may serve as a counterreference to neoliberal development. In 2002 the International Planning Committee (IPC) of the NGO Forum on Food Sovereignty (held concurrently at the FAO World Food Summit Rome +5) initiated a dialogue with FAO Director General Jacques Diouf. Via Campesina saw both potential risks and benefits in direct collaboration with the FAO:

The risks of this undertaking are the following:

- The dialogue is turned into a "public relations" act that mainly serves the interests of the institution, negatively affects our political profile and absorbs significant leadership capacities that are needed elsewhere.
- At the international level the FAO may make all kinds of interesting commitments. However, at the national level the FAO may still behave as before by supporting policies that are contrary to our objectives.

Potential advantages could be the following:

- We could use this institution to introduce important issues like food sovereignty, land reform, rights to seed, etc. into the governmental debate. This could be done by having more progressive governments introduce these issues (on our behalf) to the FAO. This would help to break the governmental consensus on the neo-liberal policies.
- We could mobilize resources for concrete initiatives at the national/regional level.
- We could generate "official" research capacity and analysis that strengthens our criticism of the current neo-liberal policies.[26]

In addition to attempting to delegitimize inflexible institutions and negotiate with potential allies, Via Campesina organizations have consistently put intensive pressure on their respective national representatives when they travel to international meetings. National agricultural ministers, for example, know that when they are off in far-off convention centers, they will have to face the masses on their ministry doorsteps when they return home.

Via Campesina is composed of thousands of rural organizations and many tens of millions of rural people, making it by far the largest social movement in the world, and one with unprecedented influence, as demonstrated in its ability to establish dialogue with the director of the FAO. Yet when I visited its international headquarters in 2004 (then located in Tegucigalpa, Honduras), it had a staff of three. In national contexts, one is often hard-pressed to locate it—perhaps its name will be called out through a bullhorn at some provincial demonstration, more often not. In most contexts it is submerged or embedded within local organizations.

Via Campesina suddenly materializes before one's eyes at international actions and events. It could be seen as the international expression of local and national movements rather than a discrete organization unto itself: it emerges from its constituent organizations when necessary, but it is still contained within them. And yet it exists with a reach and fluidity perfectly befitting the digital age. So in Via Campesina one finds a rare example of an organization with NGO-like organizational capacity, but without NGO-like divisions in leadership and analysts, without the proclivity to produce long reports, with few overhead costs, no calls for donations, and no donor agencies with long lists of criteria to satisfy. It is mass- and place-based, but also internationalist; its project is to create the conditions that will allow viable agrarian societies to emerge from within.

Slow Food

In 1989 Carlo Petrini, a leftist Italian intellectual and food journalist, founded Slow Food in reaction to the opening of a McDonald's in the center of old Rome. The group took "fast food" as its enemy; hence its use of the English "slow food." It is a network of producers, restaurateurs, retailers, and consumers of "culturally significant" foods endangered by the corporatization of food production and what it views as the homogenization of food tastes. It has from its beginnings associated quality food with traditional ingredients and preparations. Unlike most other gastronomic associations, Slow Food never went for "high" cuisine.[27] The Slow Food network sought to protect particular breeds of animals, geographically specific varieties of fruit and vegetables, and specific techniques of producing particular cheeses, honey, sausages, salt, oils, and a variety of products significant to local gastronomic tradition. Slow Food later evolved into the first "ecogastronomic movement," its initial promotion of traditional products, recipes, and food techniques deepening through understanding that the quality, and indeed the very existence, of such foods is directly linked to the wider landscapes in which they are produced.[28]

A primary vehicle for Slow Food in its early years was the wine of the Piedmont region.[29] The local winemakers were trying to improve the quality of their wine; but without an established reputation for fine wines, they found it difficult to sell at prices that would support the more careful production required. Winemakers decided they had to help people to appreciate that their local wine could match the standard of more famous wine from other regions. Slow Food concurred with this emphasis on taste education and began to promote Piedmont wines by writing about them in newspapers and hosting organized tastings. At this point, the group could be considered as a culturally conservative organization similar to many others around the world attempting to prevent the loss of traditional culture.

As the European Union constituted its powers in Brussels in the late 1990s, such questions of cultural homogenization and democratic processes came to the fore across Europe. In Italy, they crystallized around food. Slow Food was quick to grasp the significance of, and participate in, public campaigns, such as the one mounted to save *lardo* after the food was declared unhygienic by health authorities in the European Union (EU).[30] *Lardo*, a spiced pork fat cured in the dank house basements found in the central Italian "marble villages," became symbolic of localism, rusticity, and even national identity, all of which were opposed to a rationalized, homogenized, bureaucratic—and potentially *lardo*-less—new Europe. In this context, in which seemingly banal phytosanitation legislation became representative of state intrusion into everyday life, passions ran high. As one newspaper article of the time pungently framed the *lardo* conflict, "[t]he European Union ruins Italian cuisine."[31] Similarly, after the same EU body determined that all cheese in the EU market be pasteurized before sale, Slow Food mounted a campaign in defense of "raw milk" cheese (perhaps the first political campaign in history raised in defense of bacteria). According to Slow Food, there are good bacteria and bad bacteria; by killing off as many bacteria as possible, pasteurization affects the taste of a cheese, and diminishes the very flavors that make it unusual and interesting to eat in the first place. Slow Food charged that such legislation would endanger the entire field of activities associated with small-scale cheese production and consumption. Not only would the EU rules affect the kinds of cheese people could eat and enjoy (and the wider gastronomic culture of which such foods were a part), such regulation would have negative economic effect on small farmers. It would inadvertently affect the working landscapes in which such foods were produced.

It is this kind of attention to a whole field of activities, the intertwined social and ecological processes surrounding the consumption of a particular food, that distinguished Slow Food from most every other gastronomic association. Slow Food documents began to describe loss of foods not just in terms of dietary change, but in terms of "extinction."[32] When a food is lost, according to Slow Food, a whole cultural and ecological complex is at risk of extinction, including (1) the loss of food flavor itself and of the knowledge-base or culture that esteems a particular flavor; (2) loss of specific varieties of a plant or animal, and knowledge of methods of food production; (3) loss of knowledge of the environmental context and conditions associated with particular foods; and (4) loss of rural livelihoods and potentially of entire rural communities. Finally, as a consequence of all of these elements, there is (5) loss of the working landscapes in which such foods were produced and which are associated with a place and the way of life found there. In short, according to Slow Food, when traditional foods disappear, there is a subtle but profound loss of both material and immaterial culture, a smoothing-over of differences in the world, a thinning of available experience.

Slow Food has two key operations designed to preserve idiosyncratic but emblematic foods: the Ark of Taste and the presidia.[33] The presidia are the actual projects Slow Food creates to support the production and consumption of traditional foods. A presidium may simply be a project organized or coordinated by Slow Food: "Sometimes all it takes to conserve a product is to bring together surviving producers and make them visible, helping them to communicate the gastronomic excellence of their products and fetch more remunerative prices for them."[34] In other cases, Slow Food may make a more substantial intervention, such as providing some equipment or infrastructure necessary to a group of producers.

As of early 2008, there were 196 presidia in Italy and an additional 105 presidia in 41 countries around the world. One Italian presidium in support of an alpine honey demonstrates the interplay of social and ecological dynamics now of interest to Slow Food. This honey is made by bees gathering nectar in alpine pastures at an altitude of more than 1,200 meters: "[w]hen it was the custom to take livestock to graze in well looked after mountain pastures, the vegetation in general, hence the bees too, drew benefit. Today the mountains are depopulated, the pastures are less well looked after and the best shrubs have no space to grow."[35] Whether providing infrastructural support or simply promoting the specific qualities of a particular food, the goal of the presidia is to link disparate individual producers or already existing groups of producers with people who will consume artisan food products. Here it is worth noting that current Slow Food literature avoids the term "consumer," with its passive-aggressive connotation (the consumer, a category that includes most everyone on the planet, creates demand but is rarely related to the production that comes as a result). The presidia are meant to directly link individuals into the production of a product, to enroll people who eat a food and so continue to request its production, as "co-producers."

The Ark of Taste, in contrast to the discrete operations of the presidia, is a comprehensive and ongoing project; it is an atlas of endangered foods. It is composed of "[p]roducts of excellence threatened by industrial standardization, by hyper-hygienist laws and the deterioration of the environment."[36] Yet the Ark of Taste is not intended as a kind of eulogy to extinct foods; it is meant to call attention to unique foods as a kind of cultural wealth, to demonstrate the fragility of that wealth in the face of standardized diets. As in Via Campesina's seeds campaign, for Slow Food, preservation of food cultures can be achieved only through human activity in—not their absence from—environments.

The campaigns for *lardo* and raw milk cheese, the presidia, and the Ark of Taste represent the kind of savvy action characteristic of Slow Food. They select highly symbolic yet tangible issues and products likely to gain popular attention and sympathy. They use their connections in the press to publicize their actions. Slow Food has its own impressive mechanism for publicity, beginning with its Web site and office of media communication, and including a quarterly magazine and many smaller publications produced by individual *convivia* (the smallest unit of Slow Food affiliation). Despite its careful strategizing and publicity—or perhaps because of its wide success—Slow Food has had to address the suspicion that it celebrates a kind rusticated, proletarianized, hedonistic elitism. In the U.S. context, for example, food quantity has long substituted for food quality, to speak of quality or healthy food—or, more important, to look behind a particular food or dish to examine the processes involved in its production—was to be either a snob or an ascetic. Slow Food denies both charges, and it appears to have made substantial headway in the home country of the supersize diet: in 2001, there were three U.S. *convivia* (in Manhattan, New York; New Orleans, Louisiana; and the San Francisco Bay Area/Napa Valley, California); in 2008, there are more than 170, in addition to a number of similar food-based endeavors, such as the Iowa Place-Based Foods project.[37]

Slow Food communicates concern that the idiosyncratic qualities of particular places may be written out of existence from afar, but it also attempts to stop this cultural erosion through its campaign of taste education. In 2003, Slow Food required each of its *convivia* to support a school garden. This garden initiative signals Slow Food's intent to shake off its reputation as an up-market phenomenon and to work more directly and generally to improve popular appreciation of, and demand for, quality food. In the course of their actions, they have expanded the significance of food localism and the wider relevance of food-based politics.[38] One key, but easily overlooked, element in Slow Food is its celebratory character: in the view of its adherents, taking pleasure from eating well is not simply a selfish act, nor one simply linked to individual survival, but one in which wider communal and ecological relationships can be acknowledged and affirmed. In this sense, Slow Food puts the consumer front and center in the problems of conventional agriculture and attempts to assert individuals and communities as co-producers of vital social and ecological life.

THE PROBLEM OF CONTEMPORARY RURALITY

Via Campesina and Slow Food are very different organizations. Via Campesina is a mass movement: its organizations are involved in land occupations, crop burnings, and street protests; its activists and participants are sometimes subject to violent repression by the state or local shadow forces.[39] It has struggled to establish the voice of small farmers in the highly politicized arena of trade and international politics—and it has stressed in dramatic form that this struggle involves life and death. Slow Food, on the other hand, is a movement-network. It tends to eschew the highly charged settings in which Via Campesina operates, and instead it supports projects whose goal is to deepen the aesthetic experience of food. What do the two groups have in common?

Both Slow Food and Via Campesina were formed in a shifting global political context that has empowered the jurisdiction of distant, nonelected rule-making institutions at the expense of individuals and communities. Both organizations are opposed to the kind of globalization that entails relentless standardization, homogenization, and mechanization, with the marketplace elevated as the supreme adjudicator of all worthy things. Both have attempted to seize the processes of change and make them available for discussion, evaluation, and debate. In both organizations, the celebration of food culture, of the everyday and communal practices of cooking and eating, is notable. Both espouse the shared meal as the center of family and communal life, and both seek to deepen consideration, finally, about the goals that guide economic development.

Viewed synthetically, Slow Food and Via Campesina activities reveal an orientation toward the future that is both preservationist and prefigurative. Their preservationism is clear: they want to preserve themselves, their communities, their agrarian livelihoods, and their landscapes. They are not just *conservationist*. For example, in their view, the biodiversity on which all agriculture depends is not something to be conserved in seed banks, nature preserves, and the like. Instead it must be preserved through human activity—not absence—as people *make habitats* in which plants and animals can thrive. Via Campesina demonstrates that in many contexts the future of such agricultural habitats depends on small farmers having enforceable legal title to land, access to the cultural-ecological resources historically produced therein, and access to viable economies through which the value of such resources can be realized. The range of pragmatic demands that have long been at the center of agrarianism, such as access to credit, training programs, basic infrastructure, the right to unionize when working for cash, and legal recourse against poachers, encroachers, drug traffickers, and corrupt officials and their associated violence, are still valid as well.[40]

The action of each group also demonstrates the realization that the viability of their projects and movements is linked to extralocal processes and social groups. The movements are prefigurative, then, in the sense that they understand quite clearly that their cultural and economic survival requires a dense network of alliances and affiliations with all kinds of popular and private groups operating at national, regional, and international scales. They not only make pragmatic decisions to negotiate in conventional forums and operate in conventional markets, but also expend much energy in inventing new social relationships, new institutions, and new kinds of exchange. They share a general commitment to nonhierarchical, nondeterministic relationships that enable cooperative strategizing without truncating local experience. These movements have a sense that the quality of these distant alliances—and so the strength of the whole—will depend on the integrity of its individual parts.

Finally, both preservationist and prefigurative impulses are found in the attempt to create a new vision for rural places. Adequate food production and consumption can be considered as a necessary *precondition* to development (as in the discourse of "food security")[41] or as containing within it clues of the kind of social, ecological, and economic relations that define a *quality* of development. Although they can be interpreted as doing so, the campaigns and projects described here, and the wider vision for development of which they are a part, do not essentialize impoverished rurality as the authentic condition of rural peoples. Instead they seek to improve the quality of *rural life itself*. The goal is not to transform rural life into something else entirely, but to find the ideas, infrastructures, and policies that will allow this future rural life to emerge from within. While open to—and even dependent on—exchange with the outside world, Slow Food and Via Campesina pose the problem of something that in the age of free market liberalism is viewed with spitting contempt: the question of *endogenous* development.

One Southern Mexican Via Campesina peasant-activist told me that what his community was really struggling for was the space in which "to create ourselves." This seems a most simple definition of endogenous development. Yet the very idea of such an approach to development (as "alternative" or "postdevelopment") is sometimes treated with contempt, as consummate naiveté, and has led to an intellectual circumstance in which "any alternative . . . sounds like a return to past oppression or like a Utopian design for noble savages."[42] The question of contemporary rurality puts urban and rural as interdependent and mutually constitutive, even if these and other key words of development often appear as antinomies—urban versus rural, modern versus traditional, development versus conservation, agricultural production versus intact habitat. The problem in creating contemporary rurality is the problem of conceptualizing, and acting intentionally within, the actual cultural, economic, and biophysical flows that constitute places. If people have contempt for the ideas of alternative kinds of development, and so for the movements out of which such ideas emerge, the range of available solutions to the very real problems of agricultural development is diminished, and so too is understanding of human-environmental relationships, on a grand scale.

NOTES

1. Roger Bartra, *Agrarian Structure and Political Power in Mexico* (Baltimore, MD: Johns Hopkins Press, 1993).

2. Guillermo Bonfil Batalla, *Mexico Profundo: Reclaiming a Civilization* (Austin: University of Texas Press, 1996).

3. Eric Wolf, *Peasant Wars of the Twentieth Century* (New York: Harper Torchbooks, 1969).

4. James C. Scott, *The Moral Economy of the Peasant: Rebellion and Subsistence in Southeast Asia* (New Haven, CT: Yale University, 1969).

5. Ibid., 10–11.

6. Ibid., 3.

7. Alain de Janvry, *The Agrarian Question and Reformism in Latin America* (Baltimore, MD: Johns Hopkins Press, 1981); William W. Cochrane, *The Development of American Agriculture: A Historical Analysis* (Minneapolis: University of Minnesota Press, 1993); Harriet Friedmann, "What on Earth Is the Modern World-System? Foodgetting and Territory in the Modern Era and Beyond," *Journal of World-Systems Research* 11, no. 2 (2001): 480–515.

8. Paul E. Waggoner, "How Much Land Can Ten Billion People Spare for Nature?" *Proceedings, National Academy of Sciences* 125, no. 3 (1996): 73–93; Rhys E. Green et al., "Farming and the Fate of Wild Nature," *Science* 307 (2005): 550–55.

9. Harriet Friedmann, "The Political Economy of Food: The Rise and Fall of the Postwar International Food Order," *American Journal of Sociology* 88s (1982): 248–86; Harriet Friedmann and Phillip McMichael, "Agriculture and the State System: The Rise and Decline of National Agricultures," *Sociologia Ruralis* 29, no. 2 (1989): 93–117; IFAD (International Fund for Agricultural Development), *Rural Poverty Report 2001: The Challenge of Ending Rural Poverty* (Oxford: Oxford University Press, 2001).

10. "Neoliberalism" is a general term used to describe the ideology adopted by many prominent policymakers, intellectuals, and institutions in the 1980s and 1990s to do away with what they saw as inherently inefficient state-management of economic life (e.g., through social security programs, resource management programs, industrial development programs, environmental protection programs, and the like) in favor of market-based allocation of resources. In relation to agriculture, neoliberal economic arguments—that opening agricultural production up to global competition would increase production and lead to lower food prices—were used as justification for ending support programs to small farmers around the world, and for stripping down tariffs or other instruments that were seen (rightly or not) as barriers to trade.

11. Annette Aurelie Desmarais, *La Vía Campesina: Globalization and the Power of Peasants* (Halifax, NS: Fernwood Publishers, 2007).

12. Via Campesina, *Food Sovereignty: A Future without Hunger* (Rome: 1996); Via Campesina, "Final Declaration of the World Forum on Food Sovereignty" (paper presented at the Forum Mundia sobre Soberania Alimentaria, Havana, Cuba, September 3–7, 2001); Michael Windfuhr and Jennie Jonsen, *Food Sovereignty: Towards Democracy in Localized Food Systems* (Bourton-on-Dunsmore, UK: ITDG Publishing, 2005).

13. Peter Rosset, personal interview, Oaxaca, Mexico, September 5, 2004.

14. Enrique Espinoza, personal interview, Patzcuaro, Mexico, November 15, 2004.

15. See Nyelini 2007, http://www.nyeleni2007.org.

16. Via Campesina, "Seed Heritage of the People for the Good of Humanity" (from the Women (*sic*) Seed Forum in South Korea, September 4–11, 2007), http://viacampesina.

org/main_en/images/stories/pdf/seed_heritage_of_the_people_for_the_good_of_humanity. pdf (accessed August 10, 2008).

17. Espinoza, personal interview, 2004.

18. James Petras, "The New Revolutionary Peasantry: The Growth of Peasant-led Opposition to Neoliberalism," *Z Magazine*, October 1998, http://www.zcommunica tions.org/zmag/viewArticle/13452 (accessed August 10, 2008).

19. Jarius Banaji, "The Farmers' Movements: A Critique of Conservative Rural Coalitions," *Journal of Peasant Studies* 21, no. 3, 4 (1994): 228–45.

20. Via Campesina, *IV International Via Campesina Conference: Brazil, Sao Paulo, 14th to the 19th of June 2004, Themes and Issues for Discussion* (Tegucigalpa, Honduras: Secretaria Operativa de Via Campesina, n.d.).

21. Marc Edelman, *Peasants against Globalization: Rural Social Movements in Costa Rica* (Palo Alto, CA: Stanford University Press, 1999).

22. Nuria Costa, UNORCA: *Documentos para la Historia* (Mexico, DF: Costa-Amic Editores, S.A., 1989).

23. Neil Harvey, *The Chiapas Rebellion: The Struggle for Land and Democracy* (Durham, NC: Duke University Press, 1998).

24. Via Campesina, "Impact of the WTO on Peasants in Southeast Asia and East Asia," http://viacampesina.org/main_en/images/stories//lvcbooksonwto.pdf (accessed August 10, 2008).

25. Paul Nicholson, *IV International Via Campesina Conference: Brazil, Sao Paulo, 14th to the 19th of June 2004, Themes and Issues for Discussion* (Tegucigalpa, Honduras: Secretaria Operativa de Via Campesina, n.d.), 19.

26. Ibid., 21.

27. Partly due to the organization's success, though, some traditional foods can be so expensive that it amounts to the same thing.

28. Carlo Petrini, *Slow Food: The Case for Taste* (New York: Columbia University Press, 2003).

29. Piedmont is the home region of Petrini and several other founders of Slow Food, whose national and international headquarters are located in Bra, a town of about 15,000 not far from Turin.

30. Alison Leitch, "The Social Life of *Lardo*: Slow Food in Fast Times," *The Asia Pacific Journal of Anthropology* 1, no. 1 (2000): 103–18.

31. Ibid., 110.

32. Slow Food, *The Presidia* (Bra, Cuneo, Italy: Slow Food International Office, 2000).

33. Slow Food has mounted several other endeavors as well. In recent years, a biannual gala event, the TerraMadre Festival, has grown to become the signature event of Slow Food's international activities. The *convivia* are the local associations of Slow Food members; they may host events of their choosing in support of Slow Food objectives. The University of Taste offers courses in taste and food education—developing appreciation for quality foods is one of Slow Foods explicit goals, as mentioned below.

34. Slow Food, *The Presidia*, 2.

35. Ibid., 23.

36. Ibid., 2.

37. See Iowa Placed-Based Foods, http://www.iowaartscouncil.org/programs/folk-and-traditional-arts/place_based_foods/index.htm.

38. Melanie E. DuPuis and David Goodman, "Should We Go 'Home' to Eat? Toward a Reflexive Politics of Localism," *Journal of Rural Studies* 21 (2005): 359–71.

39. João Pedro Stedile, "Landless Battalions," *New Left Review* 15 (May/June 2005): 77–104; Angus Wright and Wendy Wolford, *To Inherit the Earth: The Landless*

Movement and the Struggle for a New Brazil (Oakland, CA: Food First Books, 2005); La Via Campesina, "Annual Report: Violations of Peasants' Human Rights: A Report on Cases and Patterns of Violances [sic] 2006," http://www.viacampesina.org/main_en/images/stories/annual-report-HR-2006.pdf (accessed August 10, 2008).

40. Stedile, "Landless Battalions"; Jose Bové, "Farmers against Food Chains," *New Left Review* 12 (November/December 2001): 89–101.

41. "Food security" has come to mean "the right of everyone to have access to safe and nutritious food" (see, for example, the FAO's Rome Declaration on World Food Security). "Access" is the operative term: there is no necessary or explicit attention to the conditions or kind of agricultural production.

42. Ivan Illich, *Tools for Conviviality* (London: Calder and Boyars, 1973).

RESOURCE GUIDE

Suggested Reading

Bové, Jose, and François Dufour. *The World Is Not For Sale: Farmers Against Junk Food*. London: Verso, 2001.

Cochrane, William W. *The Development of American Agriculture: A Historical Analysis*. Minneapolis: University of Minnesota Press, 1993.

Desmarais, Annette-Aurelie. *La Vía Campesina: Globalization and the Power of Peasants*. Halifax: Fernwood Publishing, 2007.

Edelman, Marc. "Transnational Peasant and Farmer Movements and Networks." In *Global Civil Society 2003*, ed. Helmut Anheier, Marlies Glasius, and Mary Kaldor, 185–220. London: Oxford University Press, 2003.

Friedmann, Harriet, and Phillip McMichael. "Agriculture and the State System: The Rise and Decline of National Agricultures." *Sociologia Ruralis* 29, no. 2 (1989): 93–117.

Petrini, Carlo. *Slow Food Nation: Why Our Food Should Be Good, Clean, and Fair*. New York: Rizzoli Ex Libris, 2007.

Stedile, João Pedro. "Landless Battalions." *New Left Review* 15 (2005): 77–104.

Wallerstein, Immanuel. "New Revolts against the System." *New Left Review* 18 (2002): 29–39.

Weiss, Tony. *The Global Food Economy: The Battle for the Future of Farming*. New York: Zed Books, 2007.

Wright, Angus, and Wendy Wolford. *To Inherit the Earth: The Landless Movement and the Struggle for a New Brazil*. Oakland: Food First Books, 2003.

Web Sites

Action Group on Erosion, Technology and Concentration, http://www.etcgroup.org/.

Focus on the Global South, http://www.focusweb.org/.

The Institute for Agriculture and Trade Policy, http://www.iatp.org/.

Land Research Action Network, http://www.landaction.net/.

Slow Food International (with links to national branches), http://www.slowfood.com/.

Via Campesina, http://www.viacampesina.org/.

10

Gender, Generations, and Commensality: Nurturing Home and the Commons

Lynn Walter

A RELATIONAL CONCEPT OF HOME

Industrial commodity production and market consolidation in prevailing agrifood systems are distancing us as consumers from the sources of food in the natural and social environments, from agricultural and culinary knowledge rooted in an ecosystem, and from our capacity as informed citizens to shape agrifood policy. The global reach and the systemic nature of these processes call for countervailing strategies that can ignite a synergy between sustainable agrifood systems and healthy people, communities, and environments. While many prospective catalysts are examined in *Critical Food Issues*, here the focus is on the significance of sharing food and commensality (i.e., eating together) to sustain intergenerational relations of care, commitment, and cooperation so vital to this synergy.

Fundamental intergenerational relations between parents and children are enacted in the sharing of food and other provisions. As parents feed their children, they create *home* as a time and place where sharing food across the generations is the norm. When we share food and eat together beyond the boundaries of everyday commensality, we expand the relations of *home* to embrace extended kin and community. In a critical sense, sharing sustenance is a practical meaning of kinship. Espousing this idea, Navajo consider that

> Just as a mother is one who gives life to her children through birth, and sustains their life by providing them with loving care, assistance, protection, and sustenance, kinsmen are those who sustain each other's life by helping one another, protecting one another, and by giving or sharing of food and other items of subsistence. Where this kind of solidarity exists, kinship exists; where it does not exist, there is no kinship.[1]

This understanding of the consequence of sharing food and commensality supports a *relational concept of home*. In this relational sense, *home* is a locus of gender and generational interests—most significantly, those of mothers and children, whose arrival initiates what Van Esterik identifies as mothers' "right to feed" and children's "right to be fed."[2] From this perspective, *home* signifies neither a nostalgic refusal to see problems within it nor a walled-off denial of interdependence with the world beyond its threshold.[3] Rather, *home* raises critical questions of gender and generational rights and responsibilities in a context that is as often filled with conflict as it is with cooperation. Moreover, it identifies those rights and responsibilities with relations enduring over the lifetimes that entwine the past, present, and future well-being of the generations. The significance of this conception of *home* for addressing critical food issues is that it relates the gender and generational rights and responsibilities to provide for one another's sustenance over time to our mutual responsibility to build on the legacy of past generations, ensure the capacity of the present generation of caretakers to share food, and nurture the commons for the well-being of future generations.

Everyday and ceremonial meals enact the gender and generational relations of home in its key formations—from the source of culinary traditions to the scene of commensality and homecooking and the heart of subsistence in the natural world. In its elemental form, *home* is oriented toward the immediate and long-term future—reproducing the next generation by providing for and socializing children. Through memory and culture, *home* is also about the past—intertwined with the cuisines of parents, grandparents, and ancestors rooted in the ecology of their home places and imbuing food with the tastes of home.

In this sense, to be *homeless* is to lack interpersonal connection to the food we eat, its history, its place in an ecosystem, the people who made it, and those with whom we might share it. To our detriment, we are becoming increasingly *homeless*. We are spending less time cooking and eating together and more time snacking while multitasking alone in cars and at work stations.[4] We are turning to highly processed industrial food and away from homecooking and hospitality. We are losing the skills needed to grow and prepare foods from our own culinary traditions and filling childhood memories of *home* with artificial flavors and colors.[5]

By themselves, these trends diminish our capacity to understand and address the impact of agrifood production, consumption, and distribution processes on the well-being of humanity and the environment.[6] Magnifying their impact are institutional constraints that (1) tie food security to having a steady job with a living wage, (2) increase time pressure and work-family conflicts on parents and children, (3) intensify the mass marketing of highly processed foods, particularly those marketed to children, and (4) reduce public resources for programs that provide some measure of security and time to families.[7]

The burden of these constraints falls disproportionately on women, especially low-income women and their children. The continuing reality is that mothers spend more time on food provisioning than fathers do; and low-income parents face greater food insecurity with less access to affordable, good-quality food and, often, less time to purchase, prepare, and share it.[8] For example, residential homelessness makes feeding their children and maintaining the relations of *home* an unbearable burden on parents.

Depending on our resources then, we confront the time bind and work-family conflicts in relationship to sharing food and eating together in disparate ways. A conventional recourse is to rely on processed foods, time management, and multitasking in efforts to create *home* out of the possibilities offered by the prevailing agrifood system. This approach ultimately relies on the work and time of low-waged, *flexible* workers in agriculture, food processing, and retailing and, thus, politically implicates all consumers in the quality of their lives. At the same time, as a strategy that distances us as consumers from food production, procurement, preparation, marketing, and the environment, it diminishes our capacity as citizens to shape agrifood policies democratically.

Significantly, women have taken leading roles in shaping agrifood production and reproduction in more democratic directions—in agricultural and retail labor movements, community food security coalitions, artisanal production of organic and local foods, community-supported agriculture, and fair-trade programs.[9] However, these alternative approaches also take time and can create a triple burden—in the labor force, in the home, and in democratic action—on those who engage them. It is in this light that strategies to promote caring, committed, and cooperative relationships through sharing food and eating together must attend to gender, generational, class, and other inequities in agrifood systems.

The balance of this chapter examines several customary and groundbreaking ways that sharing food and commensality nurture the relations of home at the intersection of class, gender, and generational rights and responsibilities. These are discussed in three sections: (1) community kitchens and gardens, (2) cohousing and ecovillages, and (3) Slow Food and Tsyunhehkwa. In different ways, each opens *home* to gender, generation, class, and other justice claims by extending the relations of home to wider commensal circles and by building on the heritage of past generations to sustain the well-being of present and future ones.

STRATEGIES FOR NURTURING HOME AND THE COMMONS

Community Kitchens

Quebec, Canada

A *community kitchen* is the general term for various types of community-based cooking programs, among which are *collective kitchens*.[10] In Quebec, *collective kitchens* are small groups, typically of five or six low-income women, who plan meals, pool their resources to buy food in bulk, and cook together in large quantities at a church, school, or a community-center kitchen. Then they take it home to feed themselves and their families or enjoy some of it together on site and take the rest home. In 1984, in Montreal single mother Jacynthe Ouellette, along with her sister-in-law and a neighbor, began to purchase food and cook it together; and in 1986 she and Diane Norman, a community nutritionist, began to promote this idea through the formal development of community kitchens in Montreal.[11] Quebec now has more than 1,330 collective kitchens[12] and Canada has as many as 2,500 collective kitchens.[13]

In 1990, further development of the collective kitchens in Quebec led to the founding of the *Regroupement des Cuisines Collectives du Québec* (RCCQ, Quebec Collective Kitchens Association), a nonprofit organization aimed at promoting collective kitchens in Quebec. The values promoted by the collective kitchens in RCCQ include "self-sufficiency, empowerment, dignity, democracy and social justice."[14] Interviewed for a recent study of community kitchens in three Canadian cities, participants reported that they experienced an increase in food security as well as learning more about cooking from scratch, becoming more informed readers of food labels, increasing the variety of foods consumed, and including more vegetables in their meals. Significantly, they appreciated the social dimension of the collective kitchens and the dignity they experienced in the collective kitchen, as opposed to the stigma attached to getting provisions from food banks.[15] In Canada, participation in collective kitchens has been associated with building networks of friendship and social support and sharing of community resources along with increased parenting skills and self-esteem.[16] In Quebec, where collective kitchens have flourished, some have spawned food-buying clubs, catering businesses, and community restaurants.[17]

Community kitchens are exemplified by groups who get together less frequently to prepare meals and learn about cooking healthy and affordable meals. Some community kitchens serve particular populations, such as people with mental health problems or new immigrants. For example, the Sahwanya Community Kitchen was created in 2007 in Vancouver by African immigrant women with HIV. During monthly gatherings, the members and their children enjoy the food that they have prepared there. After the meal, women share ideas, strength, and challenges. Their motto is to "break the chain of isolation and pull together for our common good."[18] Some leaders expressed the view that such community kitchens have eased negative stereotypes about immigrants.[19]

Lima, Peru

The organizers of collective kitchens in Quebec drew their inspiration from the *comedores populares* in the poverty-stricken barrios that ring many Latin America cities, where they have served much larger and poorer populations than in Canada.[20] Peru, like many Latin American countries in the 1980s and 1990s, experienced (1) national debt crises, (2) runaway inflation of food prices and concomitant increases in malnutrition and hunger, and (3) international creditor-mandated cutbacks in state-supported social welfare programs. As Hays-Mitchell notes, "the most vulnerable populations of Peru frequently converge in the lives—and homes—of low-income women, as their households commonly include elderly and youthful dependents."[21] These were the women who organized collective kitchens to sustain their families.

In Peru, local women, with the support of donated provisions and organizational coordination from the Catholic Church and other religious organizations, the United Nations Children's Fund (UNICEF), political parties, and national feminist organizations, have organized to promote food security and advance other forms of social provisioning and community infrastructure.[22] Among the best known examples of this grassroots mobilization by women are the collective kitchens of Lima, Peru.[23] As of 2003, there were 5,000 *comedores populares* in the Lima metropolitan area and almost 16,000 in Peru. The 5,000 collective kitchens in Lima have at least 100,000 women participants serving 480,000 food rations daily to approximately 6 percent of the population.[24] While the original goal of the members of collective kitchens in Lima was contributing to their own family food security, the women of the various collective kitchens began to organize and develop alliances across families. Some twenty to thirty women work together in each collective kitchen, taking turns in leadership, purchasing provisions, and cooking, typically in a member's kitchen. Collective kitchens were later organized into city federations and confederations by regions.[25] From collective food provisioning and in collaboration with feminist organizations, the collective kitchen members' goals expanded to nutritional and health education, women's rights, leadership development, and community planning and organizing.[26] This strategic development characterized *autonomous* collective kitchens and grassroots organizations that were less constrained from the top down by government agencies, political parties, or religious groups.[27]

Discussion

Molyneux's distinction between *practical gender interests* and *strategic gender interests* is useful for an analysis of the goals of collective kitchens.[28] Practical gender interests are derived inductively from the pressing needs of women that arise from their place in a gender division of labor. Strategic gender interests are deduced from analyses of ways to end women's subordination. In the case of the *comedores populares*, organizing to address their practical need for food for themselves and their families led members to formulate analyses of long-term strategic gender interests as well. Specifically, they have turned from the gender division of labor, which assigned personal responsibility to wives to cook for their husbands, toward a collectivized responsibility, sometimes in the face of their husbands' expressed objections. They also created new forms of cooperation among female kin, friends, and neighbors as well as new settings in which to develop their own analyses of strategic gender interests.[29] María van der Linde, an Anglican nun who helped start the first *comedores* in Peru, gave the following assessment of their impact on the women who have sustained them: "I know they will never go back to being stuck in their houses, never. They have learnt a lot, about their rights, their capabilities, about organizing. Maybe it won't be *comedores* anymore, but it will definitely be something else."[30] From "home" as a place of confinement for women, collective kitchens have opened doors to neighbors, friends, extended kin, and even strangers who come to share food together and support one another in social provisioning.

From a way to feed their families under conditions of extreme poverty to an organization capable of acting collectively, the sheer numbers of *comedores populares* and independent organizations have attracted the attention of the state and political parties. State and party have been interested in harnessing their strength by controlling the distribution of food aid. From this clientelist relationship to the state the criticism is derived that the *comedores populares* have not been able to change the prevailing political and economic power structures. Another criticism is that they do not challenge the gender role stereotype of mothers as the ones responsible for feeding their children. On the other hand, by acting collectively as women, the members gained new confidence in their own abilities as women to act independently from their husbands, a development that is especially important in situations of domestic violence.[31] Furthermore, they have used this collective power to promote their common interests within their community as a whole.

Given the much better economic and political position of women in Canada, it is telling that the collective kitchens there have confronted similar gender and class contradictions. In the Canadian community kitchens, however, there are both more male and more middle-class women members, an indication of the spread of an organizational form from low-income women to middle-class women and to men.[32]

Collective kitchens as livelihood strategies and as strategies for community development can be a catalyst for a sustainable agrifood synergy when supported by those that address low-income women's practical and strategic gender interests as well as their class interests in food security.[33] One supportive structure would be access to land and capital resources to develop income-generating activities and cooperative childcare facilities from their *comedores* either through state or nongovernmental organization (NGO) support or through microcredit programs. Another is for food aid in the form of surplus commodities to be replaced with financial assistance to purchase local food and to grow their own.[34]

Community Gardens

United Kingdom

Community gardens are typically set aside and supported by a city government for its residents to grow some of their own food. Community gardens encourage men and women, low-income people, and new immigrants to nurture the commons. Nurturing the commons is a strategy for supporting a relational concept of home that connects caring for children to caring for common resources. Like the collective kitchens of Latin America, community gardens were originally developed to address food insecurity among low-income groups. The collective kitchens of Lima, Peru, were established when people from rural areas could no longer support themselves on their small plots and moved to the city in search of jobs. This process of urbanization along with the concentration of agricultural land in the hands of fewer farmers began in Great Britain in the sixteenth century and proceeded through four centuries of enclosures—that is, confiscations by large estates of the common lands used by peasant farmers. To address the abuses, malnutrition, and civil unrest that resulted, the General Enclosure Act of 1845 called for allotments of garden plots to landless urban immigrants. Peaking during World War II at 1.4 million allotment gardens in the United Kingdom, numbers gradually declined until the 1970s, when a resurgence of interest in community gardens began.[35]

In the United Kingdom in the late 1960s, 96.8 percent of the allotment gardeners were men, many of them low-income, and by then elders, who continued to contribute to their family's well-being by providing fresh fruits and vegetables. In contrast, the renewal of interest in community gardens has been characterized by an increase in number of women gardeners from 3 percent in the 1960s to 15 percent in 1993, and much higher in some regions. An increase also has been seen in the number of low-income women from ethnic minorities. Women gardeners are more likely than men to bring their children with them to the gardens. And British women of Asian heritage are more likely to garden collectively, thereby experiencing social benefits as well as the benefits of consuming more fresh fruits and vegetables. Women community gardeners tend to use fewer herbicides and synthetic fertilizers than men, which may, in part, reflect a generational difference between men and women gardeners, who tend to be younger.[36] Nevertheless, in the United Kingdom, where women represent only 5 percent of the farmers, they constitute 50 percent of those who farm organically, a trend not uncommon throughout the organic sector in other countries.[37] This pattern of women being interested in organic gardening is found across ethnic groups and social classes in the United Kingdom.[38]

Cape Town, South Africa

In Sub-Saharan Africa, where women have long been associated with subsistence farming,[39] their ability to farm has been constrained by lack of access to land and other resources, a problem with multiple sources, including a colonial history, customary land inheritance patterns, the AIDS epidemic, war, land concentration in commercial agriculture, cuts in social services, and urbanization. Federici argues that rural development schemes that support export commodities and devalue subsistence farming have led women to shift their subsistence farming into urban areas.[40] All of these factors affected women gardeners of southern Africa.[41] Xhosa women who work "food gardens" in townships of Cape Town, South Africa, have powerful reasons for maintaining their gardens, in spite of their rather limited commercial returns. These reasons include comfort from the violence in the townships, a sense of stability, more control over household food supply, and empowerment through the development of social networks and community development.[42] Through their gardens these women were able to exert more influence over household food choices. Also, although many of their gardens are not community gardens, strictly speaking, the women nevertheless work their gardens collectively, going in turn from one to another. In this way they developed social networks that they have been able to use to address patriarchal forms of oppression. For example, they gathered together to enforce the legal prosecution of a rape case.

As their numbers grew, they attracted the attention of Abalimi Bezekhaya (Planters of the Home), a Xhosa NGO working on the development of urban agriculture and the environmental quality.[43] Through such connections, some urban gardeners have moved from survival to subsistence to livelihood gardening.[44] Christina Kaba, project coordinator for a community garden project, identified access to land and compost as their greatest constraints in this progression to livelihood gardening. In response, she and others created the Powerlines Project, which claimed unused land under the power lines.[45] Their practice reflects gender interests in both its practical and strategic forms. As an example of the strategic interest, they are beginning to question gender roles that once confined them to their home. One of the Fezeka community gardeners, Phillipina Ndamane, states, "Before the garden we were sitting in our houses . . . the garden is strengthening us; it's why we are here every day."[46] Interestingly, Kaba reports that she has started a new project that includes men gardeners, who are also eager to participate.[47]

Support for community gardens comes from the city of Cape Town, which has approved an urban agricultural policy, and from NGOs. Pat Featherstone of Soil for Life, one of the environmental NGOs helping to build township gardens, states that "[t]here's so much that goes on in these communities that makes it really difficult to garden . . . in fact, it's not about growing food, it's about growing people."[48]

Discussion

Community kitchens and community gardens reflect a relational concept of home in which sharing the labor and the fruits of cooking and gardening not only provides for women and their children, but also for neighborhoods and cities. The creation of community kitchens and gardens parallels women's collective action in establishing more interpersonal relations between farmers and consumers, as, for example, in community-supported agriculture.[49] These activities expand the relations of home by expanding the commons, the land and places where people work together to provide food for their families and communities. Furthermore, they develop the knowledge base of the participants in the skills to grow and prepare food and the connection of these processes to those of the natural environment.

For those women and men who can derive a livelihood from such strategies, time is not an insurmountable barrier to their participation. For the many who cannot derive such a livelihood, community kitchens and community gardens need the support of other social formations, like the food justice movement and city planners in Cape Town and the environmental NGOs in South Africa. These supportive structures might also include ones like *cohousing*, which make it easier to grow, cook, and share food by working together at a home place.

Cohousing and Ecovillages

Denmark

Cohousing is a living arrangement whereby private houses or apartments are connected to one another by the residents' shared stewardship of the commons and by their cooperative participation in community services, especially shopping, cooking, and cleaning up in the community dining facilities. Other community services might include childcare, laundry, and gardening. Cohouses are typically initiated, owned, worked, and managed by the residents. The key qualities of cohousing are as follows: (1) common facilities, (2) intentional neighborhood design, (3) participatory development process, and (4) total resident management.[50] In its most recent incarnation cohousing began in the 1970s in Denmark, Sweden, and the Netherlands, where it is now a part of the regular mix of housing options.[51] It has since spread throughout northern Europe and to the United States and Canada.[52] Estimates are that cohousing developments numbered 7,000 around the world by 2005.[53]

An earlier version of cohousing, known as *collective housing* in Sweden, was promoted by the prominent Swedish social welfare advocate Alva Myrdal as an answer to its population crisis of the 1930s by making it easier for women to manage the double burdens of employment as well as childcare and housework. Collective housing consisted of apartments with paid staff providing the cooking, cleaning, and childcare.[54] This type of collective house still exists, especially in senior housing. However, the more recent forms of cohousing follow the principle that all adults, men and women, be coresponsible for community duties like cooking, yard and garden work, cleaning, and childcare. Contemporary cohousing in Denmark and Sweden tends to be smaller than collective housing, typically with fifteen to fifty private household residences.[55] At first, cohousing residents were mostly middle-class because (1) cohousing was largely new greenfield construction, (2) there was little government support for it, and (3) lending agencies were reluctant to loan money when the ability to claim equity from the property seemed unclear. A 1981 Danish law permitted groups to apply for a government-sponsored loan to establish limited equity cooperative housing with a minimum of eight household units. This has diversified the population in cohousing by income and family status with more single-person and single-parent households. The entry of speculative developers into cohousing has diversified the stock of subsidized cohousing.[56]

The residents point to several factors that initially drew them to cohousing and keep them living there. One is the balance between private housing and community.[57] This balance between privacy and community may be especially important to low-income and minority families who have often experienced the outside world as threatening.[58] Parents want a way of life that not only makes it easier to care for children, but also provides an enriching experience for everyone; and many claim to have found that in cohousing. Among the benefits residents cite for cohousing is that it improves the children's capacity to be more independent, to have more friends, and to have more "parents." In fact, one of the first public rationales for cohousing was published in a 1967 newspaper editorial titled "Children Need 100 Parents."[59] No doubt, many parents would like to have one hundred co-parents, although some do complain about neighborhood children intruding into their private space. Single women and single mothers especially feel more secure living in their own home while knowing so many people all around them.[60] In Denmark a comprehensive array of supports for employed parents— public childcare, generous parental leaves, and universal health care, among other social welfare programs—places cohousing in especially fortuitous context.[61] Also, Denmark has gone further than most countries toward encouraging fathers to take equal responsibility for family meals, clean up, and childcare.

Vestbro found that the housekeeping tasks are more equally distributed between women and men in cohousing than other residential forms. He suggests that cohousing may liberate men from the psychological constraints of patriarchy, allowing them to be more attuned to their emotions and to the needs of their co-residents.[62]

Meltzer's research on environmental awareness among cohousing residents confirms that the design of the facilities, the ease of interaction, and the sharing of resources all support greater environmental awareness and the adoption of conservation practices.[63] Their collective environmental awareness has led some Danish cohousing advocates to take another step toward nurturing the capacity of the natural environment to support future generations with the creation of *ecovillages*, for example, at Munksøgard outside of Roskilde, Denmark.[64] Munksøgard was established in 2000 with environmentally sound forms of building construction and daily operation of the 100 houses.[65] Denmark may well have the most ecovillages per capita of any country. This achievement is tied to its longer experience with cohousing as well as its early adoption of alternative energy policies after the 1973 oil crisis. The Danish Association of Sustainable Communities, a network of Danish ecovillages established in 1993, counts 51 members today. One of its missions, to bring about "awareness of global interconnectedness," ties the interests of local people to the welfare of the global commons.[66]

Discussion

Cohousing addresses the time burden on mothers by extending the commensal circle to the residential community and the work of food provisioning to all adults. In its ecovillage form, cohousing situates food provisioning in the context of carework for the environment and global commons. Their success is based on a structure that respects privacy and supports the bonds between parents and children by expanding the social capital of both. For cohousing to be widely available it would have to be retrofitted to central city neighborhoods and be affordable to people in lower-income households. If the Danish experience is to serve as a model for such developments, it should be noted that cohousing and ecovillages began as grassroots rather than top-down projects and that government social welfare programs have made Denmark's overall housing patterns relatively inclusive of lower-income households.[67]

As cohousing and ecovillages expand the relations of home from household to community to the global commons, their support of the intergenerational relations between parents and children remains central to their effectiveness, just as it is with community kitchens and gardens. However, nothing in these strategies deliberately extends the intergenerational relations of home to past generations in terms of agriculinary traditions grounded in the ecosystems of home places. That they have not done so reflects patterns of urbanization and migration as well as the taken-for-granted nature of culture in general and culinary traditions in particular. As commercially processed foods replace traditional culinary practices linked through time to regional ecosystems, the accumulated legacy of agrifood knowledge that past generations have bequeathed to the well-being of the present one is eroding. Strategies that consciously connect the relations of home from past generations to present ones could strengthen the relations linking the present generation to the well-being of future ones. Transnational organizations like Slow Food and many indigenous food community programs offer strategies that build on traditional agrifood systems in ways that contribute to sustaining the intergenerational relations of home for the long-term future.

Slow Food

Slow Food stands out among alternative agrifood strategies for its recognition of the value of the contributions of past generations to the culinary heritage of the present as well as for its stress on commensality as an aspect of an aesthetic of *slow food*. Slow Food, which was established by Carlo Petrini in Bra, Italy, in 1989, has since expanded to a transnational network with more than 85,000 members in 132 countries, and with more than 1,000 local chapters, called *convivia*.[68] *Convivia*

> cultivate the appreciation of pleasure and quality in daily life by gathering regularly to share the pleasure and conviviality of meals of local food, building relationships with producers, campaigning to protect traditional foods, organizing tastings and seminars, encouraging chefs to use local foods, choosing producers to participate in international events and promoting taste education in schools.[69]

Slow Food's goals are to promote "good, clean, and fair" food in practices that connect agricultural producers with *co-producers* (i.e., consumers) and to preserve small-scale producer livelihoods based on co-producer support for their artisanal products. As part of its philosophy of *ecogastronomy*, Slow Food supports its presidia and Ark of Taste projects. The Ark of Taste consists of agrifood products certified by Slow Food as deserving of and able to benefit from their assistance in preservation. The presidia goals are to assist producers in promoting artisanal products, diverse regions, ecosystems, techniques, and crop varieties.[70]

Italy

In its original home place in Italy, Slow Food's goal of promoting closer relations between producers and co-producers, its opposition to fast food, and its call for a slower pace of life all tie the sensual qualities of food to its natural, social, and cultural context. In its *convivia* form, Slow Food also connotes the sustaining, noncommodified relationships of caring and solidarity, reinforced by commensality. Its basic *convivia* form promotes sharing food and eating together as aspects of a process that will preserve and promote good quality and good taste in food. However, because artisanal products tend to be more expensive than mass-produced ones, and food provisioning—from shopping to cooking and cleaning up—is typically more time-consuming for home cooks using "slow" ingredients and traditional culinary practices, critics have called on Slow Food to consider how these gender and class inequities might be addressed.[71] Recent Slow Food initiatives like Terre Madre, a network of "food communities," professional cooks, and universities that supports small-scale producers worldwide, indicate that, as an organization, it is broadening its approach to linking producers and co-producers within and across cultures and classes and is becoming more aligned with critical consumption.[72] Nevertheless, the fact that gender hierarchy remains relatively unexamined within Slow Food testifies to the powerful symbolic and practical association of women in Italy with familial food provisioning and men with commercial agrifood production.

Before Slow Food was created, the Italian women and men Counihan interviewed for her studies of food and family in twentieth-century Florence appreciated the pleasures of the table as part of an aesthetic of food that served intergenerational interests through carework.[73] As Counihan explains, "meals were important because they affirmed family, produced sociability, and conveyed sensual and convivial pleasure on daily and special occasions."[74] Commensality created relations of intimacy that "implied reciprocity, care, and serious commitment."[75] Clearly, Italian women have long valued and tried to maintain the relations of home through sharing food and eating together enough to devote their time to it. However, the very low birthrate (9.3 per 1,000) in Italy demonstrates the limits to the accommodations Italian women will make as individuals to maintain the relations of home—many Italian women are now having only one child. And in Italy, too, women are turning to convenience foods to save time, when they do not call on their own mothers to help make homecooking work the way it had for generations by shopping, cooking, and caring for their children and grandchildren.[76] Even in its own home place in Italy, it is clear that for Slow Food to sustain an *ecogastronomy* politics that effectively builds on the culinary legacy of past generations and traditional knowledge of artisanal agrifood production, it must also confront the gender inequities of the present and provide more support for the caretaker.

Discussion

Confronting the gender inequities in Slow Food will necessitate a reconstruction of those aspects of its cultural heritage that take homecooking and Italian women's familial carework for granted, while highlighting and celebrating the work of professional chefs and artisanal food producers. Kittay argues that supports are needed from the larger society that would make it possible for parents in whatever household forms to combine a sustainable livelihood with the care, commitment, and cooperation that it takes to sustain the relations of home.[77] The form these societal supports might take include community kitchen and gardens, cohousing and ecovillages, and feminist revisions of Slow Food, because each of these strategies places a high value on sharing food and eating together—critical practices of the relations of home. Another path is reflected in programs by indigenous nations to promote community-wide food security based on agriculinary traditions.

Tsyunhehkwa

Oneida Nation of Wisconsin

People from more community-based forms of agrifood production, like the Oneida Nation of Wisconsin, traditionally conceive of agricultural production, food provisioning for the household, sharing food, and commensality as complementary processes. The Oneida Nation of Wisconsin, a sovereign First Nation with lands in and around Oneida, Wisconsin, developed Tsyunhehkwa (pronounced, "Joon-hey-qwa"; translated, "Life Sustenance") with goals similar to Slow Food but within a cultural heritage of matrilineal kinship, egalitarian gender formations, subsistence agriculture, and community-wide patterns of food sharing.[78] Historically, women cultivated subsistence gardens while men provided game. Although nineteenth- and early twentieth-century assimilation pressures for men to take up cash-crop farming reoriented gender relations somewhat, women continued to tend the traditional corn fields.[79] And, the ideal relations of home continued to include not only the immediate household but also kin, neighbors, friends, and acquaintances in community-wide practices of sharing food and eating together.[80] This cultural heritage provided a foundation upon which to revitalize their contemporary *food community* around white corn. According to Slow Food, a *food community* is "people involved in the production, transformation, and distribution of a particular food, who are closely linked to a geographic area either historically, socially, or culturally."[81]

Like their northern neighbors, the White Earth Band of Chippewa in Minnesota, who are working to preserve their wild rice,[82] Oneida are undertaking through Tsyunhehkwa to revitalize food crops from their agricultural and culinary traditions. White corn, which is grown, processed, and distributed by Tsyunhehkwa, is one of the Three Sisters of Oneida Creation, along with beans and squash.[83] Tsyunhehkwa demonstrates ways to participate in the Three Sisters gardening, harvesting, and other agrifood projects and to improve the health status of Oneida and others. Tsyunhehkwa manager Jeff Metoxen and a staff of thirteen work with elders, youth, and others in the community to enhance food quality, community health, food security, and self-sufficiency for the nation as a whole. Tsyunhehkwa's goals are not only to reintegrate white corn into Oneida meals, but also to participate in the "rejuvenation" of an integrated agrifood, health, and well-being complex, expressed in the Three Sisters.[84] To this end, it participates in the Oneida Community Integrated Food Systems (OCIFS), which also includes the Oneida Nation Farm, Apple Orchard, Food Distribution/Pantry, Grants, and Oneida Health Center.[85]

Discussion

Since Tsyunhehkwa is a department of the Oneida Nation of Wisconsin, its intracommunity connections and links to the surrounding nonindigenous communities are more inclusive than Slow Food, even in Slow Food's home region of Piedmont. The Oneida Nation of Wisconsin relocated from their homeland in New York in a colonial process that made it increasingly difficult to provide themselves with culturally appropriate and healthy food. To overcome the food insecurity and health problems that have resulted from this past, Tsyunhehkwa and OCIFS are participating in a "healing history" to address contemporary health issues, like the extremely high diabetes rates among North American indigenous peoples, with programs that place meals in the context of holistic cultural and social traditions.[86] In this process, they participate in projects by indigenous peoples around the world to promote *food sovereignty*.

According to indigenous peoples in Atitlan, Guatemala,

> Food Sovereignty is the right of Peoples to define their own policies and strategies for the sustainable production, distribution, and consumption of food, with respect for their own cultures and their own systems of managing natural resources and rural areas, and is considered to be a precondition for Food Security.[87]

This definition, from the Declaration of Atitlan, a 2002 consultation of indigenous peoples in Atitlan, Guatemala, ties indigenous food sovereignty not only to rights in land, clean water, and other natural resources but also to the survival of cultures and communities.

Like Slow Food, Tsyunhehkwa recognizes the value of agrifood traditions and their grounding in regional ecosystems, although neither proposes to return to the past. Rather, their intent is to respect and recycle the accumulated wisdom of the past generations, build on it, and bestow it to the future.

AT HOME IN THE COMMONS

When DuPuis and Goodman ask "Should We Go Home to Eat?" they challenge advocates of localist, alternative agrifood strategies to reflect critically on issues of inequality and injustice within their home communities.[88] Underlying this challenge is the recognition that ultimately *home* cannot be a "haven in a heartless world" because it is entangled in the world and all of its problems.[89] We need *home* nonetheless, not as a nostalgic retreat from a hostile world, but as a fundamental interpersonal nexus between the generations and a primary locus of rights and responsibilities for food security. Without these relations, we are *homeless* in the most profound sense—that is, without an intergenerational nexus of support, without the interpersonal relations that connect us to past generations or to future ones. And, as Wilk notes, "In a global economy of constant flow and movement, *homeless* is *powerless*, at the mercy of the tides and currents."[90] *Homelessness*, in this sense, diminishes our capacity to fulfill the "right to food," "right to feed," and "right to be fed," rights identified with the food sharing and commensality of the relations of home.[91] The ability to realize these rights depends on the power and empowerment of those responsible for their interpersonal fulfillment.

The strategies discussed in this chapter—*community kitchens* and *gardens, cohousing* and *ecovillages, Slow Food* and *Tsyunhehkwa*—open *home* to justice claims of fairness and equality based on the value of well-being through the connections of gender and generational carework. Each one extends the commensal circles beyond the nuclear family and, by practicing more inclusive interpersonal food sharing, enhances the capacity of the relations of home to ensure food security over the generations. These examples demonstrate that *home* as the nexus of interpersonal care, commitment, and cooperation, where sharing food and commensality are critical practices, can ignite a synergy between sustainable agrifood systems and healthy people, communities, and environments. As a whole, they represent a range of strategies that nurture the relations of home in the commons.

NOTES

1. Gary Witherspoon, *Navajo Kinship and Marriage* (University of Chicago Press, 1975).

2. Penny Van Esterik, "Right to Food; Right to Feed; Right to Be Fed: The Intersection of Women's Rights and the Right to Food," *Agriculture and Human Values* 16 (1998): 225–32.

3. Power is a dimension of the relational practice of gendered intimacy expressed in homemaking. For example, meals are sometimes the scenes of patriarchal power in the form of abuse of women and children. Meals can also be the setting of female empowerment through the embodied knowledge of cooking and the practice of sharing food and children's power through demanding or refusing to be fed.

4. Alan Warde et al., "Changes in the Practice of Eating: A Comparative Analysis of Time-Use," *Acta Sociologica* 50, no. 4 (2007): 363–85.

5. Ann Vileisis, *Kitchen Literacy: How We Lost Knowledge of Where Food Comes from and Why We Need to Get it Back* (Washington, DC: Island Press, 2008).

6. Mary Story et al., "Creating Healthy Food and Eating Environments: Policy and Environmental Approaches," *Annual Review of Public Health* 29 (2008): 253–72.

7. Jerry A. Jacobs and Kathleen Gerson, *The Time Divide: Work, Family, and Gender Inequality* (Cambridge, MA: Harvard University Press, 2004); Susan Linn and Courtney L. Novosat, "Calories for Sale: Food Marketing to Children in the Twenty-First Century," *The Annals of the American Academy of Political and Social Science* 615, no. 1 (2008): 133–55.

8. Alan Warde et al., "Changes in the Practice of Eating."

9. Patricia Allen and Carolyn Sachs, "Women and Food Chains: The Gendered Politics of Food," *International Journal of Sociology of Food and Agriculture* 15, no. 1 (2007): 1–23; Silivia Federici, "Women, Land-Struggles and Globalization: An International Perspective," *Journal of Asian and African Studies* 39, no. 1, 2 (2004): 47–62.

10. Rachel Engler-Stringer and Shawna Berenbaum, "Exploring Food Security with Collective Kitchens Participants in Three Canadian Cities," *Qualitative Health Research* 17, no. 1 (2007): 75–84, 75.

11. British Colombian Institute for Co-operative Studies at the University of Victoria, "The Canadian Community Kitchen Movement," http://www.bcics.org/node/154 (accessed September 23, 2008).

12. RCCQ (*Regroupement des cuisines collectives du Québec*), http://www.rccq.org/ (accessed September 17, 2008); Kelly Ebbels, "Cooking up New Collective Kitchens," *McGill Daily*, February 16, 2007, http://www.mcgilldaily.com/view.php?aid=5464 (accessed September 23, 2008).

13. RCCQ, http://www.rccq.org/; Rachel Engler-Stringer and Shawna Berenbaum, "Exploring Food Security with Collective Kitchens Participants in Three Canadian Cities," *Qualitative Health Research* 17, no. 1 (2007): 75–84, 75.

14. RCCQ, http://www.rccq.org/.

15. Engler-Stringer and Berenbaum, "Exploring Food Security."

16. Rachel Engler-Stringer and Shawna Berenbaum, "Collective Kitchens in Canada: A Review of the Literature," *Canadian Journal of Dietetic Practice and Research* 66, no. 4 (2005): 246–51.

17. Rachel Engler-Stringer, "Collective Kitchens in Three Canadian Cities: Impacts on the Lives of Participants" (Saskatoon, CA: Community-University Institute for Social Research, 2006), http://www.usask.ca/cuisr/docs/pub_doc/health/Engler-Stringer. pdf (accessed September 12, 2008).

18. Jeanne Nzeyimana, "Sahwanya Community Kitchen: Bringing African women with HIV together in Vancouver," *Canadian Women's Health Network* Winnipeg, 10, no. 2 (2008): 22, http://www.cwhn.ca/network-reseau/10-2/10-2pg9.html (accessed September 17, 2008).

19. Engler-Stringer, "Collective Kitchen in Three Canadian Cities."

20. Lucie Frechette, "Les Cuisines collectives du Perou: 20 ans d'entraide et de developpement solidaire," *Economie et Solidarites* 29, no. 2 (1998): 124–39.

21. Maureen Hays-Mitchell, "Resisting Austerity: A Gendered Perspective on Neo-Liberal Restructuring in Peru," *Gender and Development* 10, no. 3 (2002): 71–81, 71.

22. Intermonoxfam, "Mujeres cocinando el futuro de Perú," http://www.intermonoxfam. org/es/page.asp?id=2257 (accessed September 17, 2008); Amy Lind and Emi McLaughlin, "Peru," in *The Greenwood Encyclopedia of Women's Issues Worldwide: Central and South America*, ed. Amy Lind (Westport, CT: Greenwood Press, 2003), 411–38, 419.

23. Lind and McLaughlin, "Peru."

24. Cecilia Blondet and Carolina Trevilli, *Chucharas en Alto, Del Asistencialismo a Desarollo Local: Fortaleciendo de la Participación de las Mujeres* (Lima, Perú: IEP, Instituto de Estudios Peruanos, 2004), http://www.iep.org.pe/textos/DDT/DDT135.pdf (accessed September 20, 2008).

25. Amy Lind and Martha Farmelo, "Gender and Urban Social Movements: Women's Community Responses to Restructuring and Urban Poverty" (Paper no. 76, United Nations Research Institute for Social Development, New York, 1996).

26. Annalise Moser, "Happy Heterogeneity? Feminism, Development, and the Grassroots Women's Movement in Peru," *Feminist Studies* 30, no. 1 (2004): 211–37; Maxine Molyneux, *Change and Continuity in Social Protection in Latin America: Mothers at the Service of the State?* (Gender and Development Programme, Paper No. 1, United Nations Research Institute for Social Development, New York, 2007), http://www. unrisd.org/80256B3C005BCCF9/search/BF80E0A84BE41896C12573240033C541?Open Document (accessed September 20, 2008).

27. Lind and Farmelo, "Gender and Urban."

28. Molyneux, Maxine, "Mobilization without Emancipation? Women's Interests, the State, and Revolution in Nicaragua," *Feminist Studies* 11, no. 2 (1985): 227–54.

29. Roelie Lenten, *Cooking under the Volcanoes: Communal Kitchens in the Southern Peruvian City of Arequipa* (Amsterdam: CEDLA Publication, 1993).

30. Moser, "Happy Heterogeneity?" 233.

31. Molyneux, *Change and Continuity.*

32. Ebbels, "Cooking up New Collective Kitchens."

33. Agnes R. Quisumbing et al., *Women: The Key to Food Security* (Washington, DC: Food Policy Report, the International Food Policy Research Institute, 1995).

34. Lenten, *Cooking under the Volcanoes*.

35. "Allotment History: A Brief History of Allotments in the UK," *Allotment Growing*, http://www.allotment.org.uk/articles/Allotment-History.php (accessed September 21, 2008).

36. Susan Buckingham, "Women (Re)construct the Plot: the Regen(d)eration of Urban Food Growing," *Area* 37, no. 2 (2005): 171–179, 173.

37. Buckingham, "Women (Re)construct"; Mathilde Schmitt, "Women Farmers and the Influence of Ecofeminism on the Greening of German Agriculture," in *Gender and Rurality*, ed. Sarah Whatmore, Terry Marsden, and Philip Lower (London: David Fulton Publishers, 1994), 102–116.

38. Buckingham, "Women (Re)construct."

39. FAO (Food and Agriculture Organization of the United Nations), "Women, Agriculture and Rural Development: A Synthesis Report of the Africa Region" (Rome: FAO, 1995), http://www.fao.org/docrep/x0250e/x0250e00.htm (accessed October 3, 2008).

40. Federici, "Women, Land-Struggles."

41. Rachel J. Slater, "Urban Agriculture, Gender and Empowerment: An Alternative View," *Development Southern Africa* 18, no. 5 (2001): 635–50.

42. Ibid.

43. Ibid.

44. Helen Kilbey, "South Africa: A Quiet Revolution Fuelled by Organic Vegetables," AllAfrica.com, January 9, 2008, http://allafrica.com/stories/200801090151.html (accessed October 3, 2008).

45. Sarah Ward, "Organic Gardeners Uplift Poor Communities," *AGENDA* 72 (2007): 47–49.

46. Kilbey, "South Africa"; Soil for Life, http://www.soilforlife.co.za/ (accessed October 3, 2008).

47. Ward, "Organic Gardeners."

48. Kilbey, "South Africa"; Soil for Life, http://www.soilforlife.co.za/.

49. Laura DeLind and Anne E. Ferguson, "Is This a Women's Movement? The Relationship of Gender to Community-supported Agriculture in Michigan," *Human Organization* 59, no. 2 (1999): 190–200; Betty L. Wells and Shelley Gradwell, "Gender and Resource Management: Community Supported Agriculture as Caring-Practice," *Agriculture and Human Values* 18, no. 1 (2001): 107–119.

50. Kathryn N. McCamant and Charles R. Durrett, "Cohousing in Denmark," in *New Households, New Housing*, ed. Karen A. Franck and Sherry Ahrentzen (New York: Van Nostrand Reinhold, 1989), 95–126.

51. Ibid.

52. Dick Urban Vestbro, "From Collective Housing to Cohousing: A Summary of Research," *Journal of Architectural and Planning Research* 17, no. 2 (2000): 164–78.

53. Kenneth Mulder, Robert Constanza, and Jon Erickson, "The Contribution of Built, Human, Social and Natural Capital to Quality of Life in Intentional and Unintentional Communities," *Ecological Economics* 59 (2006): 13–23.

54. Vestbro, "From Collective Housing."

55. Ibid.

56. McCamant and Durrett, "Cohousing in Denmark."

57. Clare Cooper Marcus, "Site Planning, Building Design and a Sense of Community: An Analysis of Six Cohousing Schemes in Denmark, Sweden, and the Netherlands," *Journal of Architectural and Planning Research* 17, no. 2 (2000): 146–63.

58. Sherry Ahrentzen, "Housing Alternatives for New Forms of Households," in *Under One Roof: Issues and Innovations in Shared Housing*, ed. George C. Hemmens, Charles J. Hoch, and Jana Carp (Albany: State University of New York Press, 1996), 33–48.

59. Hildur Jackson, "Children and Cohousing: The Birth of an International Social Movement," *Permaculture Magazine* 52 (Summer 2007): 27–29.

60. Megan Salhus, "Women in Co-housing Communities," *Women & Environments International Magazine* no. 70/71 (Spring/Summer 2006): 70–71; Alison Woodward, "Communal Housing in Sweden: A Remedy for the Stress of Everyday Life?" in *New Households, New Housing,* ed. Karen A. Franck and Sherry Ahrentzen (New York: Van Nostrand Reinhold, 1989), 71–94.

61. Lynn Walter, "The Future of Social Welfare in Denmark," in *Speaking Out: Women, Poverty, and Public Policy,* ed. Katherine A. Rhoades and Anne Statham (Madison: University of Wisconsin System Women's Studies Librarian, 1998), 119–28.

62. Dick Urban Vestbro, "Collective Housing for the Emancipation of Men?" (paper presented at the International Association for People-Environment Studies Conference, July 7–9, 2004), http://iaps.scix.net (accessed October 4, 2008).

63. Graham Meltzer, "Cohousing: Verifying the Importance of Community in the Application of Environmentalism," *Journal of Architectural and Planning Research* 17, no. 2 (2000): 110–32.

64. Munksøgård, http://www.munkesoegaard.dk/index.html (accessed October 4, 2008); Hildur Jackson, "From Cohousing to Ecovillages: A Global *Feminist* Vision?" *Communities* 127 (Summer 2005): 42–48.

65. Munksøgård, http://www.munkesoegaard.dk/index.html.

66. Landsforening for Økosamfund (The Danish Association for Sustainable Communities), http://losnet.dk/_ny/forside.asp (accessed October 5, 2008).

67. Matthias Till, "Assessing the Housing Dimension of Social Inclusion in Six European Countries," *Innovations* 18, no. 2 (2005): 153–81.

68. Slow Food 2008, *Welcome to Our World: Slow Food Companion,* http://www.slow food.com/about_us/img_sito/pdf/Companion08_ENG.pdf (accessed November 1, 2008).

69. Ibid., 10.

70. Slow Food, "Our Mission," http://www.slowfood.com/about_us/eng/mission.lasso (accessed November 2, 2008).

71. Janet Chrzan, "Slow Food: What, Why, and to Where?" *Food, Culture, & Society* 7, no. 2 (2004): 117–32; Lynn Walter, "Slow Food and Home Cooking: Toward a Relational Aesthetic of Food and Relational Ethic of Home" (paper presented at the 2nd International Conference on Sustainable Consumption and Alternative Agri-Food Systems, May 27–30, 2008, University of Liege, Arlon, Belgium).

72. Roberta Sassatelli and Federica Davolio, "Politicizing Food Quality: How Alternative Is Slow Food Vision of Consumption?" (paper presented at the 2nd International Conference on Sustainable Consumption and Alternative Agri-Food Systems, May 27–30, 2008, University of Liege, Arlon, Belgium).

73. Carole M. Counihan, *Around the Tuscan Table: Food, Family, and Gender in Twentieth Century Florence* (New York: Routledge, 2004).

74. Ibid., 121.

75. Ibid., 134ff.

76. Walter, "Slow Food."

77. Eva Feder Kittay, *Love's Labor: Essays on Women, Equality, and Dependency* (New York: Routledge, 1999).

78. Tsyunhehkwa, http://www.tsyunhehkwa.org/ (accessed October 25, 2008).

79. Jack Campisi, "The Wisconsin Oneidas between Disasters," in *The Oneida Indian Journey: From New York to Wisconsin, 1784–1860* (Madison: University of Wisconsin Press, 1999), 70–84.

80. Thelma McLester, "Oneida Women Leaders," in *The Oneida Indian Experience: Two Perspectives*, ed. Jack Campisi and Laurence M. Hauptman (Syracuse, NY: Syracuse University Press, 1988), 108–125.

81. Terra Madre, http://www.terramadre2006.org/pagine/rete/ (accessed November 2, 2008).

82. Save Wild Rice, http://savewildrice.org/history (accessed November 2, 2008).

83. Carol Cornelius, *Iroquois Corn in a Culture-based Curriculum: A Framework for Respectfully Teaching about Cultures* (Albany, NY: SUNY Press, 1999).

84. Diana Peterson, "Three Sisters Gardening: Rejuvenating a Traditional Food System with the Oneida Tribe of Indians of Wisconsin" (master's thesis, Environmental Science and Policy, University of Wisconsin-Green Bay, 2005).

85. Oneida Community Integrated Farm Systems, http://ocifs.oneidanation.org/ (accessed October 25, 2008).

86. Laura Wilcox, "Healing History: North America's Indigenous Peoples Look to the Past to Find Healthier Future," http://heifer.org (accessed November 2, 2008).

87. "Declaration of Atitlan, Indigenous Peoples' Consultation on the Right to Food: A Global Consultation, Atitlán, Sololá, Guatemala, April 17–19, 2002," http://www.treatycouncil.org/new_page_5241224.htm (accessed November 1, 2008).

88. E. Melanie DuPuis and David Goodman, "Should We Go Home to Eat? Toward a Reflexive Politics of Localism," *Journal of Rural Studies* 21 (2005): 359–71.

89. Christopher Lasch, *Haven in a Heartless World: The Family Besieged* (New York: W. W. Norton & Company, 1995).

90. Richard Wilk, *Home Cooking in the Global Village* (Oxford: Berg, 2006), 203.

91. Van Esterik, "Right to Food."

RESOURCE GUIDE

Suggested Reading

Allen, Patricia, and Carolyn Sachs. "Women and Food Chains: The Gendered Politics of Food." *Journal of Sociology of Food and Agriculture* 15, no. 1 (2007): 1–23.

Barndt, Deborah, ed. *Women Working the NAFTA Food Chain: Women, Food & Globalization*. Toronto: Second Story Press, 1999.

Counihan, Carole M. *Around the Tuscan Table: Food, Family, and Gender in Twentieth Century Florence*. New York: Routledge, 2004.

DeVault, Marjorie L. *Feeding the Family: The Social Organization of Caring as Gendered Work*. University of Chicago Press, 1991.

Kim, Grace. "Culture: A Retrospective of Danish Cohousing." The Co-Housing Association of the United States, 2008. Available at http://www.cohousing.org/docs/2008/denmark_retrospective.pdf.

Van Esterik, Penny. "Right to Food; Right to Feed; Right to Be Fed. The Intersection of Women's Rights and the Right to Food." *Agriculture and Human Values* 16 (1998): 225–32.

Warde, Alan, Shu-Li Cheng, Wendy Olsen, and Deal Southerton. "Changes in the Practice of Eating: A Comparative Analysis of Time-Use." *Acta Sociologica* 50, no. 4 (2007): 363–85.

Web Sites

Abalimi Bezekhaya, http://www.abalimi.org.za/ (a Xhosa urban agricultural and environmental NGO).

ECDQ.tv Catholic Church of Quebec, "Community Kitchens in Peru Video." http://www.ecdq.tv/en/videos/443cb001c138b2561a0d90720d6ce111.

Fresh Choice Kitchens, the Community Kitchen program of the Greater Vancouver Food Bank Society, http://www.communitykitchens.ca/main/?communityKitchens (community kitchens video).

Munksøgård, Danish Ecovillage, http://www.munkesoegaard.dk/index.html.

Regroupement des cuisines collectives du Québec, http://www.rccq.org/.

Slow Food, http://ww.slowfood.com.

Tsyunhehkwa, http://tsyunhehkwa.org.

11

Cultural Differences in Food Preferences

Regan A. R. Gurung

Every Saturday during the summer, the Green Bay (Wisconsin) farmer's market is awash in color: rich varieties of flowers, verdant leafy greens, and the requisite set of crafts and knick-knacks. There is a clear majority among the assembled party of farmers displaying their wares. The farmer's market is dominated by Hmong Americans, with tables overflowing with pumpkin vines, pea tendrils, amaranth, Chinese broccoli, bok choy, mustard greens, water spinach, and other herbs. The Hmong people originally lived in the hills of the Laos People's Democratic Republic in Southeast Asia. In 1975, Laos fell to communist forces, and 150,000 Hmong fled to refugee camps in Thailand and then to America. In fact, the American government promised the Hmong asylum in exchange for their help in fighting the Vietnam War. Correspondingly, thousands of Hmong men, women, and children immigrated to America and settled primarily in California, Minnesota, and Wisconsin. The Hmong were farmers in the hills of Laos and brought their traditions with them. Across America, it is not surprising to see the Hmong tending small plots of land and growing their own produce, even in the busiest of American cities. For example, in Massachusetts, Hmong and Cambodian immigrants are active beneficiaries of the New Entry Sustainable Farming Project.[1] Since 1998, the project has helped farmers access land and grow crops that are native to their homelands. Growing your own food and selling the excess to make a living is not a new idea. Before the rise of technological innovation and conglomerate food industries, most of the world subsisted in such a way.

Most of the immigrants to America brought their own food-raising traditions with them. The American Indians, earliest inhabitants of the Americas, also have a rich tradition of working the soil. In fact, looking at cultural differences in nutrition and eating habits reveals connections to the soil and between food and culture that have considerable significance for the sustainability movement. More often than not, traditional cultural dietary prescriptions, farming traditions, and diets reveal sustainable patterns. The example of the Hmong highlights the fact that some cultural groups have different relationships with food than others. The Hmong diet is primarily vegetarian and heavily dependent on what is produced in the home garden. What are other cultural differences in food preferences? What are the implications for sustainability? This chapter will focus on different cultural groups that have distinct food preferences and prescriptions for healthy eating. After clarifying how I use the term "culture," I shall briefly discuss the development of food preferences following an overview of philosophical differences to nutrition that form the underlying basis for eating behavior. Whereas the Chinese and Taoist approach focuses on balance of yin and yang foods and the Indian-Ayurvedic tradition focuses on matching food to body type and season, the Western approach aims to balance nutritional value. I will then briefly review how different religions also have different prescriptions for eating. Each section will discuss implications for how food is produced and consumed. As the globe embraces multiculturalism, migration and immigration are changing food preferences with implications for health and sustainability.

WHAT IS CULTURE?

What do your mother, your region, your best friend, and your religion have in common? They each constitute a way that you are socialized and compose elements of culture. Take parents, for example. Whether we do something because they told us to (e.g., "Eat your greens!") or exactly because they told us not to (e.g., "Don't eat too much ice cream"), they have a strong influence on us. If our friends frequent fast-food establishments, we will be more likely to do the same. Similarly, religions have different prescriptions for what individuals should and should not do. Muslims should not eat pork or drink alcohol. Hindus are prohibited from eating beef. Even where we live can determine our habits and can predict the diseases we may die from as studied in detail by the area of health geography. Parents, peers, religion, and geography are a few of the key determinants of our behaviors and are examples of what makes up our culture.

There are many definitions of culture; Soudijn, Hutschemaekers, and Van de Vijver analyzed 128 definitions.[2] Culture can be broadly defined as a dynamic, yet stable, set of goals, beliefs, and attitudes shared by a group of people.[3] Culture can include the social construction of similarities in physical characteristics (e.g., skin color), psychological characteristics (e.g., levels of hostility), and common superficial features (e.g., hair style and clothing). Culture is dynamic because some of the beliefs held by members in a culture can change with time. However, the general culture stays mostly stable because the individuals change together. These beliefs and attitudes can be implicit, learned by observation, and passed on by word of mouth, or they can be explicit, written down as laws or rules for the group to follow. The most commonly described objective cultural groups are categorized by ethnicity, race, sex, and age.

The most recent census data list the population of the United States as being around 302 million. That number can be broken down along different cultural lines. An example of a "cultural group" that most people tend to think of first is race. Of that 302 million population, approximately 13 percent are African American or black, approximately 4 percent are Asian American (including Americans of different Asian backgrounds such as Chinese, Japanese, Korean, and Indian), and approximately 1 percent are American Indians or Native Americans. The remaining

82 percent of the population are considered European American or white and include people of Latin American and Spanish ancestry. Commonly referred to as Latinos, the preferred term, or Hispanic (a term applied to this ethnic group by the U.S. government in the 1980 Census), the truth is that people in this same group have their own names for their groups depending on which part of the United States they live in and their specific country of origin. For example, *Hispanic* is preferred in the southeast and much of Texas, New Yorkers use both *Hispanic* and *Latino*, and in Chicago, *Latino* is preferred.[4] Each ethnic group has distinct cuisines and food preferences, as I shall describe later.

A second type of culture is religion. Of the 302 million Americans, the absolute majority are Christians, accounting for 84 percent (57 percent Protestant and 27 percent Catholic). The next largest percentage of Americans do not have any religious affiliation (8 percent). The rest are Jewish (2 percent) and a number of smaller groups (e.g., Hindu). Although there are different subcultures, such as age-groups, socioeconomic status, geographic regions, biological sex, and gender, ethnic and religious differences are most directly tied to differences in food preferences.

DEVELOPMENT OF FOOD PREFERENCES

Have you wondered why you like certain foods and dislike others? A part of our food preferences are biologically programmed.[5] Humans have two completely innate preferences: we innately prefer sweet and salty tastes and are adverse to sour tastes. In general, our experiences and exposure to food determine the bulk of our preferences. If the context in which you were given broccoli was positive, you probably will develop a preference for broccoli. If you always were forced to eat your beans, you probably will develop an aversion to beans. If you were raised near a cheese factory, you probably will develop a preference for cheese. Basic reward and punishment and sociocultural factors also play a large role in the development of our food preferences.[6] Children growing up in families who eat together often develop healthier eating habits (and are healthier adults too).[7] Foods used as rewards (e.g., clean your room and you get your ice cream) or paired with fun social events or holidays (e.g., Mom's spice cake at Christmas) automatically become preferred. A recent study of more than one thousand children showed that the ethnicity of the parents and correspondingly ethnic food preferences also influenced what children ate.[8] Changes in food marketing and availability are the most recent and blatant environmental factors influencing eating.[9] The fast-food industry has been "supersizing" its offerings. For a small increase in costs, fast-food chains generate a large profit from the public, many of whom like to get large servings. The influence of larger servings in restaurants is seen as one component of an industrial way of life because it tends to be localized to industrial countries. As proof of the ills of "Western living," researchers[10] compared Pima Indians in the United States with Pima Indians living in a rural part of Mexico. The U.S. Pima Indians had a mean body mass index (BMI) of 35.5. The Mexican Pima Indians had an average BMI of 25.1. Similarly, the Navajo Indians of New Mexico are experiencing rising cases of gallbladder infection and other diet-related problems.[11] How much food does a person really need? The actual amount of food in a recommended serving may surprise you.[12]

Whereas overeating and the obesity epidemic in America may not directly seem to relate to sustainability, one cannot help but wonder whether eating healthier portions would help sustainability. Evidence suggests that our biology holds within its DNA code remnants of times in our evolutionary history when food availability was not a given. Correspondingly, we evolved to eat more when food was available because we did not know when food supplies would extinguish because of drought or pestilence. Today, the ready availability of food is almost directly tied to obesity levels. Most overweight people eat more than healthy weight people and often do not even realize the quantities they consume. That said, overweight people do not eat more of just anything. A variety of social and psychological factors influence how much we eat and when.[13] For example, we eat more when we are stressed or hassled.[14] Taste and quality are particularly important. Studies suggest that overweight individuals actually prefer (and eat) more fat than healthy weight people. Be warned, though; most people eat more if they are given larger servings.[15] Furthermore, a greater variety of foods presented leads to greater quantities consumed by individual eaters.[16] If only one type of food is available at a meal, people eat a moderate amount of it. If a second food is introduced, the amount of the new food eaten will be more than if it was presented by itself. This phenomenon is called sensory-specific satiety. Even thinking that more variety is available can make you eat more. Brian Wansink showed that people will eat more jelly beans when they are mixed up (and there seems to be more variety) than when a number of varieties are served separately.[17] Simply changing the cost of foods makes a difference too.[18] The cheaper the food is, the more people will eat, which even applies to healthy items such as fruits.

These general factors associated with food preference and eating have been shown to be relatively constant worldwide; however, philosophical approaches to nutrition and eating do vary significantly. What we eat often is deeply tied to our cultural backgrounds. Throughout history, many cultures have ascribed health-promoting powers to certain foods, and many religions have followed specific dietary practices. Chinese "herbs of immortality" were a popular fad among the ancient Egyptians. These herbs have a modern manifestation in the Chinese herbs that are promoted to bodybuilders in health food stores. Different cultures have different beliefs about what should be eaten. Cultures including the Chinese believe that some foods are hot and others are cold. This belief refers to a food's influence on health and well-being, not to the temperature or spiciness of foods. Cold foods include most vegetables, tropical fruits, dairy products, and inexpensive cuts of meat (e.g., rump). Hot foods include chili peppers, garlic, onion, most grains, expensive cuts of meat, oils, and alcohol. Just as the U.S. Department of Agriculture (USDA) Food Guide Pyramid balances nutritional value, cultures such as the Chinese and the ancient Indians suggested eating foods to balance energy levels. Most non-Western cultures believe that the type of food eaten needs to balance the type or condition of the person. For example, pregnancy is considered a "hot" condition during which many Latinos typically avoid hot foods, believing this will prevent the infant from contracting a "hot" illness, such as a skin rash. In contrast to the Latino beliefs, the Chinese believe that pregnancy is a "cold" condition during which the expectant mother should consume hot foods to keep in balance and remain healthy. In the next section, I will describe three major world philosophies and their relation to eating. In each, good nutrition is seen as a valuable component of health, and I have framed the discussion of food around health.

WESTERN NUTRITION

The USDA's earliest attempts to inform consumers about how much protein, fats, and carbohydrates to consume date back to the early 1900s. The first food guide was published in 1916 and consisted of five major groups. The economic problems of the Great Depression in the 1930s greatly influenced families' buying habits as they had to balance price and nutrition. Affordable foods were often low in nutritional value. To alleviate this situation, the USDA released buying guides with 12 food groups in the 1930s. Over the next several decades, the number of food groups changed from seven in the 1940s to four in the 1950s and 1960s and then back to five in 1979 with the "Hassle-Free" Foundation diet. The Food Guide Pyramid, as seen on bread packages and cereal boxes through mid 2005, was introduced in 1984 with six food groups. The 1984 configuration was revised in the early 1990s based on the U.S. Department of Health and Human Services' (DHHS) Surgeon General's Report on Nutrition and Health. The report included the recommendations of a panel of nutritional experts selected by the USDA and the DHHS. This pyramid established the basic principles of a balanced diet designed to help people maintain or improve their general health and reduce the risk of diet-related diseases. The pyramid, although easily recognized, was not well used or well understood.

Because of problems with understanding the pyramid, cultural variations needed for it to apply to all Americans, and a large amount of new nutritional research, the pyramid as many middle-age adults knew it was discontinued. The DHHS released an updated set of nutritional guidelines for Americans in January 2005, complete with a new pictorial guide revamping the pyramid, now called MyPyramid. A modified version for older adults was released in January 2008. Key changes include explicitly urging the consumption of more whole grains, a variety of fruits and vegetables, and an increase in physical activity. Instead of the horizontal bands of the old pyramid, rainbow-colored bands now stream down. Food groups are represented by six different colors: Orange for grains, green for vegetables, red for fruits, yellow for oils, blue for milk products, and purple for meat and beans. The bands are wider for grains, vegetables, fruit, and milk products to remind people to eat more of them. Instead of one band for all, twelve individually tailored models outline the food guides for different age groups and for men versus women.

The food guides show foods typically eaten by North Americans to illustrate the USDA and DHHS recommendations. The pyramid suggests the types and amount of foods to eat each day. Four factors were considered in establishing the serving sizes (e.g., eat two to three servings of fruit): (1) typical portion sizes from food consumption surveys, (2) ease of use, (3) nutrient content, and (4) traditional uses of foods. Although a single serving of one type of fruit may have more calories than a single serving of another, the number of different serving sizes was kept to a minimum to make the pyramid easy to use.

The fourth factor, "traditional uses of food," makes you consider the fact that different cultural groups all have different traditional foods. To compensate for this fact, Oldways Preservation and Exchange Trust of Cambridge, Massachusetts, developed food pyramids for different cultural groups. The Mediterranean, Asian, and Latino diet pyramids, as well as a Native American food pyramid, incorporate habits of various ethnic groups in the United States The main difference between these pyramids and the standard USDA pyramid is that the culturally diverse pyramids illustrate proportions of food to be consumed and not exact serving sizes. Furthermore, the Oldways pyramids show foods specific to the different cultures and suggest consumption amounts over a period of two to three days, weeks, or even months, in contrast to the USDA guide.

TRADITIONAL CHINESE BELIEFS

To better understand Chinese prescriptions for eating, one needs to gain a good sense of the philosophy behind Traditional Chinese Medicine (TCM), where what you eat directly ties to your health.

Two main systems categorize the forces identified in TCM that influence health and well-being: yin and yang and the five phases. According to one Chinese philosophy, all life and the entire universe originated from a single unified source called Tao (pronounced "dow"). The main ideas about the Tao are encompassed in a 5,000-word poem called the *Tao Te Ching* written about 2,500 years ago that describes a way of life from the reign of the Yellow Emperor, Huang Ti. In fact, Chinese medicine is based on *The Yellow Emperor's Classic of Internal Medicine* (approximately 100 B.C.E.). The Tao is an integrated and undifferentiated whole with two opposing forces—the *yin* and *yang*—that combine to create everything in the universe.

In TCM, health is the balance of the yin and yang, the two complementary forces in the universe. Yin and yang are mutually interdependent, constantly interactive, and potentially interchangeable forces. Each yin and yang contains the seed of the other. The circle represents the supreme source or Tao. Yin translates to "shady side of a hill," whereas yang translates to "sunny side of the hill." Yin is traditionally thought of as darkness, the moon, cold, and female, whereas yang is thought of as light, the sun, hot, and male. In TCM, ten vital organs are divided into five pairs, each consisting of one "solid" yin organ and one "hollow" yang organ. TCM practitioners believe that the yin organs—the heart, liver, pancreas, kidney, and lungs—are more vital than the yang organs, and dysfunctions of yin organs cause the greatest health problems. The paired yang organs are the gallbladder, small intestine, large intestine, and bladder. A healthy individual has a balanced amount of yin and yang. If a person is sick, his or her forces are out of balance. Specific symptoms relate to an excess of either yin or yang. For example, if you are flushed, have a high temperature, are constipated, and have high blood pressure, you have too much yang.[19]

The yin and yang are often translated into hot and cold (two clear opposites), referring to qualities and not temperatures. To be healthy, what you eat and drink and the way you live your life should have equal amounts of hot qualities and cold ones. Balancing hot and cold is a critical element of many different cultures (e.g., Chinese, Indian, and even Mexican), although the foods that constitute each may vary across cultures. Some "hot" foods include beef, garlic, ginger, and alcohol. Some "cold" foods include honey, most green leafy vegetables, potatoes, and some fruits (e.g., melons, pears).

The five phases or elemental activities refer to specific active forces and illustrate the intricate associations that the ancient Chinese saw between human beings and nature. Energy or *qi* (pronounced "chee"), another critical aspect of TCM, moves within the body in the same pattern as it does in nature with each season and with different foods helping to optimize energy flow within the body. The five elements of wood, fire, earth, metal, and water each link to a season of the year, a specific organ, and a specific food. Each element has specific characteristics, is generated by one of the other forces, and is suppressed by another. For example, wood generates fire that turns things to earth that forms metals. The heart is ruled by fire, the liver by wood, and the kidneys by water. Fire provides qi to the heart and then passes qi onto the earth element and correspondingly the stomach, the spleen, and pancreas. Thus, what you eat can influence your different organs and your well-being in general.

AYURVEDIC NUTRITION

Many herbal supplements in use today came into prominence because of ancient Ayurvedic writings, and various health care products on the market that tout natural bases (e.g., Aveda products) have roots in Ayurveda, a traditional Indian holistic system of medicine. Although you do not see as much explicit evidence of this form of medicine in North America (i.e., you do not find Ayurveda shops in Little India parts of cities corresponding to Chinese herb shops in Chinatowns), many Americans practice forms of Ayurveda. Ayurveda originated more than 6,000 years ago in India and was considered a medicine of the masses.[20] In fact, the basic ideology underlying Ayurveda still influences how health is viewed by many of the billion inhabitants of India today. Many Indian Americans even use the prescriptions of Ayurveda in daily life (e.g., swallowing raw garlic is good for you and chewing on cloves helps toothaches), and many European Americans are using Ayurvedic practices such as yoga and natural supplements. The first two major Ayurvedic texts, the *Charaka Samhita* and the *Sushruta Samhita*, have been dated to 1000 B.C.E., although Ayurvedic practices are also referred to in the Vedas (3000 to 2000 B.C.E.), ancient Indian texts containing the wisdom of sages and sacrificial rituals. The *Charaka Samhita* has 120 chapters covering such diverse areas as the general principles of Ayurveda, the causes and symptoms of disease, physiology and medical ethics, prognosis, therapy, and pharmacy.

Ayurveda was developed by Charaka. Charaka described four causative factors in mental illness—namely, (1) diet (incompatible, vitiated, and unclean food); (2) disrespect to gods, elders, and teachers; (3) mental shock caused by emotions such as excessive fear and joy; and (4) faulty bodily activity. Thus, Ayurveda considers a biopsychosocial approach in formulating causative factors in mental disorders. Charaka, while emphasizing the need for harmony between body, mind, and soul, focused on preventive, curative, and promotive aspects of mental health. Ancient Indian court physicians further developed Ayurvedic practices and were given vast resources because the health of the king was considered equivalent to the health of the state. Ayurvedic medicine was well developed by the time of the Buddha (500 B.C.E.) and the rise of Buddhism. Jivaka, the royal physician to the Buddha, was so well known that people actually became Buddhists so he could treat them. When Alexander the Great invaded India in

326 B.C.E., he even took Ayurvedic physicians back to Greece with him. The use of Ayurveda flourished until the year 900 when Muslim invaders came into India and created a new form of medicine called Unani, a combination of Greek and Ayurvedic medicine with Arabic medicine.[21] Ayurveda continued in different forms even after European forces invaded India around 1500, bringing Western medicine with them. The use of plants and herbal remedies plays a major part in Ayurvedic medicine. About six hundred different medicinal plants are mentioned in the core Ayurvedic texts. Just knowing the name of the plant is not enough. The texts even prescribe how the plant should be grown (e.g., type of soil and water) and where. The use of plants to cure is perhaps one of the key areas in which Ayurveda is practiced in North America. Western drug companies have used a number of plants originally used in India to cure diseases. For example, psyllium seed is used for bowel problems, and other plants are used to reduce blood pressure, control diarrhea, and lessen the risk of liver or heart problems. A substance called forskolin, isolated from the *Coleus forskohlii* plant, has been used in Ayurveda for treating heart disease, and its use has now been empirically validated by Western biomedicine.

TCM and Ayurveda share many basic similarities. Ayurvedic science also uses the notion of basic elements: five great elements form the basis of the universe. Earth represents the solid state, water the liquid state, air the gaseous state, fire the power to change the state of any substance, and ether, simultaneously the source of all matter and the space in which it exists. Each of these elements can either nourish the body, balance the body serving to heal, or imbalance the body serving as a poison. Achieving the right balance of these elements in the body is critical to maintaining a healthy state. These elements also combine to form three major forces ("doshas") that influence physiological functions critical to healthy living. Ether and air combine to form the *Vata dosha*, fire and water combine to form the *Pitta dosha*, and water and earth elements combine to form the *Kapha dosha*. Vata directs nerve impulses, circulation, respiration, and elimination. Pitta is responsible for metabolism in the organ and tissue systems as well as cellular metabolism. Kapha is responsible for growth and protection. We are all made up of unique proportions of Vata, Pitta, and Kapha, which cause disease when they go out of balance. These three doshas are referred to as humors or bodily fluids and correspond to the Greek humors of phlegm (Kapha) and choler (Pitta). There is no equivalent to the Greek humor blood, nor is Vata (wind) represented in the Greek system. Similar to the meridians in TCM, the existence of these forces is demonstrated more by inference and results of their hypothesized effects than by physical observation. Vata, Pitta, and Kapha are also associated with specific body type characteristics. Of critical relevance to this chapter is that what you eat directly influences the doshas and corresponding health. The Ayurvedic philosophy has clear-cut prescriptions and nutritional guidelines based on essential body types. You determine your body type, and then eat accordingly.

Each of the three major philosophies of nutrition described above influence the eating habits of the adherents to their systems. All three philosophies are constant in suggesting moderation and both Ayurvedic and Chinese systems recommend consuming the freshest produce possible—growing it yourself is the best, and also eating small quantities of meat (the wilder the better). These major common prescriptions can be satisfied by sustainable practices. In addition to these major philosophical approaches, there are also clear-cut religious prescriptions regarding food. It is this component of culture that I turn to next.

RELIGIOUS PRESCRIPTIONS TO EATING

Two of the world's religions have strict prescriptions about what their adherents should or should not eat. Jewish and Islamic dietary laws have many similarities and both significantly influence what food is grown and how food is processed and consumed.

All Orthodox and some conservative Jews follow *Kashrut*, dietary laws set down in the Torah (Jewish written law and sacred texts) and explained in the Talmud, a record of discussions pertaining to Jewish law. Most of us are probably more familiar with the term *kosher*. This is the popular term used to signify what is "fit" for consumption according to *Kashrut*. Food that qualifies is often packaged with the kosher symbol.

There are four major categories of Kashrut dietary laws. First, there is a clear list of animals that are permitted to be eaten. Mammals that have a completely cloven foot or that regurgitates may be eaten (e.g., all cattle, deer, goats). Only fish with fins and scales are allowed (e.g., no catfish, sharks, or shellfish). In addition, certain parts such as blood and fat that is separate from flesh are not to be consumed. Second, the meat of permitted animals is only allowed if the animal is killed by a special process (*shehitah*) that is quick, relatively painless, and minimizes the amount of blood left in the body. Animals with blemishes or disease are avoided. Third, there are clear prescriptions for how food is cooked. Meat has to be prepared by removing forbidden parts and after soaking in water and covering it with kosher salt. Separate dishes and utensils are often used for meat versus dairy. Food has to be examined to ensure that it does not contain insects or worms, and processed food must be packed under the supervision of a rabbinical authority. Finally, meat and milk products are not to be eaten together. Meat can be eaten an hour after dairy products, but dairy products can only be eaten six hours after eating meat.

Islam, the second largest religious group in the world, has a similar set of strict prescriptions for eating. Documented in the *Koran*, the Islamic dietary laws are referred to as *Halal*. To Muslims, followers of the Islamic faith, eating is considered a form of worship. Consequently, there are clear prescriptions of not just what to eat but how much to eat as well. Muslims are advised to not eat more than two-thirds of their capacity. Foods that are not permitted, or *haram*, include all animals that catch their prey with their mouths and birds of prey that seize their prey with their talons. Similar to kosher prescriptions, animals must be killed in a humane way. In particular, the person killing the animal must say "In the name of God, God is great" at the time of the slaughter. Many Muslims do not eat meat if they cannot ascertain that is has been killed in the correct manner. Drinking stimulants such as coffee and tea, as well as smoking, is discouraged, and alcoholic drinks are prohibited.

Other religious groups also have dietary restrictions though not as extensive as Jews and Muslims. Many Hindus, for example, do not eat meat to avoid inflicting pain on animals. Hindu scriptures (*Laws of Manu*) do not prohibit eating meat but state that abstaining from meat and wine will be beneficial for physical, mental, and spiritual health. Although some Hindus eat meat, beef is avoided as the cow is considered sacred. Pork is rarely eaten. In direct relevance to sustainability issues, cows are raised primarily for milk and dairy needs.

CONCLUSION

The link between culture and sustainability has been made before. For example, a 1997 UNESCO (United Nations Educational, Scientific, and Cultural Organization) conference focused on culture and sustainable development in the Pacific. Speakers at that conference discussed the political and economic ramifications of fostering cultural practices in light of sustainability issues, but food and agriculture was not part of the discussion. As described in the preceding sections, there are vast differences in how food preferences develop, philosophical approaches to nutrition, and religious prescriptions regarding eating. Many of these philosophies of nutrition exist in concert with historical patterns of agricultural practices. The Hmong farmers are but one example of how agricultural practices vary by ethnicity and nationality. The other elements of culture can affect sustainability as well. As discussed, many Hindus (practitioners of Ayurveda) modify their diets based on seasons. Certain foods are recommended for each season. These foods often match what is naturally grown in that particular season and in that particular area, making these ancient prescriptions common practical sense. In the modern age, we can get carried away with trying to "eat local," while ignoring the natural growing cycle of plants, wisdom inherent to many ancient philosophies of food. For example, you may want to buy locally grown cucumbers, but if cucumbers are not native to where you live and are grown in greenhouses that require additional energy expenditure and resources, you are not doing the environment any favors. In such cases it may be prudent to buy cucumbers grown where they are naturally abundant, even if this means buying from another country. Of course, the alternative is to only eat what is in season (returning to Ayurvedic principles).

The notion of eating what is in season also resonates clearly with the TCM approach to eating and health. According to the Chinese, it is important to live in concert with nature. Health is best achieved when human beings are acting in concert with the seasons, that is, eating what is seasonal. In fact, both the Chinese and Indian traditions suggest that optimal health and balance is achieved only when we are eating what is in season. This consequently precludes the use of aggressive chemical fertilizer and artificial means for growing. It also advocates the use of sustainable farming, which is thought to produce the healthiest produce.

I have focused on a few specific cultures, the Chinese and Indian traditional systems in particular, but many more examples demonstrate ways that food, culture, and sustainability interact. Patricia Klindienst spent three years traveling the United States gathering the stories of immigrants who used their gardens to retain their cultural heritages. In growing their own produce, her interviewees are prime examples of how cultural traditions can foster sustainable agriculture. Whether Mexican Americans in New Mexico, Gullah elders in South Carolina, Polish and Japanese Americans in Washington State, or Indian and Italian Americans in California, Klindienst's gardeners are prototypes of how sustainability can be made operational.[22]

Although universities and colleges in North America have offered courses and programs in food and culture for some time now, the link to sustainability has yet to be made. It is but a short step from cultural differences in nutrition and eating to the basic agricultural practices that vary as a consequence. Perhaps a closer look at the differences in ethnic and religious practices as described in this chapter can provide fertile ground for the development of interventions to bolster sustainable agriculture. If we can capitalize on culturally diverse nutritional practices that are naturally sustainable and support the reemergence of these practices, we add a new dimension to food studies and set the stage for a more sustainable pattern of living.

NOTES

1. Sustainable Agriculture Research and Education, http://www.sare.org/publica tions/limited-resource/profile2.htm.

2. Regan A. R. Gurung, *Health Psychology: A Cultural Approach* (San Francisco: Cengage, 2010).

3. David Matsumoto, "Key Issues in Culture," in *Getting Culture: Incorporating Diversity Across the Curriculum*, ed. Regan A. R. Gurung and Loretto Prieto (Arlington, VA: Stylus, 2009).

4. Earl Shorris, *Latinos: A Biography of the People* (New York: Norton, 1992).

5. Linda M. Bartoshuk, "The Biological Basis of Food Perception and Acceptance," *Food Quality and Preference* 4 (1993): 21–32.

6. Rickelle Richards and Cherry Smith, "Environmental, Parental, and Personal Influences on Food Choice, Access, and Overweight Status among Homeless Children," *Social Science and Medicine* 65 (2007): 1572–583; Graham Finlayson, Neil King, and John Blundell, "The Role of Implicit Wanting in Relation to Explicit Liking and Wanting for Food: Implications for Appetite Control," *Appetite* 50, no. 1 (2008): 120–27; Lucy Cooke, "The Importance of Exposure for Healthy Eating in Childhood: A Review," *Journal of Human Nutrition and Dietetics* 20 (2007): 294–301.

7. Debra L. Franko et al., "What Mediates the Relationship Between Family Meals and Adolescent Health Issues," *Health Psychology* 27, no. 2 (2008): S109–S117.

8. Mozhdeh B. Bruss et al., "Ethnicity and Diet of Children: Development of Culturally Sensitive Measures," *Health Education and Behavior* 34 (2007): 735–47.

9. Susan Linn and Courtney L. Novosat, "Calories for Sale: Food Marketing to Children in the Twenty-First Century," *Annals of the American Academy of Political and Social Science* 615 (2008): 133–55; Corrina Hawkes, "Regulating Food Marketing to Young People Worldwide: Trends and Policy Drivers," *American Journal of Public Health* 97 (2007): 1962–1973.

10. Gurung, *Health Psychology*.

11. Lori Alvord and Elizabeth Cohen Van Pelt, *The Scalpel and the Silver Bear: The First Navajo Woman Surgeon Combines Western Medicine and Traditional Healing* (New York: Bantam, 2000).

12. USDA (U.S. Department of Agriculture), http://www.mypyramid.gov/.

13. Wolfgang Stroebe, *Dieting, Overweight, and Obesity: Self-Regulation in a Food-Rich Environment* (Washington, DC: American Psychological Association, 2008).

14. Daryl. B. O'Connor et al., "Effects of Daily Hassles and Eating Style on Eating Behavior," *Health Psychology* 27 (2008): S20–S31.

15. Brian Wansink, Koert van Ittersum, and James E. Painter, "Ice Cream Illusions Bowls, Spoons, and Self-Served Portion Sizes," *American Journal of Preventive Medicine* 31 (2006): 240–43.

16. Brian Wansink and Jeffrey Sobal, "Mindless Eating: The 200 Daily Food Decisions We Overlook," *Environment and Behavior* 39 (2007): 106–123.

17. Brian Wansink, *Mindless Eating: Why We Eat More Than We Think* (New York: Bantam, 2007).

18. Myles S. Faith et al., "Toward the Reduction of Population Obesity: Macrolevel Environmental Approaches to the Problems of Food, Eating, and Obesity," *Psychological Bulletin* 133, no. 2 (2007): 205–226.

19. Ted, J Kaptchuk, *The Web That Has No Weaver: Understanding Chinese Medicine* (New York: McGraw-Hill, 2000).

20. Robert E. Svoboda, *Ayurveda: Life, Health, and Longevity* (New Delhi: Penguin Press, 2004).

21. Farokh Erach Udwadia, *Man and Medicine: A History* (New Delhi: Oxford University Press, 2000).

22. Klindienst, Patricia, *The Earth Knows My Name: Food, Culture, and Sustainability in the Gardens of Ethnic Americans* (Boston: Beacon Press, 2006).

RESOURCE GUIDE

Suggested Reading

Anderson, Eugene Newton. *Everyone Eats: Understanding Food and Culture*. New York University Press, 2005.

Civitello, Linda. *Cuisine and Culture: A History of Food and People*. Hoboken, NJ: Wiley & Sons, 2008.

Counihan, Carole, and Penny Van Esterik, Eds. *Food and Culture: A Reader*. London: Routledge, 1997.

Gabaccia, Donna R. *We Are What We Eat: Ethnic Food and the Making of Americans*. Cambridge, MA: Harvard University Press, 1998.

Goodall, Jane, Gary McAvoy, and Gail Hudson. *Harvest for Hope: A Guide for Mindful Eating*. New York: Time Warner, 2006.

Goyan Kittler, Pamela, and Kathryn P. Sucher. *Food and Culture: A Nutritional Handbook*. San Francisco: Wadsworth, 2000.

Klindienst, Patricia. *The Earth Knows My Name: Food, Culture, and Sustainability in the Gardens of Ethnic Americans*. Boston: Beacon Press, 2006.

Menzel, Peter, and Faith D'Aluisio. *What the World Eats*. Berkeley, CA: Tricycle Press, 2008.

Root, Waverly, and Richard De Rochemont. *Eating in America*. Hoboken, NJ: Ecco Press, 1995.

Web Sites

Eating in America, http://www.eatinginamerica.de/.

Ohio State University, College of Food, Agricultural, and Environmental Sciences, "Cultural Diversity: Eating in America Hmong," http://ohioline.osu.edu/hyg Fact/5000/5254.html.

Ohio State University, College of Food, Agricultural, and Environmental Sciences, "Cultural Diversity, Eating in America Amish," http://ohioline.osu.edu/hyg-Fact/5000/5251.html.

12

Images of Sustenance in Contemporary Literature

Aeron Haynie

There was just enough headroom for him to stand. He ducked under a lantern with a green metal shade hanging from a hook. He held the boy by the hand and they went along the rows of stenciled cartons. Chile, corn, stew, soup, spaghetti sauce. The richness of a vanished world. Why is this here? The boy said. Is it real?

The Road, Cormac McCarthy[1]

Food is essential for human life and has been an integral part of the stories we tell, from the lotus eaters and heroic feasts in Homer's *Odyssey* to Oliver Twist's plaintive request for more gruel to McCarthy's description of the miraculous appearance of generic canned food in a postapocalyptic America. Food is a primal motivation, a method of characterization, a form of symbolism, a rich source of metaphor, and a way of making characters' lives more textured, more real to readers. Novels about food—which take place in the mind, but evoke the reader's physical appetite—challenge Western philosophers' views that "human existence is bifurcated into two realms or substances: the bodily, on the one hand; the mental or spiritual, on the other."[2] Representations of food often make literary characters' lives more concrete, more material. Eating is both a common ground and a site of difference: we all eat, but *what* we eat and *how* we eat can demonstrate our ethnicity, religious beliefs, gender, or social status. Food is so central to Western culture that food metaphors are used to describe every aspect of life: from Sappho's description of love as "bittersweet" to the simile "as American as apple pie." As literary critic Mary Ann Schofield argues, food can be used to transform the abstract into the concrete, to articulate things that are difficult to express; "the food rhetoric objectifies the ineffable qualities of life."[3] Literature about food has a long and rich history.

The popularity in the United States of recent nonfiction about food, such as Michael Pollan's *Omnivore's Dilemma*, Eric Schlosser's *Fast Food Nation*, and the film *Supersize Me*, indicates a growing concern about what we eat. At the same time, representations of food in literature have begun to reflect concerns about the politics of hunger, environmental threats to the source of food production, and the necessity of protecting our food sources.[4] How can we farm more sustainably? What pressures do farmers face from agribusiness? What happens to children around the world who do not have enough to eat? What would it be like to live in a radically destroyed environment? As this chapter will demonstrate, literature does not merely report (often dire) conditions of hunger, migration, and environmental damage; it has the ability to imaginatively transform, creating possibilities and celebrating alternatives. In this chapter, I will discuss five recent American novels that powerfully imagine contemporary food issues: Barbara Kingsolver's *Prodigal Summer*, Ruth Ozeki's *All Over Creation*, Cormac McCarthy's *The Road*, Dave Eggers's *What Is the What*, and Louise Murphy's *The True Story of Hansel and Gretel*. Only two of these novels—Kingsolver's and Ozeki's—could be classified "environmental novels"; thus, these novels demonstrate the importance of food as a subject in mainstream (critically acclaimed, popular) contemporary literature, not merely in environmental literature. Obviously, this list is not exhaustive, as food has become an increasingly popular topic in fiction today.[5] Each of these novels proposes that the solution to global food problems lies in creating communities of commensality, or ideal societies of nonbiological extended families in which everyone is fed. In addition to illustrating hunger, migration, and environmental damage, each of these novels figures absent mothers, yet each imagines substitutes for the traditional mother figure, signaling a need to think creatively if we wish to sustain ourselves.

At first glance, these novels seem topically unrelated; after all, what does Eggers's novel about a Sudanese "lost boy" have in common with Ozeki's narrative about an Idaho potato farmer and his estranged daughter? Yet despite the range of subject matter—postapocalyptic America, Sudanese refugees, family farming, and World War II—each novel represents food as a central motivating force, and all are permeated by anxieties of scarcity and moments of surprising abundance. Ultimately, these novels illustrate radical possibilities—some horrifying, some uplifting, some domestic, some global in scope—of what the future of food might mean.

Barbara Kingsolver has addressed environmental and political issues in all of her fictional works.[6] *Prodigal Summer* is her recent novel and the most explicit in its environmentalism. The novel weaves the stories of three sets of characters: Deanna, a middle-age wildlife biologist cut off from human society; Lusa, a young widow who inherits her new husband's farm after he tragically dies; and Garnett, an elderly widower passionate about saving the American chestnut tree. While each of these characters has a vital relationship with the natural environment, at the beginning of the novel, each character is profoundly alone. In the course of one profligate summer each character's relationship to nature beguiles them into lasting human contact: Deanna has a passionate affair with a much younger hunter, Lusa becomes a part of her late husband's rural family, and Garnett finally claims his grandchildren (and discovers the surprising charms of his combative, organic-farming neighbor). Throughout the novel, images of producing and consuming food symbolize the characters' movements toward community and wholeness.

In the sections titled "Moth Love," Lusa feels alienated from the rural farming family she has recently married into. Newly widowed after less than one year of marriage, she feels rejected by her rural in-laws. Lusa is not sure she wants to take charge of running the family farm, and she certainly doesn't want to grow tobacco, the one reliable cash crop. However, Lusa becomes more and more connected to this tightly knit extended family and to the land which was so treasured by her husband. These connections are represented, in large part, through scenes of preparing and consuming food. Many conversations occur in Lusa's kitchen as she cans fruits and vegetables from her prolific garden. Although seen by her in-laws as a citified outsider, Lusa has a natural affinity for growing things:

> Red and yellow peppers glowed like ornaments on their dark bushes, and the glossy purple eggplants had the stately look of expensive gifts. Even the onions were putting up pink globes of flower. During all the years of childhood she'd spent sprouting seeds in pots on a patio, she'd been dreaming of this.[7]

Lusa becomes an expert gardener, even develops a radical plan to raise goats that actually proves profitable, eventually earns respect from the farming community, and learns to appreciate their less-educated wisdom.

Lusa's first real relationship in this new environment is with her sister-in-law, Jewel, an exhausted single mother. Jewel's first act of intimacy is to ask Lusa to feed her two kids when she works late. Thus, Lusa's ability to grow food allows her to nurture her husband's niece and nephew: " 'I've got tomatoes put up, spaghetti sauce—maybe twenty quarts—and I'm freezing broccoli, cauliflower, you name it. Tons of corn. Your kids ate their own weight each in corn last night, by the way.' "[8] Feeding children is a primary act of nurturing in all of the novels discussed in this chapter and Lusa's care of Jewel's children incorporates her into this extended family. At the end of the novel, Lusa plans to legally adopt these children when Jewel dies of cancer. Surrogate motherhood is one of the many ways that the novel implies that inclusion and diversity are necessary to sustain an ecosystem. The novel shows how the introduction of nonnative elements, while sometimes destructive—two of the deaths in the novel may have been caused by the use of insecticides—can produce a healthier community, as when Lusa resurrects the Widener family farm.

Deanna Wolfe—whose chapters are titled Predator"—is a 47-year-old divorced wildlife biologist who lives alone in a primitive cabin high in the mountains. After her affair with a young hunter, she unexpectedly becomes pregnant. This pregnancy symbolizes the abundance of nature and challenges the separation between scientist and animal. In Kingsolver's novel, people's lives are part of the life cycle of nature. As Suzanne Jones has argued, "Kingsolver's greatest success in this novel is in helping readers to see the human and nonhuman interdependencies in an ecosystem. . . . The similarity between humans and animals that Kingsolver calls attention to here is repeated in multiple ways throughout the novel."[9] Initially, Deanna is attune to the wildlife around her and is able to accurately analyze animal scat, but unable to recognize her own body's hungers. She subsists on a minimalist diet and often forgets to eat: "[She] ate cold ravioli out of a can while she finished recording her notes. To hell with the body's cravings."[10] Deanna's physical desire for a young hunter upsets her quiet existence and proves that she is subject to natural mating laws as well: "It was the body's decision, a body with no more choice of its natural history than an orchid has, or the bee it needs."[11]

Although this bird-and-the-bees explanation of human reproduction is clichéd, Kingsolver's detailed, scientifically accurate descriptions of nature—the habits of moths' reproduction, morel growing, goat farming, and the flora and fauna of southern Appalachia—make this novel rich with the specificity of place. Just as people are described in animal terms, the natural landscape is personified, as when she describes the particular presence of the mountains in southern Appalachia:

> People in Appalachia insisted that the mountains breathed, and it was true: the steep hollow behind the farmhouse took up one long, slow inhalation every morning and let it back down through their open windows and across the fields throughout every evening—just one full, deep breath each day.[12]

Although occasionally lyrical, Kingsolver's prose does not romanticize the environment; with her background in evolutionary biology and ecology she is too knowledgeable an author to present a naïvely idealized view of the natural world. For example, Lusa realizes that the pretty honeysuckle growing on her barn must be torn down, and Deanna discovers the snake that she defended has eaten a nest of baby birds.

The title "Prodigal" clearly refers to nature's abundance, yet also recalls the biblical parable of the prodigal son who returns after squandering his inheritance and is joyously welcomed by his father. Tellingly, the prodigal son's poverty while he is away is described in terms of a lack of food. When he returns, expecting nothing, his father instead orders his servants to kill the fatted calf and prepare a feast to welcome his son home.[13] Similarly, the three main characters in Kingsolver's novel are welcomed back into the lives they once rejected: Lusa returns to the farming ways of her ancestors; Deanna becomes a mother at 47 and comes down from the mountain to join her childhood community; Garnett is reunited with the grandchildren of the son he had rejected. Each character experiences rebirth and renewal through connections to the land and human community; thus the novel suggests that if we return to earlier forms of farming, we will be welcomed with a bounteous feast. All three narratives also stress the importance of parenting, and motherhood in particular. Yet *Prodigal Summer* does not romanticize farming nor suggest a return to the traditional, nuclear family; the families established at the end of the novel are nonbiological, extended, and somewhat unconventional.

This linking of human and environmental ecosystems also occurs in Ruth Ozeki's recent novel, *All Over Creation*. Composed of an even more diverse group of characters, Ozeki's novel illustrates the struggles of beleaguered small farms and the economic pressures they face, the toxic danger of modern agribusiness practices, and the complex network of human relations involved in farming. This human ecosystem includes Lloyd Fuller, a potato farmer in Liberty Falls, Idaho; his Japanese wife, Momoko, who raises exotic plants and heirloom seeds; their estranged daughter, Yumi, and her three children; their farmer neighbors the Quinns; "The Seeds," an itinerant group of anarcho-environmental activists; a public relations man working for a corrupt agribusiness; and assorted townspeople. The narrative threads are numerous, but all of the characters finally converge, literally and figuratively, at Lloyd Fuller's farm.

All Over Creation is not as celebratory as *Prodigal Summer*; it is set in Idaho, a farming landscape that is less lush and more spare and unrelenting. The plot, although madly comical in places, can also be darker. We learn that Lloyd Fuller's prodigal daughter, Yumi, left home at 14 after getting pregnant by her high school teacher. Too afraid to tell her parents she was pregnant, Yumi was subtly coerced by her teacher into having an abortion and then was cast out by her father. When she returns years later with her three children to care for her dying father, it is clear that he still judges her decision to terminate her pregnancy (instead of seeing her as a victim). When an environmentalist describes agribusiness's plans to create a "plant [that] kills its own embryo," Lloyd replies pointedly: "A life is a life. . . . It is God's gift! How can you be so careless?"[14] This is a conservative character's view, and not necessarily the view endorsed by the novel itself. However, Yumi is portrayed as a negligent mother who is reprimanded by her neighbor, Cass Quinn, a farmer's wife who is unable to have children,

> I just think you're being a really lousy mother to them right now. They way you carry on, it's like you forget they even exist. You don't know how lucky you are, and I just can't stand to watch you treat such a blessing with such . . . such carelessness.[15]

It is hard not to read this as an anti-abortion message, when babies are likened to the precious heirloom seeds that must be protected. However, Ozeki's novel refuses easy moral judgments; every character has flaws, yet the novel treats them with compassion (even, to a small extent, Yumi's former teacher). Like *Prodigal Summer*, this novel's representation of families is inclusive; Cass finally adopts the baby of one of the environmentalists after his girlfriend dies, suggesting that unexpected alliances can be the most generative and that the best families are not always biologically determined.

All Over Creation offers a message that is similar to the one found in *Prodigal Summer*: rid the land of harmful pesticides and genetically engineered crops and preserve biodiversity. The novel shows how a coalition of traditional farmers, counterculture environmentalists, and committed gardeners can be formed. The moment of greatest community occurs during the July 4th Idaho Potato Party at Lloyd's farm when traditional farmers and hippie activists come together. Part "Be-In," part Boston tea party, and part farmers' convention, this gathering is a wonderfully utopian vision of how diverse groups might come together to take back control of the nation's agriculture. At this gathering, Lloyd gives an impassioned speech about the dangers of tampering with the natural processes of reproduction: "I have always assumed that whatever base corruptions man has inflicted upon nature, there were certain of our Maker's laws, sacred and inviolable, that even man could not breach. In this assumption we have been sadly mistaken."[16] Ozeki's novel thus warns of technology's potential for permanently destroying the environment, while also demonstrating the ways that people can change to become more responsible and knowledgeable stewards of the land.

If Ozeki's novel warns against the dangers of tampering with nature, Cormac McCarthy's Pulitzer Prize–winning novel, *The Road*, describes in horrific detail what it might be like to live on an environmentally devastated Earth. In this savage vision of the future, a nameless father and son struggle to stay alive in a post-apocalyptic American landscape. In this barren future, nothing grows, and those left alive are reduced to scavenging among the ashy ruins of the former civilization for sustenance. The rich environment of the Earth has been made "barren, silent, godless,"[17] a "cauterized terrain . . . cold [enough] to crack stones."[18] No full explanation is given of the event that destroyed the Earth, just the father's memory of "a long shear of light and then a series of low concussions [and] . . . a dull rose glow in the windowglass."[19] The few survivors exist in a primitive state of bare subsistence, many becoming bands of lawless cannibals.

Amidst this novel's grand questions of the nature of evil, the destruction of the Earth, and the possibility for human tenderness, food is the central focus of the main characters. The father and his young son travel down an endless road with little hope for survival: "Mostly he worried about their shoes. That and food. Always food."[20] All contemporary judgments about the quality of food have been leveled; in this novel all food is precious, whether it is a lone morel mushroom or a can of Coca-Cola. Food is both a relic of the lost richness of the Earth and a reminder of the civilization that has vanished. Most of all, food is evidence of the love between the father and his son, a love that separates the characters from the brutality around them.

Because the planet has been destroyed, finding food is a small, unexpected miracle. In one such scene, after witnessing unspeakable horrors, the father stumbles across a hidden bunker filled with canned food:

> Crate upon crate of canned goods. Tomatoes, peaches, beans, apricots. Canned hams. Corned beef. Hundreds of gallons of water in ten gallon plastic jerry jugs. Paper towels, toiletpaper, paper plates. Plastic trashbags stuffed with blankets. He held his forehead in his hand. Oh my God, he said.[21]

At first the boy cannot comprehend the appearance of so much food: "Why is this here? The boy said. Is it real?"[22] Because the novel so compellingly describes a world with no sustenance, these simple cans of ordinary food become miraculous to the reader as well. By putting these objects into this particular context, McCarthy has managed to transform food into the uncanny. McCarthy's prose, with its alliterative consonants, transforms this list into an incantation.

In a land where nothing grows, humans have become food to other humans. McCarthy expertly evokes human's primal fears of cannibalism. As the father and his son grow unbearably hungry, we feel the danger of others' hunger. Critic Margaret Vissers argues that the fear of cannibalism lies behind many of our elaborate food rituals:

> Somewhere at the back of our minds, carefully walled off from the ordinary consideration and discourse, lies the idea of cannibalism—that human beings might become food, eaters of each other. . . . Behind every rule of table etiquette lurks the determination of each person present to be diner, not a dish. It is one of the chief roles of etiquette to keep the lid on the violence which the meal being eaten presupposes.[23]

This threat of violence permeates McCarthy's novel, and each new encounter offers the possibility of either life-giving food, or unspeakable horrors. In one of the most horrifying moments in the novel, the father and son stumble upon a "charred human infant headless and gutted and blackening on [a] spit."[24] The scene hints that the cannibals are purposely breeding women to harvest this human crop. This gruesome scene echoes an earlier scene where the boy and his father stumble upon dried ham in an old smokehouse, which is described as "like something fetched from a tomb."[25] The similarity in the description of the infant's corpse and the ham blurs the line between carnivores and cannibals, and suggest the inherent violence involved in all meat consumption. However, the boy and his father—who are never given names in the novel—staunchly define themselves as noncannibals:

> We wouldn't ever eat anybody, would we? [The boy asks]
> No. Of course not.
> Even if we were starving?
> We're starving now.[26]

Their decision not to become cannibals sets them apart, as if they alone stay human. Critic Maggie Kilgour has argued, "'the cannibal is the individual's 'alien' against which he constructs his identity."[27] Although the father does kill to defend his son and refuses to help a child they encounter, his assertion that they will not eat people marks them as moral. Seemingly the only noncannibals alive, the father and son create a minisociety of two, "each the other's world entire."[28] We learn that the boy's mother committed suicide rather than face this horrifying new world, thus there is no maternal presence, and this seems fitting in this barren world. He and his father's refusal to eat other humans could also be read as a refusal to incorporate outsiders. In one uncharacteristic exchange, the boy insists that they help a blind man they encounter on the road and give him some of their food. Giving food to this man is this only nonviolent encounter they have with other humans until the end of the novel. Tellingly, the father and his son do not share a meal with this man; they merely give him food, since to break bread with him would imply a greater bond. It is only after the father's death that the son joins another group of survivors, thus allowing himself to be absorbed into a larger community (which includes a surrogate mother).

McCarthy's novel, although futuristic and imaginative in its depiction of brutality, seems aware that the horrors it describes are not just imaginary. In the middle of the novel, the boy is described as "something out of a deathcamp."[29] The father and son in *The Road* are survivors of a type of holocaust, and the poignancy of the father-son bond echoes Eli Wiesel's Holocaust memoir, *Night*. In both texts, the love between the fathers and sons allows them to cling to life beyond hope. Each book also ends with the death of the father and the son's entrance into a new, questionable future.[30] It is tempting to read McCarthy's novel as "speculative fiction," as an attempt to imagine the future. However, although a nuclear holocaust has not occurred, McCarthy's description of a journey through brutal violence and extreme deprivation is already occurring in parts of the world, as Dave Eggers' provocative and profoundly moving novel, *What Is the What*, shows.

Although most of the novels discussed in this chapter have been set in the United States, it is now imperative to connect national and international food issues. Dave Eggers, a noted American writer of ultrahip, writerly texts, has done just this. He has written a novel that broadens the often narrow scope of American concerns. Although classified as fiction, this novel is based on the real experiences of a Sudanese man, Valentino Achak Deng, who collaborated with Eggers[31] to describe his experiences as one of the "Lost Boys." Abruptly orphaned and entirely alone during a violent civil war, thousands of boys in southern Sudan were forced to survive alone in a hostile environment, and these boys are some of the most traumatized war victims in history.[32] Around 3,800 of these Lost Boys were relocated to the United States, and many have told their stories. Because Deng was only seven when he was forced to flee his village, and thus could not recall every, conversation or detail, he and Eggers decided to craft the novel as fiction. Eggers's ability to imaginatively recreate Deng's childhood perspective is a testament to his powers of invention and empathy, and the novel allows Western readers to identify with a character in radically different circumstances.

Separated from his parents after militiamen burn his village, Deng ventures across a hostile landscape in an extraordinary journey that, similar to McCarthy's narrative, seems almost too horrific to be borne. During the journey, the children are preyed on by soldiers, lions, landmines, militia, and even crocodiles. Like the characters in McCarthy's novel, Deng's journey becomes an effort to survive unlivable circumstances, and many of the boys he traveled with did die from violence, disease, or starvation. Even in the refugee camps (where Deng lived for 13 years), food is still scarce: people are given only one meal a day. Deng matter-of-factly describes the effects of an inadequate food supply: "We young people went to school, tried to stay awake and concentrate on one meal a day."[33] Similarly, in McCarthy's novel, we see the painful process of starvation as the father and son fail to find enough food: "The boy's candlecolored skin was all but translucent. With his great staring eyes he'd the look of an alien."[34] In both books, starvation makes the characters appear less human.

In Sudanese culture, sharing food is expected. One of the fallouts of the violent civil wars is the disruption of traditional habits of sharing food. As the boys pass through villages, they have grown so thin that they no longer look human; and some of the villagers mock them, referring to their emaciated shapes as "eggs sitting on top of twigs" and "spoons walking."[35] Strangely, even these descriptions of starvation utilize food metaphors. Still, their traditions of sharing food are so engrained that the leader of the boys asks each village chief for a meal. In one village the chief, afraid that the boys are rebels, refuses to feed them and violence ensues. During their arduous trek to the promise of safety in Ethiopia, the boys become scavengers, eating elephant meat, baby birds from nests, and whatever else they find.

Both McCarthy's and Eggers's novels contain a couple of hopeful scenes when characters find food. In *What Is the What*, Deng is temporarily taken in by a mysterious man who feeds him groundnuts from a secret hole under his carpet. As he leaves, the man gives Deng a "perfectly round and fresh" orange; and oranges become part of Deng's fantasy of the abundance he will find in Ethiopia: "As we drew closer to the border, my expectations had come to include homes for each of us, new families, tall buildings, glass, waterfalls, bowls of bright oranges set upon clean tables."[36] As one can imagine, Ethiopia proves a severe disappointment. While the boys are safer, the conditions are harsh. Even relocating to Atlanta proves hazardous, thus proving true the Dinka creation myth that choosing the unknown leads to misery.

The title of the novel comes from a Dinka creation myth in which god offers mankind a choice between a known quantity (cattle) and an unknown possibility. According to the myth, the Dinka choose the cattle, which they knew would provide them with nourishing food and which "carried something godlike within themselves."[37]

> So the first man and woman knew they would be fools to pass up the cattle for this idea of the What. So the man chose cattle. . . . [God] was testing the man, to see if he could appreciate what he had been given, if he could take pleasure in the bounty before him, rather than trade it for the unknown.[38]

This myth foreshadows Deng's descent into the "what," or the unknown, after his village is destroyed and traditional society unravels. Similar to Christian myths of the land of milk and honey, this Dinka myth centers on a stable source of food: an ideal society is one in which people are fed. As Barbara Kingsolver has argued, "The decision to attend to the health of one's habitat and food chain is a spiritual choice. It's also a political choice, a scientific one, a personal and convivial one."[39] Eggers's telling of Deng's story transforms an abstract political situation into a personal, lived experience. Eggers's novel, like McCarthy's, distills the complex social-historical problems into a clear, persistent question: who will feed this child?

The images of unprotected children in *The Road* and *What Is the What* are horrifying. Both texts represent worlds in which the parents cannot fulfill the primal act of parenthood: feeding their child and keeping him from being prey. This ultimate crime of abandoning one's child and leaving him to be cannibalized is depicted in the classic fairy tale, "Hansel and Gretel." In the original Grimm brothers' tale, a famine leads a father and mother to abandon their son and daughter in the forest. The most memorable part of the story is, of course, the children's discovery of a house made of gingerbread and candy. After gorging on this nonnutritious food, the children are taken in by a witch who attempts to cook them in her oven. Later versions of the tale change the mother into a stepmother, suggesting that the image of a mother abandoning her children was intolerable. Some critics, such as Bruno Bettelheim and Jack Zipes, have argued that the mother and the witch both represent the mother figure, a projection of a child's worst fear. Both the witch and the mother forsake their roles as nurturers and instead selfishly choose to assuage their own hunger by sacrificing the children.

Louise Murphy's novel, *The True Story of Hansel and Gretel: A Novel of War and Survival,* is a retelling of the story of Hansel and Gretel. In this novel Hansel and Gretel are the assumed names of two Jewish children who are sent into the woods of Poland by their father and stepmother to avoid capture by the Nazis during World War II. This novel modernizes the classic fairy tale, and it challenges the negative stereotype of the stepmother and the old woman. In Murphy's novel, after their parents drop them off in the woods, urging them never to reveal their identities as Jews, the children discover a tiny house in the forest. They are taken in by Magda, whom the villagers call a witch, an old woman who lives in a hut in the primeval Bialowieza forest, one of the oldest in Europe, filled with bison, wild boar, lynx, wolf, fox, and numerous bats.[40]

Magda's chapters, titled "The Witch," begin and end the novel, giving her authority in this version of the story: "The story has been told over and over by liars and it must be retold."[41] Her rustic house is not made of gingerbread; instead she feeds the children her own simple fare of wartime Poland: "potatoes and bread and . . . hot water with ground rye in it."[42] Her folk knowledge and distance from the village help save the children, who eventually are reunited with their father. In Murphy's novel, mother-figures are prevented from nurturing the children by the hardships of war, prejudice, and violence, and their deaths are not punishment but self-sacrifice. As in the original fairy tale, the children blame the stepmother for their abandonment, but the novel presents the stepmother as a more complicated figure, a pragmatic and fierce woman who ultimately proves heroic.

The most extreme revision of the original fairy tale is when the "witch's" oven becomes the children's refuge. Magda hides them inside it when the Nazis storm her house. Initially fearful, the children trust Magda and sit carefully in the hot oven, trying to keep their backs from burning on the metal sides. After the Nazis leave, the children flee the burning house and travel through the woods until they eventually are reunited with their father. As in the original fairy tale, the stepmother has died, only in Murphy's novel the reader knows that the stepmother died trying to save her stepdaughter's life.

Meanwhile, the "witch," Magda, is killed in the ovens of the concentration camp; and her gruesome death makes real the horror of the original fairy tale, in which Gretel pushes the witch into her own oven and leaves her to die: "The air was full of something that burned her skin and lungs. She kept opening her mouth and taking air in, but the air wasn't air anymore."[43]

In Murphy's novel, the oven is still a place of death, but it is also a place of maternal safety and nourishment, the womb of the surrogate mother. These double images—of the cottage's oven and the concentration camp ovens—mirror the original fairy tale's mixing of the magical and the deadly, the candy house and the cannibal. Even Murphy's prose is evocative of the fairy tale's supernaturalism, as shown in Magda's last thoughts: "Wild ponies. A kiss salted by tears. The scent of raspberry syrup in a bottle. Oranges. Two lost children who come to your house in the dark forest."[44] In this novel, particular foods, not abstract concepts of goodness or love, represent the joy of living.

In switching perspectives from child to adult, Murphy's novel shifts the original fairy tale's perspective from that of the abandoned children to the stepmother and the woman who takes them in. Both women enter into surrogate motherhood involuntarily during a time when caring for these children threatened their own lives.

The loss of the mother permeates each of the books discussed in this chapter. *Prodigal Summer* contains two sets of motherless children; *All Over Creation* contains the tragic death of a newborn's mother; in *What Is the What*, Deng is separated from his mother; in *The Road*, the mother commits suicide rather than watch her child die. These mothers' absences are profound and signal the importance of the maternal. It would be facile to read this emphasis on the material as merely symbolizing a concern for "mother Earth." Instead, I propose that each novel's imaginative representation of surrogate motherhood—Lusa feeding Jewel's children in *Prodigal Summer*; Cass adopting Charmey's baby in *All Over Creation*; the boy in *The Road* being taken in by another family; the representation of Deng's various humanitarian foster parents in *What Is the What*; as well as Magda and the stepmother's bravery in *The True Story of Hansel and Gretel*—suggests broadening the definition of motherhood to include our global responsibility to feed all children.

Literature allows readers to imagine themselves as different characters in various time periods and settings, often in a more visceral way than by reading nonfiction. Through reading these recent novels about food, we are able to experience life as a farmer, an activist, and a Sudanese refugee. For just a few days, we immerse ourselves in an alternate reality that can broaden our awareness of contemporary food issues. These novels also imagine the consequences of current food policies, and offer hopeful possibilities for solutions.

NOTES

The author is grateful for the research assistance of Morgan Bloohm.

1. Cormac McCarthy, *The Road* (New York: Vintage Books, 2006), 139.

2. Susan Bordo, *Anorexia Nervosa: Psychopathology as the Crystallization of Culture*, ed. Carole Counihan (New York: Routledge, 1997), 230.

3. Mary Anne Schofield, *Cooking By the Book* (Bowling Green: Bowling Green State University Popular Press, 1989), 2.

4. Food production has been represented in novels before, most notably in Upton Sinclair's *The Jungle* (1906), but it has not been as popular a focus as in today's novels.

5. Most notably, this chapter will not discuss the many novels that examine the gender issues of food, such as Judith Moore's *Fat Girl*, Laura Esquivel's *Like Water for Chocolate*, Tsitsi Dangarembga's *Nervous Conditions*, many novels by Margaret Atwood, and Michael Cunningham's *The Hours*.

6. Most recently, in *Animal, Vegetable, Mineral*, Kingsolver chronicles her family's year of eating locally.

7. Ibid., 374–75.

8. Ibid., 375.

9. Suzanne Jones, "The Southern Family Farm as Endangered Species: Possibilities for Survival in Barbara Kingsolver's *Prodigal Summer*," *The Southern Literary Journal* 39, no. 1 (Fall 2006): 83–97.

10. Kingsolver, 65.

11. Ibid., 24.

12. Ibid., 31.

13. *Bible* (Luke 15:11-32).

14. Ruth Ozeki, *All Over Creation* (New York: Penguin, 2003), 266–67.

15. Ibid., 390.

16. Ibid., 301.

17. Ibid., 4.

18. Ibid., 14.

19. Ibid., 52.

20. Ibid., 17.

21. Ibid, 138.

22. Ibid., 139.

23. Margaret Vissers, *The Rituals of Dinner* (New York: Penguin, 1991), 34.

24. McCarthy, *The Road*, 198.

25. Ibid., 17.

26. Ibid., 128.

27. Maggie Kilgour, *From Communion to Cannibalism* (Princeton, NJ: Princeton University Press, 1990).

28. McCarthy, *The Road*, 6.

29. Ibid., 116.

30. The end of McCarthy's novel contains many parallels to Weisel's memoir: the sons' inability to give their fathers proper burials and the son's rejection of traditional religion are contained in both.

31. Proceeds of *What Is the What* are used for Deng's college education, and the rest go to improving the lives of Sudanese.

32. Between 1983 and 2005, the civil war of Sudan killed roughly 2 million civilians and displaced 4 million. More than 200,000 children and women were enslaved, and many young boys escaped into jungles and made the long journey alone to refugee camps.

33. Dave Eggers, *What Is the What: The Autobiography of Valentino Achek Deng* (New York: Vintage, 2007), 371.

34. Ibid., 129.

35. Ibid., 143.

36. Ibid., 256.

37. Ibid., 62.

38. Ibid., 62.

39. Kingsolver, Foreword to *The Essential Agrarian Reader*, ed. Norman Wirzba (Lexington: University Press of Kentucky, 2003), xvii.

40. Bialowieski National Park, http://www.staff.amu.edu.pl/~zbzw/ph/pnp/bial.htm.

41. Louise Murphy, *The True Story of Hansel and Gretel: A Novel of War and Survival* (New York: Penguin, 2003), 1.

42. Ibid., 41.

43. Ibid., 252.

44. Ibid., 297.

RESOURCE GUIDE

Suggested Reading

Carver, Raymond. *A Small, Good Thing, Where I'm Calling From.* New York: Vintage, 1989.

Eggers, Dave. *What Is the What: The Autobiography of Valentino Achek Deng.* New York: Vintage, 2007.

Esquivel, Laura. *Like Water for Chocolate: A Novel in Monthly Installments with Recipes, Romances, and Home Remedies.* New York: Doubleday, 1992.

Gilbert, Elizabeth. *Eat, Pray, Love: One Woman's Search for Everything across Italy, India and Indonesia.* New York: Viking, 2006.

Kingsolver, Barbara. *Prodigal Summer.* New York: HarperCollins, 2000.

McCarthy, Cormac. *The Road.* New York: Vintage Books, 2006.

Moore, Judith. *Fat Girl: A True Story.* New York: Plume, 2006.

Murphy, Louise. *The True Story of Hansel and Gretel: A Novel of War and Survival.* New York: Penguin, 2003.

Ozeki, Ruth. *All Over Creation.* New York: Penguin, 2003.

Web Sites

Alimentum, The Literature of Food, http://www.alimentumjournal.com/.

College English, Special Topic: Food, http://www.ncte.org/pubs/journals/ce/contents/125133.htm.

The Guild of Food Writers, http://www.gfw.co.uk/.

PBS, The Meaning of Food, http://www.pbs.org/opb/meaningoffood/.

Research Centre for the History of Food and Drink, http://www.arts.adelaide.edu.au/centrefooddrink/.

13

Indigenous Knowledge Systems

Esther Katz

With globalization, industrial foods are now reaching even remote places in the world. Yet, the tendency to make diets more uniform throughout the planet has generated opposite movements that promote indigenous traditions of food production and consumption.

FOOD "DELOCALIZATION" AND ITS CONSEQUENCES

In the early 1980s, the anthropologists Gretel and Pertti Pelto pointed out the process of food "delocalization," the fact that food items are consumed far away from the place where they are produced.[1] The process is not new, as markets and exchanges have always existed. However, since the nineteenth century, delocalization has been expanding, along with industrialization and improvements in transportation that have led to larger, more complex distribution networks, increasing levels of migration, and the development of a money-based economy and agroindustry.

Food delocalization has been accelerating even more rapidly since the early 1980s. According to the sociologist Claude Fischler,[2] consumers who are confronted with foods they cannot easily identify (industrial foods in particular), because they have not seen them growing or being processed, suffer from what he called "gastro-anomy." Since "you are what you eat," the consumer questions his own identity. The lack of control by the consumer over food production and its origin has raised fears in recent decades, in particular with the case of Bovine Spongiform Encephalopathy (BSE, "mad cow disease"). The question of taste has also been raised, especially in Southern European countries. Fruits and vegetables, which are transported over long distances, even within the same country, are often picked green, kept in cold chambers, and matured with gas. They are far from being as tasty as fruits and vegetables that were picked ripe and consumed the same day. Efforts have been made to improve the taste of industrially produced foods, but their taste still does not compare to the taste of fresh, local food.

Gretel and Pertti Pelto showed that, in most cases, the new foods make the wealthy people's diet richer and the poor's poorer, since the new foods tend to replace—and displace—more nutritious traditional foods, thus leading to health problems, made even more serious by the reduction in physical activity. The industrial foods, in particular, usually contain more carbohydrates and fats that have dramatic consequences on the health of millions of people, causing them to be overweight or obese and leading to diabetes and cardiovascular diseases. These epidemiological problems have increased tremendously in the last two decades. The population of the United States had already been exposed to these problems before other countries. Industrial foods and drinks have been available in the United States for several decades, and most cities are designed in such a way that people use their cars for transportation instead of walking. Now, Mexico and Brazil are second and third in rank for obesity, and many countries are facing these same public health problems. In the United States, minorities with lower income are the most exposed to diseases linked to poor nutrition, in particular black Americans, Hispanics, and Native Americans. In Mexico, where the increase in the rate of such problems has been tremendous, urban populations have been more exposed than rural populations have, but obesity and diabetes have been reported in rural areas too, and even in Indian communities in recent years, sometimes linked to migration to the United States.[3]

REINVIGORATING LOCAL FOOD KNOWLEDGE SYSTEMS IN WESTERN EUROPE

At the end of the 1970s in Western Europe, several types of movements arose that became even more important in the 1990s. These movements were reactions against food uniformity and industrialisation; they drew support for their critiques from the 1992 Rio de Janeiro Convention on Biodiversity and from public response to several food scandals, such as BSE.

For example, associations and actions emerged that aimed at the promotion and conservation of biodiversity, including the Apple Munchers Association (*L'Association des Croqueurs de Pommes*). In Western Europe, there is an extensive diversity of apples and pears cultivated in individual gardens, while no more than ten varieties are widely commercialized. In 1978, when a terrible frost caused the loss of old orchards in Eastern France, an amateur gardener founded this association, as he realized that a whole heritage was at risk of disappearing. The association was composed of 6,000 voluntary members in 2005. Only 6 percent of these members have a profession linked to agriculture or fruit tree cultivation, but most do engage in cultivating at least one local variety of fruit tree in their region. The association is based on voluntary work. It organizes free courses on fruit tree cultivation, promotes agricultural trade shows and events, publishes technical bulletins, diffuses information on the risks of genetic erosion and the conservation of fruit tree biodiversity, and has contributed to the creation of conservatory orchards (*vergers conservatoires*).[4]

A few marginal farmers affiliated with the Farming Seed Network (*Réseau Semences Paysannes*) are reviving the cultivation of old varieties of wheat that they produce organically and process and sell locally (as "baker-farmers"). They exchange seeds and agricultural knowledge through this network, which includes old farmers who have retained some of this knowledge, farmers who experiment with the cultivation of different varieties of wheat, and scientists. They oppose the French law that does not allow the commercialization of seeds and plant varieties not registered in the "Common Catalogue of Varieties of Agricultural Plant Species." They lobby for the preservation of agrobiodiversity and for a change in the legislation.[5]

The Slow Food® association also promotes food biodiversity, which describes itself as

> a non-profit, eco-gastronomic member-supported organization that was founded in Italy in 1989 to counteract fast food and fast life, the disappearance of local food traditions and people's dwindling interest in the food they eat, where it comes from, how it tastes and how our food choices affect the rest of the world.[6]

It calls upon people to "rediscover the flavors and savors of regional cooking and banish the degrading effects of *Fast Food*."[7] Its forerunner organization, Arcigola, was created in 1986 to resist the opening of a MacDonald's fast-food restaurant in the historical city center of Rome. Today, it has more than 85,000 members in 132 countries. An office was opened in 2000 in the United States. The last Terra Madre (Mother Earth) Slow Food festival occurred in Brazil in 2007. Globally, Slow Food promotes local artisans, local farmers, and local flavors through regional events such as *Taste Workshops*, wine tastings, and farmers markets. It promotes taste education and informs citizens about the risks of fast food, monoculture, and reliance on too few varieties and about the drawbacks of commercial agribusiness. It lobbies for the inclusion of organic farming concerns within agricultural policy and against the use of pesticides and genetic engineering. It encourages ethical buying in local marketplaces. Slow Food created the University of Gastronomic Sciences in northern Italy. Slow Food instituted two types of labels for outstanding food products: the Ark of Taste (to safeguard biodiversity, like Noah's Ark) and the presidia. Since the Slow Food association has grown so large, some people now criticize it. They claim that Slow Food is no longer representative of local people and that its main goal has shifted to self-promotion.[8]

The use of Geographical Indications, more familiarly known as labels of origin (*appellations d'origine*), is reinvigorating local food production and knowledge systems.[9] These labels, which originated in France at the beginning of the twentieth century from a law against origin fraud, were adopted by the European Union in 1992 and drew the interest of non-European countries after the Convention on Biological Diversity was signed. The primary aim of the 1905 law was to protect the production and commercialization of wines and liquors. It was established, for instance, that a Champagne wine could only be produced in the region of Champagne and other sparkly wines should be designated by another name. The labels of origin were later applied to cheese, meat products, and other food productions.

Although labels of origin are legislated by state governments, European food producers have a hand in the process of designation. A producers' union has to request that their product be labeled, and they have to define the characteristics of their product: its area of production, the type of production system (that has implications for the landscape), the traditional knowledge involved in its production and processing, and its characteristics and gustative qualities. The producers' request goes through a heavy bureaucratic process, involving research and taste panels representing the interests of the consumers. The certification requirement (*cahier des charges*) of the product is a result of a consensus between the producers and the other stakeholders. In France and other European countries, labels of origin have contributed to the preservation of rural heritage and the maintenance of agricultural landscapes. They enhanced local identities. They helped to maintain agricultural profitability in zones considered to be marginal, both through production and tourism. They helped traditional products remain in production, when they might have disappeared otherwise, thus preserving food diversity.[10]

The 1992 Convention on Biological Diversity declared that local communities and farmers should be granted specific rights to the genetic resources that they have developed. Several countries have found Geographical Indications a good tool to protect biodiversity, because it does not apply to the protection of a specific form of indigenous knowledge linked to the use of resources—which could grant rights to an ethnic group or a local community whose status would be difficult to define—but rather applies it to actual products linked to a territory.[11] So far, in Mexico and Brazil, it has mainly been applied to agricultural products that are not in the hands of small farmers, such as coffee, wines, and liquors. The Brazilian Ministry of Agriculture is now trying to identify regional small-scale production items for which this type of certification would be appropriate. So far, this action by the ministry is totally unknown to producers and does not appear to consider the cultural aspects of the knowledge systems. In Mexico, the label of origin was granted to tequila as early as 1974. A recent study showed that the labeling has had rather negative impacts on the sustainability of production and on the economy of small farmers.[12]

REINVIGORATING LOCAL FOOD KNOWLEDGE SYSTEMS ON THE AMERICAN CONTINENT

In the United States, Native American associations have been trying to rejuvenate their traditional knowledge systems to return to better health and nutrition. Across the continent, First Nations have raised their voices, especially since the 1980s, but the phenomenon of promoting local knowledge and culinary heritage has occurred mainly in places where it had been lost.

The nutritional status of Native Americans is dire in most American countries, including industrial countries like the United States and Canada, where poor nutrition and its consequences (obesity and diabetes) are serious problems.[13]

In Mexico and the Andes, the best lands were taken by the colonizers, while indigenous populations remained in the steepest or highest lands, with a limited access to permanent land tenure rights. They are struck by poverty in a higher proportion than nonindigenous and often suffer malnutrition.[14] Nevertheless, they have retained a rich knowledge of their environment and, in particular, a rich agricultural knowledge. Both areas are centers of plant domestication and diversification. Mexico is known for its diversity in maize, beans, and chili pepper, and the Andes is known for its maize and potatoes and indigenous plants such *quinoa, kiwicha, oca,* and *ullucu*. The nutritional value of these plants has been rediscovered; *quinoa*, for instance, is now widely exported, and Peruvian chefs are creating elaborate dishes with Andean products in a *Nouvelle Cuisine* style, called *Cocina novo-andina*.

In Mexico, indigenous people's food is often seen as poor people's food or abominable food—since they consume insects—but the national cuisine is actually based on indigenous diet. Corn tortillas, beans, and chilli pepper are the core of the diet of all Mexican people. These are the basic foods of Indian and *mestizo* farmers and lower-income people, but they also are present in the meals of most middle-class people, although the middle-class diet may be richer or include more meat.[15] Indigenous festive foods, such as meat cooked in earth ovens (*barbacoa*), *mole* (a thick chilli pepper sauce usually served with meat), or *tamales* (steamed corn dough often stuffed with meat and chilli pepper sauce) are also national festive foods. Because they are appreciated all over the country, they are still commonly eaten.[16] In a protest against the establishment of a MacDonald's fast-food restaurant in the center of the colonial city of Oaxaca in 2003, local people chose to counteract this symbol of North American capitalism and poor nutrition by an "orgy of *tamales*," representing tasty food and Mexican heritage.[17]

It does not seem that indigenous people are otherwise trying to promote their local food, but they have not lost it yet. The North American Free Trade Agreement (NAFTA), which was signed in 1992 between the United States, Canada, and Mexico, has had negative impacts on Mexican agriculture, as more North American products are being imported. Many Mexican indigenous and nonindigenous farmers have been migrating to the United States. Remittances sent by migrants from the United States are inducing change in food habits: rural people are eating more imported corn and beans, more meat, more industrial products, and fewer wild greens and locally grown fruit and vegetables.[18] Emigration may lead to a loss of local agricultural knowledge and biodiversity. In Mexican cities, about 10 years ago, hot dogs, pizzas, and hamburgers started to replace *tacos* and *tamales* in street food stands. Poor nutrition has become a more serious public health problem than malnutrition. In these conditions, movements for the reinvigoration of healthy local food products are likely to appear.

In the Amazon, natural resources are usually more abundant than in the highlands, and population density is much lower. In some areas, people may suffer hunger, but on the whole, local populations are better off than in the mountainous areas. Fishing and hunting contribute much larger portions of the people's diet than in Mexico or the Andes, where consumption of animal proteins is fairly low. Many wild plants are available, and agricultural diversity is high, especially for fruit trees. In the multiethnic region of the Middle Rio Negro, for instance, about one hundred food plant species have been reported, including seventy-five varieties of cassava and different varieties of chilli pepper, pineapple, and yams.[19] A nutritional research study in 2004 in an Awajun (Aguaruna) community in Peru demonstrated that this Indian population had a satisfactory diet, based on the exploitation of natural resources. Their diet was composed of boiled or grilled sweet cassava, plantain, peach palm, tubers, greens, mushrooms, insects, eggs, meat and fish, lightly fermented drinks of cassava, plantain or peach palm, as well as palm hearts and many fruits. They consumed only minimal quantities of purchased foods (less than 1 percent). In those Awajun communities where rice monocropping was practiced and had partly displaced traditional agriculture, an overall decrease in diet quality was observed.[20] In forest communities of the Rio Negro, the quality of the diet may be compared to that of the Awajun. It is mainly based on fish and bitter cassava products. Chilli pepper, tubers, peach palm, and other palm fruits are often consumed as well as many other fruit species, insects, river turtles, and game. People have easier access to outside food than the Awajun do, but they do not often purchase it, and they consume more on weekends or at festivals. It does not really threaten the local diet yet.[21]

The situation is different in towns of the same region. Presently, according to the national statistics, about 65 percent of the population of the Brazilian Amazon is urban.[22] The population of the regional towns doubled or tripled in the last 15 years. Many people used to fish for an hour or two in the late afternoon, but now they do not find fish easily, so fishing is more in the hands of professional or semiprofessional fishermen who have to go farther to find fish. Agriculture is still practiced around the urban areas, but not every family has members engaged in this activity. Because agricultural products are rarely traded but rather exchanged, families who do not have members practicing agriculture and are short of time when involved in a salary work have a more limited access to fruit and tubers. They tend to purchase more outside food such as rice and beans, which are culti- vated thousands of miles away in the south of the country, as well as pasta, canned fish and meat, salted beef, frozen chicken, bread, butter, and coffee, that is, food items of much lower nutritional quality. Moreover, urban dwellers have access to television and have often been educated in the Catholic missionary schools where they got used to "white people's food." Therefore, they place a higher value on this food and consume it on festive occasions.[23] This situation has not yet induced a movement to reappropriate local knowledge systems, because these systems are still alive, but it has raised concerns among some inhabitants who long for foods they used to eat more often. The local indigenous associations are interested in applying to a registration of the local agricultural knowledge (including food knowledge) as part of the intangible heritage at the National Institute of the Historical and Artistic Heritage (IPHAN).[24] This heritage label, in the food domain, has so far been applied to the knowledge of processing certain food products, such as Bahian *acarajé*, but not yet to a whole agricultural and food system.

Other societies in the Amazon have lost part of their knowledge and their tra- ditional diet. This is the case of the Xavante Indians of the Mato Grosso, who suf- fered a drastic change in food production and consumption in the seventies. They passed from horticulture, hunting, and gathering to rice cultivation. By stopping hunting and gathering, they dramatically reduced both their physical activity and the consumption of a great variety of wild plants. On the other hand, they increased their consumption of fat (with industrial oil) and carbohydrates (with locally cultivated rice and industrial sugar). According to a nutritional study con- ducted in the 1990s, the rates of overweight people, obesity, and diabetes were high in the communities that had gone through these changes in their subsist- ence.[25] Some nongovernmental organizations (NGOs) and scientists are now working with these communities to recuperate their sweet potato varieties and their edible wild plants.

In southern temperate Brazil, the situation of the Guarani Indians is even more dramatic. Their lands have been encroached upon by cattle raisers and soybean producers. Their ancestral territories have been deforested, they often do not have enough land to cultivate, and they have lost varieties of corn, peanuts, and other food plants. Several Guarani groups now live on food aid from the state. It is obvious that, in these precarious conditions, they are struggling just to survive and to recuperate their lands. The reviving of their food knowledge depends on their access to land.[26]

Throughout the United States, in the last half of the twentieth century, indigenous food systems went through drastic changes. The effects of the destruction of an indigenous food system cannot be seen more clearly than in the case of the Tohono O'odham (Papago) community. We draw substantially on an article by Tristan Reader about this community's nutritional situation and their action to rejuvenate their traditional food system.[27]

The Tohono O'odham, whose name means the "Desert People," have lived for centuries in the Sonoran Desert of Arizona and Mexico. Over countless generations their seminomadic ancestors depended upon customary subsistence practices of dryland farming, food storage, and harvesting the wild plants and animals to support their families in this arid environment. This way of life successfully sustained them as late as the 1920s when they were still farming over 10,000 acres using indigenous agricultural methods. According to Gary Nabhan, in his book *The Desert Smells like Rain*, from the 1920s the number of acres farmed using traditional techniques rapidly declined to 2,500 acres in 1949 to fewer than 100 acres today.[28] At the same time, the Tohono O'odham also abandoned their customary foraging and food storage practices.

The loss of their indigenous food system has had devastating consequences for the health of contemporary Tohono O'odham people. Traditional desert foods like tepary beans, mesquite beans, cactus buds, and chia seeds, which scientific studies have shown help regulate blood sugar levels, are no longer consumed. As they began to rely on federal food aid programs and processed food, their rates of adult-onset diabetes skyrocketed. Today, at a rate of over 50 percent of the population, they have the tragic distinction of being the people with the highest incidence in the world of this debilitating disease.

These changes in diet and subsistence base are correlated with destructive changes in their culture. Because Tohono O'odham culture is intricately intertwined with their subsistence practice, the decline of the latter has led to the loss of language, ceremonies, and ancient knowledge. The decline of the saguaro harvest and wine ceremony, a ceremony that brought forth the rain that made traditional agriculture possible, is a direct result of the Tohono O'odham people's loss of a traditional local food system. As Tristan Reader, codirector of Tohono O'odham Community Action, notes regretfully, "there is no longer a reason to learn the songs which bring down the rain, no reason to bless the ground . . . no reason for a key element of Tohono O'odham culture to continue."[29]

This pattern of the loss of traditional foods, subsistence, and culture to be correlated with declines in health status is not uncommon in indigenous communities throughout the United States. Encouragingly, many Native people in the United States, including the Tohono O'odham, are developing programs to "rejuvenate" traditional food systems. For example, the Tohono O'odham Community Food System, in conjunction with Tohono O'odham Community Action and various individuals, families, and organizations within the community, has begun to develop a program that builds upon the traditional agrifood system with new organizational forms. Their projects include: (1) establishing community gardens where traditional crops, farming methods, and traditions can be relearned and taught to the next generation, (2) supporting programs to help families grow traditional crops in their own gardens, (3) organizing trips to collect traditional wild foods and teach about their use, (4) "revitalizing" ancient flood plain fields, (5) sponsoring cultural events based upon traditional food practices, and (6) developing markets to distribute traditional foods to local people and others. The various levels of these projects—from private family actions, to small enterprises and community institutions such as schools, hospitals, and elder care—provide various entry points into a renewal process that Tristan Reader states is intended to nurture "body and spirit for generations."[30]

The Tohono O'odham Community Association is a member of the Indigenous Seed Sovereignty Network. This is a network of organizations that includes the Traditional Native American Farmers Association, Tsyunhehkwa Project at Oneida,[31] New Mexico Acequia Association,[32] Tesuque Pueblo, White Earth Land Recovery Project, and Native Hawaiian Farmers. Like the European associations described above, these organizations have been inspired by a growing worldwide movement, active in India and Bangladesh and other places, for food and seed sovereignty based on culturally and ecologically sustainable agriculture.[33]

Together, the associations of this network "are broadening and enriching their discussions related to traditional foods, diabetes, and community food systems."[34] They are working to restore traditional food knowledge and to create local food economies on the basis of traditional agricultural methods and seeds. They oppose efforts to genetically modify their traditional crops actively and the biopiracy of medicinal and other plants. According to Native Harvest, "From rescue of traditional corn and squash varieties and food preservation techniques at Oneida to broad-based political campaigns in the New Mexico State Legislature, to ongoing programs with our youth and elders, the Network is taking a leading role in preparing for truly sustainable local food economies."[35]

One of the most visible associations of this network is the Traditional Native American Farmers Association (TNAFA). Based in New Mexico, it also develops projects outside of the United States with Mayan Indians of Belize. The aim of TNAFA is "revitalizing traditional agriculture for spiritual and human need."[36] TNAFA members believe that "family oriented farming is the best approach in developing a sound future in agriculture, which has always been at the heart of the community's economy."[37] They encourage farmers to go back to the land and farm organically, using traditional methods. They provide training in permaculture, organic farming, and traditional seed saving and develop educational programs that demonstrate sustainable agricultural methods and the threats of GMO (genetically modified organisms) to native seeds.[38] TNAFA was established in 1992 with the help of the Native Seeds/Search (NSS) association, based in Tucson, Arizona, and acting in the southwestern United States and northwestern Mexico. NSS aims to preserve the crop genetic diversity of the region, through both *ex situ* (a regional seed bank) and *in situ* conservation programs, and it promotes the recuperation of lost varieties through their free exchange. At the regional level, NSS links scientists, indigenous and nonindigenous gardeners and farmers, and other associations such as the Tohono O'odham Community Association and TNAFA.

CONCLUSION

Through this short panorama of traditional food revival in Europe and America, we have seen that globalization is leading to the same types of problems around the world with the loss of local varieties of plants and constantly increasing consumption of less-nutritious "delocalized" and industrial foods. People have to confront the growing importance of GMO and seeds produced by large multinational companies. Unfortunately, in spite of supposedly promoting the conservation of genetic resources, some governments do not permit the free cultivation, circulation, and exchange of native seeds. The civil society, cultivators, and even amateur gardeners are essential for conserving food biodiversity. The role of scientists in demonstrating the importance of traditional knowledge and supporting these actions is crucial, too. On the American continent, indigenous people are holding rich knowledge on the environment and agrobiodiversity. As minorities, they have often suffered from the loss of land and poverty and from a lower status in the national societies. In the United States in particular, these groups are losing traditional ways of subsistence, which has led to dramatic increases in nutritional and health problems. Over the last decades, on the whole continent, indigenous people's associations have been taking strength, exchanging experiences, and reviving their traditional knowledge. Their actions are not only for themselves but for humanity as a whole.

NOTES

1. Gretel Pelto and Pertti Pelto, "Diet and Delocalization: Dietary Change since 1750," *Journal of Interdisciplinary History* 14 (1983): 507–28.

2. Claude Fischler, *L'Homnivore* (Paris: Odile Jacob, 1990).

3. G. Olaiz et al., eds., *Encuesta Nacional de Salud y Nutrición 2006* (México: Instituto Nacional de Salud Pública/Secretaria de Salud, 2006); Miriam Bertran, *Cambio Alimentario e Identidad de los Indígenas Mexicanos* (México: Universidad Nacional Autónoma de México, 2005).

4. Les Croqueurs de Pommes, http://www.croqueurs-de-pommes.asso.fr/ (accessed January 30, 2009); Claude Scribe, "*Les Croqueurs de Pommes* (Apple Munchers Association)," in *Biodiversity and Local Ecological Knowledge in France*, ed. Laurence Bérard et al. (Paris: INRA/CIRAD/IDDRI/IFB, 2005), 138–40.

5. Réseau Semences Paysannes, www.semencespaysannes.org/ (accessed January 30, 2009); Élise Demeulenaere, "Préface. Initiatives paysannes autour de la semence de blé: De la réhabilitation des variétés anciennes à la pratique collective d'une sélection paysanne," in *Voyage autour des blés paysans* (Réseau Semences Paysannes, 2008), 4–13; Guy Kastler, "The *Réseau Semences Paysannes* (Farming Seed Network)," in *Biodiversity and Local Ecological Knowledge*, 148–50.

6. Slow Food, http://www.slowfood.com/ (accessed January 29, 2009).

7. Ibid.

8. Slow Food, http://www.slowfood.com/; Wikipedia, "Slow Food," http://en.wikipedia.org/wiki/Slow_Food#cite_note-4; Didier Chabrol, "Slow Food: Protecting and Promoting Taste," in *Biodiversity and Local Ecological Knowledge*, 209–212.

9. "A geographical indication is a sign used on goods that have a specific geographical origin and possess qualities or a reputation that are due to that place of origin. Most commonly, a geographical indication consists of the name of the place of origin of the goods. Agricultural products typically have qualities that derive from their place of production and are influenced by specific local factors, such as climate and soil. Whether a sign functions as a geographical indication is a matter of national law and consumer perception. Geographical indications may be used for a wide variety of agricultural products." World Intellectual Property Organization (WIPO), http://www.wipo.int/geo_indications/en/about.html (accessed January 24, 2009).

10. François Roncin, "The Birth of a Protection and Promotion Policy: The INAO Experience," in *Biodiversity and Local Ecological Knowledge*, 175–80; Elisabeth Barham, "Translating *Terroir*: The Global Challenge of French AOC Labeling," *Journal of Rural Studies* 19 (2003): 127–38.

11. Valérie Boisvert, "International Protection of GIs: Challenges and Opportunities for Southern Countries," in *Biodiversity and Local Ecological Knowledge*, 229–35.

12. Sarah Bowen and Ana Valenzuela Zapata, "Geographical Indications, *Terroir*, and Socio-Economic and Ecological Sustainability: The Case of Tequila," *Journal of Rural Studies* 25 (2009): 108–119.

13. Harriet V. Kuhnlein and Olivier Receveur, "Dietary Change and Traditional Food Systems of Indigenous People," *Annual Review of Nutrition* 16 (1996): 417–42.

14. Bertran, *Cambio Alimentario*.

15. Esther Katz, "Tortillas, haricots et sauce piquante: l'alimentation au Mexique," *Savoirs Partagés* (Agropolis Muséum, Montpellier, 2004), http://museum.agropolis.fr/ (accessed January 30, 2009).

16. Esther Katz, "Alimentação indígena na América Latina: Comida invisível, comida de pobres ou patrimônio culinário?" *Mesa Redonda 13, A Comida e o comer na sociedade contemporânea: desigualdade, diversidade e diferença*, (26th Reunião Brasileira de Antropologia [RBA], Porto Seguro, Bahia, Brazil, June 1–4, 2008), http://www.abant.org.br/.

17. UITA, "El camino correcto. Pobladores de Oaxaca protestan contra MacDonald's con orgía de tamales" (UITA, Montevideo, August 28, 2002), http://www.rel-uita.org/old/companias/mac%20donald/mexico.htm (accessed January 30, 2009).

18. Esther Katz, "Emigration, mutations sociales et changements culinaires dans le haut pays mixtèque (Oaxaca, Mexique)," *Anthropology of Food* S4, *Modèles alimentaires et recompositions sociales en Amérique Latine* (2008), http://aof.revues.org/ (accessed January 30, 2009).

19. Laure Emperaire et al., "Diversité agricole et patrimoine sur le Moyen Rio Negro" (Paris: Actes du Bureau des Ressources Génétiques 7, 2008), 139–53.

20. M. L. Roche, H. M. Creed-Kanashiro, I. Tuesta, and H. V. Kuhnlein, "Traditional Food System Provides Dietary Quality for the Awajun in the Peruvian Amazon," *Ecology of Food and Nutrition* 46, no. 5 (2007): 377–99.

21. Esther Katz, fieldnotes, 2007–2009.

22. Instituto Brasileiro de Geografia e Estatística, www.ibge.gov.br.

23. Esther Katz, fieldnotes, 2007–2009; Katz, "Emigration, mutations sociales"; Ludivine Eloy, "Diversité alimentaire et urbanisation: le rôle des mobilités circulaires des amérindiens dans le Nord-Ouest amazonien," *Anthropology of Food* S4, *Modèles alimentaires et recompositions sociales en Amérique Latine* (2008), http://aof.revues.org/.

24. Laure Emperaire, Lucia van Velthem, and Ana Gita de Oliveira, "Patrimônio cultural immaterial e sistema agrícola: o manejo da diversidade agrícola no médio Rio Negro, Amazonas" (26th Reunião de Antropologia [RBA], Porto Seguro, Bahia, Brazil, June 1–4, 2008), http://www.abant.org.br/ (accessed January 30, 2009).

25. Sílvia Gugelmin and Ricardo Ventura Santos, "Ecologia humana e antropometria nutricional de adultos Xavánte, Mato Grosso, Brasil," *Cadernos de Saúde Pública* 17, no. 2 (2001): 313–22.

26. Sylvia Bahri, personal communication, 2008; Martin Tempass, "A Distribucão de 'Cestas Básicas' para Os Mbyá-Guarani: Impactos e Representacões" (26th Reunião Brasileira de Antropologia [RBA], Porto Seguro, Bahia, Brazil, June 1–4, 2008), http://www.abant.org.br/ (accessed January 30, 2009).

27. Tristan Reader, "Reviving Native Foods, Health, and Culture: The Tohono O'odham Community Food System," Oxfam America, February 3, 2003, http://www.oxfamamerica.org/whatwedo/where_we_work/united_states/news_publications/art4144.html (accessed January 30, 2009).

28. Gary Paul Nabhan, *The Desert Smells like Rain: A Naturalist in O'odham Country* (Tucson: University of Arizona Press, 2002).

29. Reader, "Reviving Native Foods."

30. Ibid.

31. Association of the Oneida Indians of Wisconsin. In the Oneida language, *Tsyunhehkwa* means "life sustenance." The white corn is very important in their culture. Tsyunhehkwa, http://www.oneidanation.org/tsyunhehkwa/.

32. New Mexico Acequia Association, http://www.lasacequias.org/2006/12/.

33. See Navdanya, founded by Vandana Shiva, an Indian scientist and a prominent figure in the alter-globalization movement. "Navdanya is actively involved in the rejuvenation of indigenous knowledge and culture. It has created awareness on the hazards of genetic engineering, defended people's knowledge from biopiracy and food rights in the face of globalization." (http://navdanya.org/ [accessed January 30, 2009]).

34. Native Harvest, http://nativeharvest.com/node/244.

35. Ibid.

36. Native Harvest, "Traditional Native American Farmers' Association," http://nativeharvest.com/tnafa.

37. Ibid.

38. Ibid.

RESOURCE GUIDE

Suggested Reading

Bérard, Laurence, et al. *Biodiversity and Local Ecological Knowledge in France*. Paris: INRA/CIRAD/IDDRI/IFB, 2005.

Kuhnlein, Harriet V., and Olivier Receveur. "Dietary Change and Traditional Food Systems of Indigenous People." *Annual Review of Nutrition* 16 (1996): 417–42.

Lentz, Carola. "Changing Food Habits: An Introduction." *Food and Foodways* 5, no. 1 (1991): 1–13.

Nabhan, Gary Paul. *The Desert Smells like Rain: A Naturalist in O'odham Country*. Tucson: University of Arizona Press, 2002.

Pelto, Gretel, and Pertti Pelto. "Diet and Delocalization: Dietary Change since 1750." *Journal of Interdisciplinary History* 14 (1983): 507–28.

Reader, Tristan. "Reviving Native Foods, Health, and Culture: the Tohono O'odham Community Food System." Oxfam America, February 3, 2003. Available at http://www.oxfamamerica.org/whatwedo/where_we_work/united_states/news_publications/art4144.html.

Shiva, Vandana. *Stolen Harvest: The Highjacking of the Global Food Supply*. Cambridge, MA: South End Press, 2000.

PART III

Ethics

14

Food Security: Three Conceptions of Access—Charity, Rights, and Coresponsibility

Lisa Heldke

What does it mean for a community to guarantee all members—of every bodily configuration, economic position, race, ethnicity, and religion—access to genuinely adequate food—food that meets not only each person's daily nutritional requirements, but also their cultural, religious, environmental, and other commitments? In the United States, more than 10 percent of the population experiences "low" or "very low" food security. Among African American and Latino households, and households with children headed by a woman, those percentages climb; more than 30 percent of woman-headed households and more than 20 percent of African American households experience some level of food insecurity at some point during the year each year.[1] While the United States does not experience mass starvation or other, more dramatic forms of hunger, lack of access to food is a deep, prevalent, and serious threat to the health and well-being of the population as a whole, and of children in particular. This chapter examines the question from the perspective of three different social paradigms or frameworks, which I label "charity," "human rights," and "coresponsibility."

When access to food is considered in the contemporary United States, obstacles to adequate access are usually presumed to be economic; people do not have the food they need and want because they are poor or economically struggling. When I discuss the concept of access in this chapter, my focus is much broader; I mean it to include the particular kinds of obstacles or challenges faced by persons with disabilities; persons of minority faiths, races, and ethnicities; persons with allergies or sensitivities; and persons with particular moral, ethical, or nutritional commitments. Indeed, my understanding of access is intended to draw attention to the fact that *each of us* encounters such systematic obstacles to access, and would do well to understand our needs and wants as intimately related to those of other community members. Access, in short, is something that concerns us all. I contend that attending to these other kinds of access will create a deeper, more robust sense of genuine food justice, by linking people's interests together and challenging the "us/them" thinking that prevails whenever we conceive of access as a problem or concern only for those on the margins of society.

In this chapter, I ask how each of the three paradigms conceptualizes access. The first two—charity and rights—are familiar and are invoked daily, for example, on the pages of newspapers in the United States. More specifically, the rights paradigm conceptually undergirds "antipoverty" or "antihunger" models of food access. Despite some obvious advantages the rights paradigm holds over charity, I will argue that the two are actually linked in a way that makes rights an inadequate framework for developing a robustly just notion of accessibility. The third paradigm is my own invention.[2] I believe it offers the best way to conceptualize access, "best" in the sense that it is most able to promote genuine social justice by conceptually linking the needs and interests of persons from across societies. I will ultimately suggest that this paradigm provides some much-needed conceptual undergirding for an alternative movement for adequate food access, namely, the community food security (CFS) movement.[3]

DISABILITY AND FOOD INSECURITY

Before examining the paradigms, I define two other terms that provide important background for my discussion here, namely, "disability" and "food insecurity." Accessibility is often understood as that which mitigates disability; I am interested in thinking about how the concept of disability can help conceive food insecurity. To be disabled means that one cannot, in the words of disability theorist Susan Wendell, "perform activities to an extent or in a way that is either necessary for survival in an environment or necessary to participate in some major aspect of life in a given society."[4] By extension, one is food insecure when one's diet specifically leaves one unable to "perform activities to an extent or in a way that is either necessary for survival in an environment or necessary to participate in some major aspect of life in a given society." Borrowing and modifying Wendell's definition illuminates conceptual ties between these two kinds of circumstances; it also invites us to reflect on the concrete and practical ties that exist between disability and food insecurity.

A note is in order here about my choice to speak of food insecurity, rather than poverty. The U.S. Department of Agriculture has come under criticism for its decision to replace the word "hunger" with the expression "extremely low food security," an expression that critics believe "sugarcoat[s] a national shame."[5] I may seem guilty of a similar sugarcoating, in choosing not to pair hunger (or perhaps poverty) with disability. Each of these terms—hunger and food insecurity—acts as a magnet or lens, to draw our attention to different phenomena in a society and to link them via different features. Neither term should be seen as a replacement for the other; rather, they serve as complementary or overlapping forms of analysis, both of which can usefully be employed to illustrate different aspects of the relevant terrain. Hunger focuses our attention on economic inequality. I focus on food insecurity because I am interested in paying attention to the diversity of forms food insecurity can take—including forms that are experienced even by people of considerable economic means, such as access to safe food, or culturally appropriate food (in the case of cultural minorities). I do so to disrupt the "us versus them" dynamic that too often characterizes discussions about access, especially when those discussions are framed in terms of charity or rights. To see these different kinds of insecurity as related to each other in significant ways need *not* blunt the impact of the problem of "real hunger," but might instead create links of solidarity among persons across the economic spectrum, as they come to understand their own food vulnerabilities as part of a network that leaves all at risk in one way or another.

THE THREE PARADIGMS

In examining each paradigm, I consider the following questions: (1) What are the key principles upon which each is built? (2) How are persons conceived on this paradigm? (3) How do we understand access on this paradigm—that is, how does this paradigm secure for everyone the ability to perform duties or participate in major aspects of society? (4) What are the limitations of this paradigm, specifically with respect to the matter of access for disabled or food-insecure persons? Ultimately, I will argue that rights and charity paradigms *share* what is known as an "atomistic" (i.e., individualistic and self-contained) conception of personhood; a conception that does not work, whether it is being applied to the issue of disability or to food insecurity. The coresponsible paradigm, by contrast, understands persons *relationally*. Thus, this paradigm enables us to see relationships *among* different forms of marginalization (such as disability and food insecurity) and also to understand various forms of food insecurity as interrelated. The net result is a conception of access that is more useful for, and more productive of, deep and broad justice.

Paradigm 1: Charity

According to an everyday understanding of the concept, charity is voluntary, though some givers might understand themselves to be morally obligated (e.g., by religion) to provide for those "less fortunate." On a charity paradigm, regardless of the obligations *givers* may have, *recipients* are not morally entitled to what they receive. The appropriate response to charity from recipients is gratitude for the benevolence of others.

A hierarchical relation holds between benefactors and recipients; recipients are beholden (and thus often considered morally inferior) to their benefactors. Individuals may be morally motivated by altruism (a moral position in which one acts without regard to the benefits one may accrue) or egoism (a position on which all moral actions are understood to benefit the actor, either directly or indirectly). Egoism and altruism are here understood as polar opposites of each other, such that the presence of one motivation "dilutes" the other; charity is the ultimate altruism. On a charity paradigm, the moral worth of an action is tainted if one acts in the hopes of benefiting from it.

The charity paradigm tends to treat conditions like poverty and disability as individual misfortunes that simply befall some unlucky people. No structural or systemic injustice calls for redress; only accident, bad luck, or moral laxity leaves some persons unable to "do for themselves." Because these misfortunes are in no way the fault of society, it is not the responsibility of society to fix them. The choice of individuals or organizations in society to do so is *supererogatory*—above and beyond any reasonable call of duty.

Access

Given such an understanding of disability and food insecurity, the concept of *access* does not really belong in the vocabulary of the paradigm. To speak of access presumes persons are *entitled* to goods or services, but this is just what the charity model does *not* grant to everyone. The charity model tends to clump those unable to provide for themselves into two groups: the "deserving" and the "undeserving." The former are given *gifts* (not entitlements) to meet basic needs; the undeserving are left to fend for themselves—or are helped by the feckless, by those who are just too good for their own good, or (in some societies) by the government.

Recalling Wendell's definition of disability, we might observe that, in a just state, it is particularly the "major aspects of life" to which all members ought to have adequate access. The charity model could acknowledge the existence of such aspects, but it recognizes no particular *right* to participate in them, and decidedly no societal *obligation* for other members to enable you to exercise your right to participate. On the charity paradigm, disability and food insecurity are individual misfortunes that it is not the job of society to redress.[6] It is your problem—and any loss society may experience because of your inability to participate goes unmentioned.

Rather than access, the charity paradigm posits that disabled persons have "special needs," where the meaning of "special" is defined against an often-unstated conception of "normal" personhood and of the "normal" responsibilities of a community. (Normal people ambulate with their own legs, for instance.) Others in the community have a "charitable duty" (or "opportunity") to meet those needs (by providing transportation for those who cannot walk). Poor people also have "special needs" that arise because they happen not to have money. Charitable workers help them out of their own goodness. They hope that "the poor" are *also* "good" and therefore deserving, though at present in the United States, many sectors of the population harbor a strong suspicion that the poor are lazy and undeserving.[7] (Note that in the United States, even so-named *entitlement* programs such as food stamps are viewed as charity; "government handouts" to people too lazy to "do an honest day's work.")

In sum, a genuine notion of access has no real place on a charity model. Or, more precisely, those assumed to be "normal members of society" have all the access they need, and thus the notion is built right into what it means to be a "normal person." Normal or ordinary persons are those who can freely access the goods and services of society to participate in the major aspects of life. Access, then, is just what everyone who is "normal" already has.[8] "Special gifts, favors, and benefits" are what everyone who is not "normal" gets.

Limitations

The inadequacies of this concept, from a justice perspective, are evident. Charity does not set itself up to afford real justice for all members of a society; it gives us *noblesse oblige*. Charity offers no *guarantee* that marginalized persons will be able to participate in the activities that enable them to survive, or that constitute what Wendell calls the "major aspects of life." Instead, it invites, encourages, or (rarely) demands some subset of society to *grant* them means of participation—through, for instance, "emergency" food providers. Their inability to participate fully in a society, and the failure of the charity paradigm to *guarantee* their participation by implementing structural social change, combine to leave marginalized persons second-class citizens at best.

A second limitation is this: because benevolent gifts are just that—*gifts*—benefactors labor under no obligation to include recipients in decisions about the form gifts should take. It is up to *them* to decide how to extend their largesse.[9] While I may choose to pay attention to your cultural needs when stocking food in the emergency pantry, it is an act of benevolence for me to do so; as a recipient of charity, you have no "right" to expect culturally appropriate food—or nutritionally high-quality food.

These limitations to the charity paradigm derive in part from the fact that it does not conceive of individuals' well-being as necessarily and essentially connected to that of others—specifically, it does not see the well-being of a society's privileged members as linked to that of its marginalized members. It is not conceptually required to acknowledge a loss—to the community or to its "normal" members—when other of its members are systematically incapable of participating in the life of that community, because, for example, they do not have access to safe and culturally appropriate food.

Recognizing this limitation leads me to some observations about the conception of personhood embodied in the charity paradigm—a conception it shares with the rights paradigm. The fact that they conceive of personhood in similar ways is the chief reason I believe the rights paradigm is also incapable of supporting a notion of access that robustly advances justice—despite its association with the antipoverty-antihunger movement.

Personhood on the Charity and Rights Paradigms

Who or what counts as a person shifts over time; in the United States, for instance, the number considered "full persons" has expanded since our founding, but many people are still regarded as only "partial persons," with rights not fully guaranteed by law, or not treated particularly seriously in practice. Being or failing to be a "full person" is directly connected to the rights one may or may not claim for oneself—in particular, the rights of access to those goods and services that enable one to function in society.[10]

Charity and rights frameworks share a conception of personhood rooted in the tradition of liberal individualism. We see its character in the charity model's sharp division between egoism and altruism. The self is individual, atomic, and substantial, where "substantial" means it is an independent, free-standing substance possessed of certain essential attributes from which it cannot be separated.

Relations among atomistic individuals are only indirectly relevant to their identity; to *be*, to exist, is not predicated on being in relation to others; relations are accidental, not essential aspects of persons. As philosopher Eva Kittay puts it, the exemplar or standard bearer of this model of personhood is the independent adult. All others are exceptions to their "rule," with needs that must be understood derivatively. Of course all of us some of the time and some of us all of the time *are* exceptions to this state. Babies, old people, disabled people, people asleep, people who do not know how to grow their own food; all of us are dependent on others—most of the time, as it turns out. Despite its being held up as the standard on this paradigm, independence is in fact the anomaly.

These two paradigms only adequately account for freely chosen relations between independent equals. As philosopher Annette Baier points out,

> Relationships between those who are clearly unequal in power, such as parents and children . . . , doctors and patients, the well and the ill . . . , have had to be shunted to the bottom of the agenda and then dealt with by some sort of "promotion" of the weaker, so that an appearance of virtual equality is achieved.[11]

In the charity paradigm, such promotions are voluntary, not mandatory. In the rights paradigm, they end up being mandatory, but the effect is much the same—the sense that one's "equality" has an asterisk after it, indicating it is a special, "derived" equality, granted to one who does not come by it "naturally."

This model of the self contributes directly to the ways these two paradigms can conceptualize access, and the obligations of society to provide it. If personhood means independence, self-containedness, and equality with other persons, then full participation in a society will expect as much from all those who claim personhood. Charity and rights paradigms differ primarily with respect to the matter of what to do with persons who are not able to "measure up." Conceptions of persons as disabled, for example, are rooted in highly contingent notions of "normal human bodies" (no one who does not have legs—but no Supermen either), and also in beliefs, understandings, and expectations about what a "normal society" should be expected to provide for all its citizens. On a charity paradigm, there is no need to provide *either* wheelchair ramps, *or* Superman-strong doors except as a "courtesy to our customers." Once we established the Americans with Disabilities Act—an act embodying the view that disabled persons have a *right* to access—ramps are necessary to comply with the law, but there is no real budging on the notion that there is a set of things that "normal humans" need, and then a separate set of "special needs" items. The whiff of the supererogatory—the "above and beyond the call of duty"—remains about these items even when they are taken as rights; societies that provide them as a matter of course are "generous," even "noble."

When it comes to food, we find similarly contingent, often ethnocentric senses of what count as a "normal" diet and "normal" human nutrition; likewise, there is a tendency to dismiss as "unnecessary" any dietary demands that are not part of the "normal perceiver's" own frame of reference. Thus, a "normal" human may need a certain number of calories per day—but there is no "normal" need for those calories to be vegetarian, for instance, or to contain rice or millet—or, for heaven's sakes, for them to be organic or fair trade. To demand such things is to demand "special privileges," which "subnormal" or "provisionally normal" persons ought not do.

Armed with this understanding of the notion of personhood it shares with charity, I turn now to examine the rights paradigm, and the conception of access it produces.

Paradigm 2: Rights

A rights paradigm rests upon the notion that those defined as persons deserve some set of goods and other benefits essential to human flourishing. Those who count as persons are all "interchangeable," insofar as the very same rights—but no more—extend to each one of them. Rights entail corresponding responsibilities, including those assigned to the society to ensure that all persons can exercise their guaranteed rights. With regard to access, this element of social responsibility is the chief difference between charity and rights paradigms.

We see the rights paradigm embodied in documents like the U.S. Bill of Rights and the United Nations Declaration of Human Rights.[12] Two features derive from it:

a model of justice that conceives of justice as equality (understood to mean "sameness of treatment"), and a concept of universality or universal applicability that is the flip-side of equality. On this paradigm, we are all guaranteed access to the set of benefits deemed necessary for persons.

A just society is one in which all persons are equally able to realize or act on their full range of universally recognized rights. Philosopher Martha Nussbaum uses the notion of "capacities" to describe this sense of justice, suggesting that all community members must have the opportunity to develop their human capacities (irrespective of whether they choose to do so).[13] Many versions of this liberal individualist paradigm also hold that that the matters of *who* counts as a person and *what* count as foundational rights are themselves open to reevaluation and expansion. Indeed, this paradigm emphasizes that the demands of justice require us constantly to reevaluate the reasons that certain groups of beings are or are not granted full personhood status. This expansion clause distinguishes rights from charity; the rights paradigm is (often) invested in increasing the numbers of those who deserve full rights, and guaranteeing their ability to exercise them. This feature of the rights paradigm connects to its concept of access.

Access

If all those defined as persons are to be regarded as equals in society—that is, interchangeable and deserving of a universal set of rights—then those so designated must be able to move within that society, unfettered by the "peculiarities" or "nonstandard features" of their personhood. To bring in Wendell's definition again, they must be able to participate in the major aspects of society (to the extent that they are interested) regardless of the configurations of their bodies or their minds or their bank balances. Access, on this liberal, rights-based definition, aims at making "nonstandard" persons "the same" in relevant respects, so that they are able to exercise their rights and participate in society to the extent that they want. My metaphor for this conception of access is the booster seat, a device that is intended, quite literally, to level the "eating field" at the dining room table. Booster seats make short children the "same" as adults—in one relevant respect. Examples of such social "booster seats" include, variously, wheelchair ramps, affordable festive foods for ethnic and religious holidays, large print texts, buses to grocery stores, and culturally appropriate nutrition assistance programs. Rights-based thinking explicitly underlies the antipoverty-antihunger approach to food security, as can be seen in the work of Patricia Allen, Julie Guthmann, and Elaine Power.[14]

Obviously there is much to praise in this conception of access—and much has been accomplished in its name. As I have already suggested above in my discussion of personhood, however, the paradigm is limited.

Limitations

The conception of access as universal and uniform that characterizes many defenses of a rights-based, welfare-state model of justice is untenable for a variety of reasons, the chief of which is that one size *does not* fit all. Such defenses tend to emphasize the importance of universal access, uniformity, and anonymity.[15] However, uniformity can turn out to be just as much a problem as it is a solution.

Sameness of access is an inappropriate goal to set with respect to participation in the meaningful institutions of our society; we need *appropriateness* of access. To use "sameness" and "universality" as our starting points only builds them into the system as problems that must be resolved further down the line.[16] Why? Because they create the presumption that, as humans, we are all "alike"—or should/could be—and thus that we all have the same needs. To the degree that your needs are bigger than, or different from, what I take to be the "norm," I will resent you for taking up more than your share of resources to be "brought" to my "level." With respect to anonymity, I agree that one kind of fairness and justice is enjoyed by the anonymous user of a universal, impersonal system; a fairness that is clearly evident when contrasting such a system to a personalized charity model that metes out benefits according to its own notions of who "deserves" such benefits. But to suppose that anonymity is all and only a benefit, and will always serve the interests of justice, is to ignore the fact that knowledge of the circumstances of particular individuals' lives *can* be used to promote greater fairness, for example for those whose needs are particularly unusual, marginal, or otherwise easily overlooked or neglected.

Upon what grounds can we build a conception of access with a deeper and more expansive sense of justice? In the final section of this chapter, I present my alternative social paradigm, the coresponsible option.

Paradigm 3: Coresponsibility

Overcoming the limitations shared by the rights and charity paradigms requires, at minimum, a different conception of personhood and also of the relation between person and society. The alternative paradigm I offer is a "fellow traveler" with other frameworks for social change that define persons as *relational* and that adopt a dynamic, fluid understanding of the relation between individual and community. This alternative conception of personhood (a conception that more accurately represents actual humans' actual conditions) gives rise, in turn, to a different conception of justice and access.

Personhood

Central to the Coresponsible Option is its conception of persons as deeply relational—as quite literally constituted through and by their relations with others. To *be* is to be *in relation*, and relations take all sorts of forms. Eva Kittay identifies one significant form, namely, that of mother to child. As she puts it, everyone is, literally, some mother's child, dependent on and—to greater or lesser extents—worthy of "a certain amount of care and connection."[17] Other dependency relations connect us to other humans, and to the rest of the natural world; most profoundly, every human depends on other living things for nourishment. The crucial point is that, unlike either rights-based or charity-based thinking, the coresponsible option makes relationality an *essential* feature of personhood, with independence a secondary or derived state.

Because relationality in general—and dependence in particular—characterize every aspect of human being, this paradigm does not posit some standard-issue, independent "normal" human, with some "ordinary" set of human needs, as its "model person," nor does it define all those who are *perceived as* failing to achieve this (mythical, impossible) independence as "special needs" or "extraordinary" or "lazy and waiting for a handout." (Of course, we *all* fail to achieve this independence. Only *some* of us are perceived to do so. For others, the strings of our dependence are rendered invisible, courtesy of the design of the system.) By starting from the fact of human dependence—by recognizing that, from cradle to grave, we all vitally depend on others in myriad ways—the paradigm makes room for all kinds of "normal" human being. We are all dependent—and we all have capabilities. These facts twine together in far more complicated ways than an atomistic sense of self, with its presumption of independence, allows us even to conceptualize.

These recognitions lead to an understanding that who and what and how *I* am are matters complicatedly and inextricably linked to *your* identity—including your health and well-being. This claim is not meant to sound tidy and neat, as if the interests of such intertwined persons will always harmonically converge; they do not. The goal of rejecting an atomistic notion of personhood is not to eliminate conflicts and competitions, but rather to put them on a different footing—to understand them inside a different context. Such reframing will enable us to think about access differently. Rather than a kind of zero-sum calculus of interests, in which every "special requirement" *you* have results in a debit from *my* "ordinary needs," a relational model of self performs the calculation quite differently.

Access

The coresponsible option acknowledges all humans' reliance on others, rejecting the imaginary "autonomous person" as its model. Using Wendell's definition, this means that, to the degree that any of us is "able bodied" or "food secure," we are so *only* because we are already enmeshed in networks of support and assistance; only the presence of such networks enables us "to participate in [the] major aspect[s] of life in a given society."[18] Coresponsibility starts from this fact, and begins all consideration of access by acknowledging the dependency systems that already make possible our functioning—or, to put it more starkly, *that mitigate our potential disability.* Take one example: were I plunked into a fishing community, I would immediately become food insecure; in my present world, my inability to fish or otherwise produce my own food is neatly mediated by my relations to retail food providers.[19]

Coresponsibility rejects the notion that access should make all persons the "same" as some imaginary independent individual (the ethical and political norm of personhood). Instead of universality or sameness, coresponsibility goes for *appropriateness* of access. Appropriate access may well not look much like sameness at all.

Conflicts over limited resources do not *disappear* in a coresponsible conception of access—the reason for choosing this paradigm is not that it eliminates dispute. Rather, the paradigm situates conflicts in a different context, one that moves away from "us versus them" thinking focused on competition for limited resources. By replacing independence and autonomy with dependence and relationality, by rejecting sameness as the goal of access, coresponsibility rejects the zero-sum calculus that turns all "special" needs into drains on the resources available for "normal" people. In its place, it understands the social context as one in which all persons recognize their well-being as complexly intertwined, such that others' gains are just as likely to be *their* gains as well. This alternative calculus already can be seen at work, for example, in the acknowledgment that ensuring all children adequate nutrition results in a host of long-term benefits for us as a society. Well-nourished children have a better opportunity to develop their physical, mental, and emotional well-being, which in turn enables them to participate in the life of their communities to the greatest degree possible.

Appropriateness of access leads to a kind of "family resemblance" sense of what a society must provide for its members—and what they must provide for each other.[20] Projects to guarantee access share no single underlying feature or goal. Instead, different approaches to access share different traits, much as members of a family share different, overlapping sets of traits with each other. This feature of the coresponsible option leads me to suggest that this paradigm provides the conceptual undergirding required by the CFS movement, which that has been criticized for lacking such a foundation.[21]

The CFS Coalition defines community food security as a movement

> dedicated to building strong, sustainable, local and regional food systems that ensure access to affordable, nutritious, and culturally appropriate food for all people at all times. We seek to develop self-reliance among all communities in obtaining their food and to create a system of growing, manufacturing, processing, making available, and selling food that is regionally based and grounded in the principles of justice, democracy, and sustainability.[22]

The coresponsible option allows us to understand CFS as a family-resemblance model that links groups, interests, and challenges in irreducible ways. CFS draws our attention to the many ways people can be food insecure; it rests *not* on a list of fundamental capabilities or rights that "normal" human should have, but rather on a recognition of the linked, nested, intertwining ways in which we depend on each other. Recognizing the ways that all members of a community are affected by food insecurity of various forms can, in turn, lead to creative efforts to form coalitions that work for food security on multiple fronts simultaneously—that is, to resist "us versus them" thinking, in favor of a much more complicated understanding of who "we" are.

CONCLUSION

Because charity and rights share a general notion of what it is to be a person, and because that notion rests on self-contained independence of body, mind, finances, and so on, the taint of *noblesse oblige* that infuses the charity model continues to permeate the rights model. Even here, guarantees of access for those deemed "nonstandard" are treated as special "add-ons" that enable people to "reach the bar" of normalcy. I submit that this taint will not easily go away on any liberal individualist model, which is why we need a different way to understand personhood. The paradigm of coresponsibility provides the framework needed for this alternative model. Budding illustrations of the coresponsible model might be seen in the work of such organizations as Missoula, Montana's Garden City Harvest program and Boston's Food Project. Both projects take a multifaceted approach to creating food-secure communities: growing food for area emergency food providers, offering garden plots for community members, creating training for youth in both gardening and leadership, and, for all who live in the community, producing sustainably-grown high-quality fresh vegetables.

NOTES

1. USDA (U.S. Department of Agriculture), Economic Research Service, "Food Security in the United States: Conditions and Trends," *Food Security in the United States*, http://www.ers.usda.gov/Briefing/FoodSecurity/trends.htm (accessed July 1, 2008).

2. See my "Food Politics, Political Food," in *Cooking, Eating, Thinking: Transformative Philosophies of Food*, ed. Deane Curtin and Lisa Heldke (Bloomington: Indiana University, 1992), 303–327.

3. For information about the CFS movement, consult the Community Food Security Coalition Web site, http://www.foodsecurity.org (accessed July 1, 2008).

4. Susan Wendell, *The Rejected Body: Feminist Philosophical Reflections on Disability* (New York: Routledge, 1996), 23.

5. Elizabeth Williamson, "Some Americans Lack Food, but USDA Won't Call Them Hungry," *Washington Post*, Sec. A, November 16, 2006, http://www.washington post.com/wp-dyn/content/article/2006/11/15/AR2006111501621.html (accessed June 26, 2008).

6. Elaine Power notes that some versions of sustainable food systems intended to be progressive end up reinscribing the charity model—particularly its tendency to blame the victim—by stripping away the universal guarantees of welfare benefits and replacing them with options that "reinforce the individualistic ideology of neoconservative policies" ("Combining Social Justice and Sustainability," in *For Hunger-Proof Cities: Sustainable Urban Food Systems*, ed. Mustafa Koc et al. (Ottowa: International Development Resource Center, 1999), http://www.idrc.ca/en/ev-30587-201-1-DO_TOPIC.html (accessed June 28, 2008)). Similarly, Patricia Allen and Julie Guthman criticize farm-to-school programs (understood as a part of the CFS movement), for their revival of neoliberal ideologies ("From 'Old School' to 'Farm-to-School: Neoliberalization from the Ground Up," *Agriculture and Human Values* 23 (2006): 401–415).
It is important to pay attention to the ways in which any move to dismantle social welfare systems and replace them with more progressive and just alternatives can end up unwittingly doing just the reverse—the charge Allen and Guthman lay against farm-to-school programs. But I would argue that such results are by no means necessary; CFS efforts and sustainable food systems are not intrinsically linked to charity and neoliberalism.

7. The disabled have been seen as undeserving, in various ways. Historically, many disabilities were understood as God's justice wrought upon a person. Today, there is a sense that many people "on disability" are "just faking it," and are simply too lazy to work.

8. This claim sounds odd—and it should. Access tends to be used *only* to describe something that persons *do not presently have*—not to characterize something one already possesses unproblematically.

9. For more on this point, see Janet Poppendieck, "Charity, Justice and Emergency Food," *The Vincentian Center for Church and Society*, http://www.vincenter.org/99/poppen. html (accessed June 28, 2008).

10. Loosely connected, conceptually, to the matter of who counts as a person is the matter of dessert; who deserves what. Even though the rights model is predicated on the assertion that rights attach to all persons *as* persons, in fact, even under its rule, the notion that people do or do not deserve their rights often holds sway. Thus, for example, entitlement programs in this country are treated as "handouts," not as entitlements. The notion that people have a right to these things is only a thin veneer over a deep, often resentful, belief that "those people" are just getting "special favors," whether it is accessible buses or food stamps.

11. Annette Baier, "The Need for More than Justice," in *Feminist Theory: A Philo-sophical Anthology*, ed. Ann E. Cudd and Robin O. Andreasen (Malden, MA: Black-well, 2005): 243–50, 248.

12. A recent theoretical expression of the rights paradigm can be found in the "capabilities approach" developed by Martha Nussbaum. Nussbaum presents a list of 10 "central human functional capabilities all citizens should have" to flourish with dignity. See "Women and Cultural Universals," in *Feminist Theory: A Philosophical Anthology*, eds. Ann E. Cudd and Robin O. Andreasen (Malden, MA: Blackwell, 2005): 302–324, 310.

13. Nussbaum, "Women and Cultural Universals."

14. Power, "Combining"; Allen and Guthman, in "From 'Old School' "; and Patricia Allen, "Reweaving the Food Security Safety Net: Mediating Entitlement and Entrepreneurship," *Agriculture and Human Values* 16 (1999): 117–29.

15. See Power, "Combining"; Nussbaum, "Women and Cultural Universals"; and Allen, "Reweaving," for examples of this. Allen and Guthman, in "From 'Old School,' " also revive the call for universals. They criticize CFS programs for their neoliberalism, a charge that is not without merit. Nevertheless, their advocacy of antipoverty and antihunger approaches sends us back to *another* form of liberalism, when they empha-size a "universal right to education," equity, and universal access, an approach that is rooted in classical liberalism in ways that are every bit as problematic as the neoliberal-ism they believe is present in CFS.

16. I do not reject the possibility of anything like universals, but the universals for which this paradigm allows are the *consequences* of our social investigations, not the *preconditions* of them. We do not begin by assuming everyone is "the same" in some crucial respect; rather, we *conclude* that they are, and we do so on the basis of an inves-tigation. See Alain Locke, "Cultural Pluralism," in *American Philosophies: An Anthology*, ed. Leonard Harris, Scott L. Pratt, and Anne S. Waters (Malden, MA: Blackwell, 2002): 433–45.

17. Eva Kittay, "Vulnerability and the Moral Nature of Dependency Relations," in *Feminist Theory: A Philosophical Anthology*, ed. Ann E. Cudd and Robin O. Andreasen (Malden, MA: Blackwell, 2005): 264–79, 274.

18. Wendell, *The Rejected Body*, 23.

19. The painter Paul Gauguin presents a vivid picture of the degree to which our abilities and our securities are context-dependent—and also of the degree to which we can tend to be oblivious to their context-dependence, and instead can mistake our-selves for independent, self-sufficient atomic units. When Gauguin moved to Tahiti for a time to paint, he found himself vulnerable in very short order: "two days later, I had exhausted my provisions; I had assumed that with money I would find all the food that I needed." Paul Gauguin, *The Writings of a Savage*, ed. Daniel Guerrin, trans. Eleanor Levieux (New York: Viking, 1978), 81. Interestingly, this experience does *not* lead Gauguin to reassess his assumptions about the degree of his own independence and self-sufficiency.

20. "Family resemblance" comes from philosopher Ludwig Wittgenstein. See *Philo-sophical Investigations*, 2nd ed., trans. G. E. M. Anscombe (Malden, MA: Blackwell, 1997), 32e.

21. See, for example, Sharon Lezberg, "Finding Common Ground Between Food Security and Sustainable Food Systems" (paper presented at the Association for the Study of Food and Society/Agriculture, Food and Human Values Society Conference, June 1999): 24; Power, "Combining," 5; and Allen and Guthman, "From 'Old School.' "

22. Community Food Security Coalition, http://www.foodsecurity.org/.

RESOURCE GUIDE

Suggested Reading

Allen, Patricia. "Reweaving the Food Security Safety Net: Mediating Entitlement and Entrepreneurship." *Agriculture and Human Values* 16 (1999): 117–29.

Allen, Patricia, and Julie Guthman. "From 'Old School' to 'Farm-to-School': Neoliberalization from the Ground Up." *Agriculture and Human Values* 23 (2006): 401–415.

Buchanan, Allen. "Charity, Justice, and the Idea of Moral Progress." In *Giving: Western Ideas of Philanthropy*, ed. Jerome B. Schneewind. Bloomington: Indiana University Press, 1996.

Heldke, Lisa. "Food Politics, Political Food." In *Cooking, Eating, Thinking: Transformative Philosophies of Food*, ed. Deane Curtin and Lisa Heldke. Bloomington: Indiana University Press, 1992.

Koc, Mustafa, Rod MacRae, Luc J. A. Mougeot, and Jennifer Welsh. *For Hunger-Proof Cities: Sustainable Urban Food Systems*. Ottawa: International Development Resource Center, 1999. Available at http://www.idrc.ca/en/ev-9394-201-1-DO_TOPIC.html.

Lezberg, Sharon. "Finding Common Ground between Food Security and Sustainable Food Systems." Paper presented at the Association for the Study of Food and Society/Agriculture, Food and Human Values Society Conference, June 1999.

Poppendieck, Janet. "Charity, Justice and Emergency Food." The Vincentian Center for Church and Society. Available at http://www.vincenter.org/99/poppen.html, 1999.

Poppendieck, Janet. *Sweet Charity? Emergency Food and the End of Entitlements*. New York: Viking, 1998.

Wendell, Susan. *The Rejected Body: Feminist Philosophical Reflections on Disability*. New York: Routledge, 1996.

Web Sites

Community Food Security Coalition, http://www.foodsecurity.org/.

The Food Project, http://www.thefoodproject.org/.

Garden City Harvest, http://gardencityharvest.org.

Institute for Food and Development Policy/Food First, http://www.foodfirst.org/.

La Via Campesina, http://viacampesina.org/main_en/index.php.

15

Animal Welfare

Andrew Fiala

Concern for farm animal welfare is growing. In 2004, the state of California passed
legislation banning the production and sale of foie gras, a delicacy produced by force
feeding geese until their livers become diseased. In June of 2008—in response to
videos of inhumane treatment of cattle made public by the Humane Society—Ed
Schaffer, the U.S. secretary of agriculture, called for a ban on the slaughter of non-
ambulatory or "downer" cattle. In Europe, concern for animal welfare is even more
mainstream. In 2004, David Byrne, the European commissioner for Health and
Consumer Protection, stated that animal welfare can be improved with minimal
cost. "The experience within Europe has shown that in many cases there are no significant additional costs in improving animal protection."[1] Indeed, the European
Union (EU) has given a central place to animal welfare. The Treaty of Amsterdam
in 1997 officially recognized farm animals as sentient beings whose welfare matters.
Recent legislative efforts in the European Union are based upon this idea. And the
European Union acknowledges the so-called five freedoms for farm animals:[2]

- Freedom from hunger and thirst
- Freedom from discomfort
- Freedom from pain, injury, and disease
- Freedom to express normal behavior
- Freedom from fear and distress

Traditional animal husbandry practices took care to provide for animal welfare,
as defined in this way.[3] But the economic pressures of the global economy have
made it more difficult to sustain traditional animal husbandry. So the intensive
animal agriculture of the factory farm has created conditions in which concern for
animal welfare is subordinated to the demand for increased productivity. In
response, organic farmers and advocates of traditional husbandry have staged a
minirevolution of sorts in the last decade. This movement produces free-range
meat and eggs, organic milk, and so on. At the other end of the food production

line, organic restaurants and chains, such as Chipotle, and stores such as Whole Foods provide cruelty-free animal products.[4]

This developing concern for animal welfare comes as demand for cheap and nutritious meat is growing at a rapid pace. In North America and Europe, seventeen billion animals are killed every year for food. Americans alone kill more than eight billion animals per year for food. Every day in the United States, twenty-three million chickens, pigs, cows, and other assorted animals are slaughtered. That amounts to per capita annual consumption of: 51 pounds of chicken, 15 pounds of turkey, 63 pounds of beef, 45 pounds of pork, 1 pound of veal, and 1 pound of lamb. If we focus on pigs alone, we should note that demand for pork has been soaring in the United States and abroad. Eight million or so hogs are slaughtered every day around the globe.[5] To satisfy our craving for meat, meat production must be intensified. And thus the vast majority of meat is produced via industrial animal agriculture, that is, on the factory farm.

As industrial animal agriculture grows, activists concerned about animal welfare focus their energies in a variety of ways. The Humane Society is dedicated to the prevention of cruelty to animals, including the confinement and crating practices of the factory farm.[6] More radical animal welfare activist groups include People for the Ethical Treatment of Animals (PETA) and the Animal Liberation Front. These groups take direct action aimed at eliminating animal cruelty—from street theater to raids on animal laboratories. One novel sort of activism occurred in spring of 2008, when PETA offered a $1 million prize to anyone who could bring to market chicken meat grown in a test tube. The goal is to produce meat for human consumption without actually using animals. Now this may sound like a quixotic or even oxymoronic endeavor. But it points to the central problem of animal welfare. Contemporary animal husbandry uses sentient animals in a way that produces suffering. Until it is possible to produce meat without animals, then animal welfare will continue to be a central concern for all.

Animal welfare is a broad topic. It includes questions about hunting and habitat preservation; animal entertainment, including horseracing, dog-fighting, and circuses; raising animals for furs; using animals in biomedical research; and breeding pets. Our focus here is animal agriculture, especially the intensive livestock operations or "factory farms" that provide the majority of our food. Intensive animal agriculture generates a number of ethical problems. Factory farms produce air and water pollution. They make use of controversial biotechnologies: from antibiotics and hormones to genetic engineering and cloning. And factory farms create labor and economic dislocations as they replace more traditional family farms. But factory farming also creates serious questions about the welfare of individual farm animals.

There are two basic approaches to animal welfare: an instrumentalist or anthropocentric approach and a deeper, nonanthropocentric or animal-centered approach.

The instrumental or anthropocentric approach is concerned with animal welfare only to the extent that animals serve human interests or satisfy human needs. Farmers are concerned with animal welfare in this sense because livestock represent capital investment and future profit. And consumers are concerned with animal welfare in this sense because they want cheap and nutritious meat. From this point of view, our duties to animals are at best indirect.

The nonanthropocentric or animal-centered approach assumes that it makes sense to consider things from an individual animal's point of view. Animal-centered approaches hold that human beings have some sort of direct moral obligation to consider the well-being of individual farm animals. And this approach maintains that it makes sense to be concerned with animals for their sake and not merely for ours. This is explained in terms of concern to prevent cruelty or reduce suffering. The most radical form of the animal-centered approach wants to extend the idea of legal and moral rights to animals.

We will consider here the sorts of assumptions that are made about morality and about animals on both sides. As we shall see, anthropocentric approaches to animal welfare can be used to justify intensive animal agriculture, while animal-centered approaches tend to maintain that factory farming—and meat consumption—is immoral.

THE FACTORY FARM AND ETHICAL VEGETARIANISM

Everyone who consumes meat and makes a profit from its production has an interest in animal welfare: consumers and producers want meat that comes from healthy animals. Animal welfare in the mainstream is anthropocentric: it is focused exclusively on the production of cheap, tasty, and nutritious meat. Farmers want their livestock to live healthy lives, put on weight, and reproduce so that they might bring their products to market. And consumers want meat that is free from disease.

The anthropocentric or instrumentalist conception of animal welfare found in the mainstream is concerned with the well-being of animals only to maximize return on investment and to satisfy the human desire for meat. Factory farms do provide for animal welfare. They keep animals safe from predators and parasites. They provide heat in the winter, plentiful food, and substantial doses of antibiotics. But this is all in an effort to keep animals healthy so that they might be turned from animals into meat.

A deeper, more animal-centered approach to animal welfare concerns itself with the welfare of animals from a perspective that takes up the animal's point of view. From this point of view, the concern is not cheap and plentiful meat. Rather the concern of deep animal welfare is in the quality of the lives lived by individual animals. From this perspective, the cheap meat of the factory farm comes at a substantial price in cruelty. Factory farms are not set up to deliberately torture animals. The cruelty of the factory farm is not sadistic or malicious. Industrial livestock operations are designed to produce cheap meat; and sadism or cruelty provide no profit. But the industrial production of cheap meat requires a drastic alteration in the natural life cycle of the animals on the factory farm.

Those who are concerned with animal welfare in its deepest sense—authors such as Tom Regan, Peter Singer, and groups such as PETA—claim that the entire process is cruel insofar as it prevents farm animals from living normal or natural lives. From the animal's perspective, the factory farm is an unnatural and cruel place because the factory farm is designed to prevent animals from acting on natural instincts and from satisfying basic drives. Farm animals are locked in cages, kept out of the sunshine, and prevented from touching the Earth. They are—contrary to their own natural tendencies—forced into proximity with others animals and are unable to escape from the stench of their own excrement. Even reproduction and birth are controlled by the use of artificial insemination and farrowing crates.

Moreover, animal agriculturalists are quite interested in creative breeding, genetic engineering, and cloning. And the resultant animals can be warped versions of natural animals: for example, animals bred to be so large that they eventually cannot stand up. Animals are also subjected to other more routine indignities and minor cruelties. Cattle are branded. Male pigs and cows are castrated without anesthesia. Chickens are debeaked and declawed to prevent them from injuring themselves and each other. And some animals—such as veal cattle and poultry raised for foie gras—are kept in complete confinement and are force fed diets that cause disease.

When the time for slaughter comes, animals are crowded in trucks and moved in conditions that often result in such significant stress that many thousands of animals die yearly in transport.[7] On the killing floor, these animals are stunned, hooked, hoisted, bled out, and skinned. The slaughter assembly line can cause significant damage to animals before they are dead: legs are often dislocated, poultry and swine are occasionally scalded alive, and downer cattle are dragged or forklifted into place. Although the law requires that mammals (with the exception of rabbits) be stunned before killing, 5 percent of the time the stunning fails and animals are hung, cut, and bled while still conscious.[8] Even though industrial standards are aimed at minimizing cruelty when animals are killed, in an industrial process focused on speed and efficiency, mistakes are made and shortcuts are taken.

Some people opt out of the animal economy altogether, choosing instead vegetarianism. Ethical vegetarians choose to avoid meat for principled moral reasons (unlike those who renounce meat for health reasons). Principled vegetarianism has grown in the Western Hemisphere in opposition to the development of factory farming. Although Eastern Hemisphere traditions such as Buddhism, Jainism, and some varieties of Hinduism have long held that it was virtuous to abstain from meat, industrial nations have a much deeper commitment to meat eating. Traditional Western agriculture was grounded on a stewardship or good husbandry model in which the farmer's duty was to care for the animals and to be thankful for the goods that the animals provided in return. In the Judeo-Christian tradition, God created the animals and gave them to humanity to care for and to use. Indeed, vegetarianism was often associated with pagan or heretical views that venerated nature in a way that was deemed antithetical to Christian orthodoxy. But the factory farm leads us away from the stewardship model of animal welfare and pushes us in an instrumental direction in which animals are merely commodities to be used without care or thanksgiving.

Some critics of contemporary animal agriculture choose to eat only animal products that are grown organically or that are produced under humane or "cruelty-free" conditions. Vegetarians avoid meat entirely. And vegans also avoid eggs and dairy. There are a variety of principled reasons to be a vegetarian.[9] Some follow Regan and Singer in rejecting meat eating altogether, on the principle that killing animals is wrong. Others, such as Martha Nussbaum, are less concerned with killing itself than with the systematic cruelty of the factory farm and its perversion of the idea of stewardship. Other vegetarians are more concerned with the negative environmental impact of meat eating: meat production creates water and air pollution, including greenhouse gases. In 2006, a UN report claimed that "the livestock sector" produced more greenhouse gases than did transportation and that livestock operations contributed to habitat loss and environmental degradation. In 2008, the head of the Intergovernmental Panel on Climate Change claimed that the world should convert to a vegetarian diet to combat global warming.[10] Others are concerned with the negative impact that intensive animal agriculture has on native animal species: concerned, for example, with the way the cattle industry in the American West has systematically destroyed wolf, bison, and prairie dog populations and habitats. Still others choose to eat lower on the food chain to leave a smaller footprint and to leave more grain and food available to fight hunger.[11] And some feminists give up meat because they link meat to male dominance and the oppression of women.[12] Vegetarians of all sorts agree that meat eating is simply not necessary for human health—since there are readily available nutritious alternatives. And if meat eating is not necessary for health, then there is no good reason to support an industry based on cruelty that produces what is basically a luxury good: meat.

In response, meat eaters and producers will defend meat eating by claiming that meat and dairy are cheap and nutritious components of a healthy human diet. They will also claim that human beings are justified in using animals as food— especially if farming and slaughtering practices are undertaken with concern for animal welfare. Let us turn, then, to the justification of using animals and the anthropocentric versions of animal welfare.

FOUR PRINCIPLED DEFENSES OF ANTHROPOCENTRISM

There are four principled ways to respond to the ethical concerns raised by vegetarians. That is, there are four basic ways to support the anthropocentric and merely instrumentalist approach to animal welfare.

Ontological Claims

The first response is to deny that animals are the sorts of beings who can suffer. This view is often associated with the early modern philosopher René Descartes, who famously claimed that animals were merely mechanical bodies—what he called machines or automatons.[13] From this perspective, although animals exhibit pain behavior, this does not indicate any sort of mental or spiritual disturbance. It is "mere pain" without understanding or, as Peter Carruthers has described it, "unconscious pain." From this point of view, animals cannot be said to "suffer," where suffering is thought to mean the presence of pain plus other affective states such as anxiety and fear, as well as the idea that pain is not justified or desired.

Descartes' view makes sense in the context of Christian theology, which denies that animals have souls. While the stewardship model of the Christian tradition holds that animals have value insofar as they are created by God, the stewardship model also holds that there is an unbridgeable ontological difference between human beings and animals: animals are made for human uses and only human beings have eternal souls. From this point of view, those who claim that animal welfare matters in a nonanthropocentric sense make a category mistake. From their perspective, animals are simply not the sorts of things that have "welfare" in the human sense of the term. Indeed, we have a word for this category mistake: "anthropomorphism," which is the tendency to project human features onto non-human objects. Defenders of a Cartesian sort of view—which denies that animals suffer—will claim that it is a mistaken anthropomorphism that makes us think that animals care about the quality of their lives or that animals can suffer from conditions such as we find on the factory farm.

Claims about Moral Concern

Closely related to this is the second response, which claims that animal "suffering," if we choose to call it such, is simply not a matter of moral concern. The Cartesian view can seem quite odd, especially for those who recognize that animal bodies and minds are quite similar to human bodies and minds. Animals bleed when cut. They feel hunger when left unfed. They can exhibit fear behaviors in response to smells, sounds, and threats. And social animals like dogs and horses can appear lonely, anxious, and so on. Indeed, animal experimentation in human biomedicine—including psychological and neurological experiments—assumes that animal physiology is similar to ours in these obvious ways. The second approach need not deny this sort of similarity. But it does deny that these elements of animal experience have moral import.

The most influential proponent of this sort of approach is Immanuel Kant.[14] Kant admits that it is possible to be cruel to animals. But on his view, morality is exclusively focused on human beings. We have direct duties only to other human beings. And any moral duty we have to animals is only indirect: the treatment of animals matters only when it has impacts on our behavior toward other humans. For Kant, cruelty to animals is wrong because it tends to encourage cruelty toward humans.

Such an anthropocentric ethical theory will tell us that we have no moral obligation to take animal pain and suffering seriously. Anthropocentric ethics maintains a simple distinction: we are obliged to care directly about humans but not about animals. This sort of view can in fact result in a quite positive assessment of factory farming: factory farming is good if it fulfills the needs and desires of the human population. Contemporary theorists who defend this point of view include libertarians such as Tibor Machan, who argues that we only have obligations to ourselves (and to our kin and fellow humans); and that we have no obligations to other species.[15]

Claims about the Order of Nature

Related to this is a third principled response, which holds some version of the view that animals are literally given to human beings for their consumption. This view can be traced back, in the Western tradition, to the idea found in Genesis, that God creates the animals for human usage. A more naturalistic or Darwinian approach would maintain that the struggle for survival that has led us to dominate the animals also entitles us to use them for our own purposes. According to proponents of this way of thinking, it might be true that animals suffer, and we might even feel compelled to minimize animal suffering (out of respect for God's creation or out of a spirit of kinship with the animals). But from this perspective, animal suffering should not prevent us from making use of animals for our own benefit. A version of this theory can be found in Friedrich Nietzsche's idea that predatory animals—including human animals—love their prey because they are good to eat.[16]

This view is anthropocentric in the sense that it claims that human beings are the focal point of creation or of evolutionary progress. From this perspective, it is our right (and maybe even our duty) to celebrate our dominion over the animals. Some take this view to an extreme that claims that human beings are by nature carnivorous hunters and that meat eating satisfies some deep primal desire in the human psyche.[17] But even hunters are concerned with animal welfare, albeit in an anthropocentric sense. Hunting clubs such as Ducks Unlimited protect wild animal habitat. And the ethics of hunting emphasize that a kill should be as clean as possible and that the meat and hides should be put to good use.

Utilitarianism

Perhaps the most sophisticated and complex way of articulating an anthropocentric approach to animal welfare is found in utilitarianism. Utilitarianism can be employed in defense of current agricultural practices. Utilitarian moral philosophy is based on the idea that it is good, as John Stuart Mill put it, to produce the greatest happiness for the greatest number.

A utilitarian would emphasize that intensive animal agriculture has produced vast benefits for human beings (and even for farm animals that would not exist, if it were not for farming).[18] Humans live longer and healthier lives now than at any time in history, and the human population continues to grow, arguably as a result of an ongoing revolution in animal farming practices. Moreover, utilitarians might argue—as Mill does—that humans are capable of higher pleasures: only human beings can enjoy art, philosophy, and politics. Even our gustatory experiences consist of more complex and subtle pleasures than animals can ever experience—as witnessed by gourmet cooking and the rich social and psychological pleasures of fine dining. From this point of view, the savory taste of bacon, hamburger, and fried chicken—not to mention the subtle flavors of veal, lamb, or foie gras—provide for important human pleasures. Moreover, the protein and calories that come from animals make such an important contribution to human happiness and productivity, that the suffering caused by meat production is justified.

ANIMAL-CENTERED RESPONSES

In response to these anthropocentric ideas, defenders of a more animal-centered approach to animal welfare can respond in a variety of ways. We will consider four responses here.

The Darwinian Approach

Defenders of animal welfare will argue that the anthropocentric claim that animals do not suffer runs counter to what we know about animal physiology and about the connections between and among species. Animal brains and bodies are similar to human brains and bodies. This similarity is assumed by those who use animal models in biomedical research. Moreover, the reason for this similarity has to do with our evolutionary connection. Mammals share much in common. Even the fishes and the birds share much in common with mammals.

If one takes the Darwinian approach seriously, then the Cartesian argument that focuses on a deep ontological difference between humans and animals must be rejected. In the *Descent of Man*, Darwin himself argues that the differences between humans and animals are matters of degree and not of kind. Given our similar physiology and evolutionary heritage—as well as the adaptive advantage of the ability to experience pain and suffering—sufficient evidence warrants the assertion that animals experience pain, anxiety, and fear, and that they suffer from it.

David DeGrazia has concluded after an extensive review of the scientific and philosophical literature, "the available evidence suggests that most or all vertebrates, and perhaps some invertebrates, can suffer."[19]

An obvious piece of evidence used to support this point of view is the fact that farm animal health does suffer under the stress of the factory farm and in transport from farm to slaughterhouse. Obvious signs of stress include chickens who peck each other to death, if their beaks are not removed; pigs who gnaw at the bars of their cages and bite each other's tails out of boredom and frustration; and veal calves who crave iron to such an extent that they would lick their own urine if they were permitted to turn around.[20]

Animals have evolved in such a way that their brains and physiology are well adapted for certain conditions, and poorly adapted for others. In general, the predecessors of farm animal species have spent millions of years adapting to the wild and domesticated species several thousands of years adapting to captivity and cultivation. The changes in environment and behavior found in the factory farm represent a radical departure from the conditions for which evolution has bred farm animals. This gives us good reason to suspect that factory farming causes significant stress and suffering for the animals raised there.

Moreover, some have argued that the Darwinian perspective can be used to undermine anthropocentric claims that humans are unique and special. James Rachels has argued in this way in support of a point of view that he calls "moral individualism." Rachels' idea is that species membership is an irrelevant factor in morality. He contends that, "how an individual should be treated depends on his or her own particular characteristics, rather than on whether he or she is a member of some preferred group—even the 'group' of human beings."[21] For example, humans with cognitive disability may have capacities that make them more similar to animals than to other humans. Rachels claims that if differences in basic capacities of individual members of a species are recognized, we will see that anthropocentrism is an unjustified prejudice.

Utilitarianism

We saw above that utilitarian approaches to ethics can in fact be used to justify meat eating and the factory farm, especially if utilitarianism is constrained in an anthropocentric way to focus primarily on the greatest happiness for the greatest number of humans. But utilitarians have long admitted that animal suffering matters ethically. If pain and pleasure are key indicators of morality, and animals experience pain and pleasure, then animal pains and pleasures should be included in any utilitarian calculation. We mentioned above that John Stuart Mill thought that human pleasures were qualitatively superior to animal pleasures. But other utilitarians have called this idea into question and have argued for equal consideration of animal pain and pleasure.

Jeremy Bentham proposed a radical revision of our view of animals a few decades before Mill, by focusing on the capabilities possessed by individual animals and humans.

> A full grown horse or dog is beyond comparison a more rational, as well as a more conversable animal, than an infant of a day or a week, or even a month, old. But suppose they were otherwise, what would it avail? The question is not, Can they *reason*? Nor Can they *talk*? But Can they *suffer*?[22]

If animals can suffer, then their suffering should be taken account of in any utilitarian calculation.

Many contemporary utilitarians end up arguing against factory farming and in favor of vegetarianism because they maintain that the cost in animal cruelty is not outweighed by the benefit of meat consumption. This is especially true if the supposed benefits of meat eating are minor gustatory pleasures. In other words, if there are easy and nutritious meat substitutes, then there is no good reason to cause animal suffering in the production of meat. Peter Singer is the most famous contemporary utilitarian proponent of vegetarianism and critic of factory farming. Singer's now classic book, *Animal Liberation* (first published in 1975), makes just such an argument. In a recent defense of his ideas, Singer states his view quite clearly:

> The only acceptable limit to our moral concern is the point at which there is no awareness of pain or pleasure and no conscious preferences of any kind. That is why pigs are objects of moral concern, but lettuces are not. Pigs can feel pain and pleasure, they can enjoy their lives, or want to escape from distressing conditions. To the best of our knowledge, lettuces can't. We should give the same weight to the pain and distress of pigs as we would give to a similar amount of pain and distress suffered by a human being.[23]

Singer argues that animals deserve what he calls "equal consideration," which means that animal pain and pleasure would have to be included in any calculation of "the greatest happiness for the greatest number." Utilitarian defenders of industrial animal agriculture will either have to claim that the human pleasure of eating meat outweighs the animal suffering caused on the factory farm. Or, they can resort to denying that animals feel pain or suffer. Animal welfare advocates such as Singer claim that we have a moral obligation to give equal consideration to the interests and well-being of animals. If we fail to give equal consideration in this way, we are guilty of what Singer maligns as "speciesism." Singer explains speciesism as "a prejudice or attitude of bias toward the interests of members of one's own species and against those of members of other species."[24] Anthropocentric approaches to animal welfare remain speciesist because they do not give equal consideration to animal suffering.

The Aristotelian Approach

One of the problems of the utilitarian approach is found in the sorts of cross-species comparisons that Bentham, Singer, and others end up making. Their ideas can lead to odd conclusions in which some animals are treated better than some humans. For example, Bentham suggests that horses may be of more concern than infants. And Singer is notorious for condemning factory farming while also arguing that euthanasia for retarded human infants might be permissible. One of the problems here is the focus on equal consideration and moral individualism.

In response to this problem, we might focus on understanding "species typical function," and thus base our treatment on the natural norm for members of a given species. The idea of species typical function fits more closely with an Aristotelian approach to the issue. This approach looks into the normal or natural function of a species and is not focused on the capacities of individuals. This approach still results in a radical critique of factory farming.

Unlike the utilitarian approach that looks at pain and suffering, the Aristotelian account attempts to make sense of a broader conception of welfare or well-being. Anthropocentric accounts will tend to argue that welfare is a concept that only makes sense with regard to human beings: only humans have an interest in concepts such as well-being or quality of life because such concepts matter to us in a subjective way. But an Aristotelian approach is concerned with an objective inquiry into the question of whether a human being or an animal is living well. For the Aristotelian, objective criteria for well-being matter as much as subjective experience.

Welfare literally means to fare well, do well, thrive, or flourish. Philosophers have reflected on this concept at least since the time of the ancient Greeks.[25] Aristotle claims that happiness or flourishing occurs when a creature actualizes its purpose or function (Greek: *telos*). For Aristotle, a thing's purpose or function is defined by its nature. So to understand welfare or well-being, we have to inquire into the natural capacities of the thing. A plant flourishes when it grows, flowers, fruits, and spreads its seeds. A human being flourishes when it actualizes its capacities as a rational, political animal. In the same way, we could say that a social animal, such as a pig, flourishes when it actualizes its natural capacities: when it grows, socializes, and reproduces.

Bernard Rollin has made use of this sort of idea in his work on farm animal welfare. Rollin is quite sympathetic to the idea of good husbandry and the stewardship view of animal welfare. Traditional animal husbandry is supposed to help animals flourish in this Aristotelian sense. This view of animal welfare can still allow for a firm ontological distinction between animals and humans, because humans and animals have different natures. Nonetheless, Rollin describes a sort of human-animal "social contract" that was typical of good husbandry practices for thousands of years. Human farmers helped their farm animals to thrive by protecting them from predators and weather, providing them with nutritious food, and so on. In exchange, the animals provided the farmer with food, fiber, and toil. Rollin maintains that in traditional husbandry, animal interests and human interests coincided. It was in the interests of humans to help the animals fulfill their natural functions, to satisfy their own animal interests, and to provide for their welfare. Traditional husbandry decried cruelty to animals and even appointed rest days—the Sabbath—for animal laborers. The credo of traditional agriculture was, according to Rollin, "we take care of the animals—and the animals take care of us."[26] But Rollin argues that the factory farm has changed this equation in radical ways by preventing animals from fulfilling their natural functions.

A further elaboration of this sort of idea can be found in the recent work of Martha Nussbaum. Nussbaum is sympathetic to Singer's utilitarian approach. But her point of view is closer to Rollin's view. Nussbaum asks us explicitly to return to Aristotle in trying to make sense of animal welfare. Aristotle was one of the first philosophers to take up the systematic study of animal life. He tells us that each of the wide variety of animals is marvelous, beautiful, and wonder-inspiring, because each is the embodiment of some unique purpose or function.[27] From this perspective Nussbaum claims that sentient animals should be given the opportunity to live according to what she calls the natural "dignity of their species." Nussbaum concludes: "No sentient animal should be cut off from the chance for a flourishing life, a life with the type of dignity relevant to that species … all sentient animals should enjoy certain positive opportunities to flourish."[28] Like Rollin, Nussbaum is reluctant to completely condemn the system of intensive agriculture. Instead, Nussbaum concludes with a compromise position that attempts to include concern for animal welfare and global utilitarian concern for human health.[29] Such a compromise would be criticized by Singer and others who argue that human health can be sustained by a purely vegetarian diet.

The Kantian and Animal Rights Approach

Moderate conclusions of the sort we find in Rollin or Nussbaum will appear insufficient for those committed to a more demanding idea of animal welfare. The Aristotelian approach can allow killing and consuming animals for food, so long as animals are raised in a way that affords them dignity and allows them to fulfill their natural capacities. And utilitarians such as Singer could allow for animals to be used if it turned out that there were serious human needs to be fulfilled by eating meat (say if there were no alternative sources of protein available). But all of this can seem insufficient if one believes that animals have rights that simply cannot be violated.

Nussbaum derives her idea of dignity and respect for nature from the Aristotelian view that sees wonder and purpose in the natural world and its diverse species. But ideas about dignity and respect can be pushed even deeper. Concepts such as dignity and respect are often associated with a Kantian or deontological approach to ethics. We have seen that Kant claims—following upon insights that connect him to Descartes and to the history of the Christian tradition—that only human beings have dignity and are worthy of respect.

But some philosophers have argued that animals are in fact the sorts of beings that are deserving of respect in the deepest sense of this term. The most famous proponent of such a view is Tom Regan, who first published his *Case for Animal Rights* in 1983. Regan claims that at least some animals are "subjects of a life," by which he means that animals have the sorts of interior lives that allow them to understand themselves and to have an interest in their own continued existence. Another way of putting this is to claim that animals have a kind of intrinsic value, which means that it is wrong to use them for our purposes. When this sort of assumption is made, quite radical conclusions follow. Regan calls for the abolition of animal agriculture and animal testing in the laboratory: "the rights view will not be satisfied with anything less than the total dissolution of the animal industry as we know it."[30] If what Regan says about the intrinsic value of animals is true, then vegetarianism becomes obligatory; and it is not merely a personal choice: "Merely to content oneself with personal abstention is to become part of the problem rather than part of the solution."[31]

Regan's radical views have inspired the sorts of direct action taken by members of the Animal Liberation Front and others. But also within the legal system, the concept of animal rights has led some to argue for changes in the law. Steven Wise, for example, has called for the extension of the "legal convention" of rights to animals—especially for higher animals such as chimpanzees.[32] Without this legal basis, authors such as Francione claim that it is impossible to press animal welfare claims.[33] The worry is that anticruelty laws that are based on merely indirect duties to animals will ultimately be ineffective. If obligations to animals are completely indirect and derivative of human ownership rights, then the owners of animals can simply claim that they can do whatever they want with their own property. It is true, of course, that we do have anticruelty and animal protection laws that make it illegal for humans to do certain things to their own animals. But these laws are usually directed at animals commonly kept as pets. And anticruelty statutes in most states are often written so that there are exemptions for "common farming practices," including the use of confinement, farrowing crates, and so on.[34] Proponents of the animal rights approach will claim that the only solution to the problem of animal cruelty is to give animals more obvious and strenuous protection under the law.

CONCLUSION

Animal welfare activists can cite some recent successes, as noted at the outset, in expanding concern for animal welfare. But these successes are often met with strong resistance from those who make money from cheap meat as well as those who enjoy eating it. Self-interest is often at work in those who are resistant to thinking critically about animal welfare—perhaps more so than deep philosophical disagreements about the concept of animal welfare. Further progress must be made on both fronts: encouraging people to think more critically about the animals they consume, while also enabling people to imagine profitable and nutritious alternatives to factory farming.

In the long run, humans must take the issue of animal welfare seriously. As our population grows and as the taste for meat spreads around the globe, more and more animals will become part of the meat production line. Even those whose concern for animals is entirely anthropocentric must realize the risks of meat production in terms of diseases such as E. coli and bird flu and in terms of pollution and other negative impacts that directly affect human health. The factory farm can indeed be criticized from an anthropocentric perspective. It also seems that we must take seriously the nonanthropocentric concern for animal welfare: animals experience pain and it makes good sense to talk about the quality of an animal's life. Traditional animal husbandry acknowledged this. Traditional farmers and herdsmen directly cared for the animals that fed and clothed them. But in the age of industrial animal agriculture, we are disconnected from the animals that support us. Concern for animal welfare is thus an important part of a larger attempt to be mindful of what we are eating. Once we realize that billions of animals per year are raised in inhumane conditions and slaughtered for the minor human pleasure of tasty meat, once we see that nutritious alternatives to meat are readily available, then it becomes more difficult to justify the cost in cruelty of contemporary animal agriculture.

NOTES

1. David Byrne, Speech at the World Organization for Animal Health (OIE), Paris, February 23, 2004, European Directorate for Health and Consumers, http://europa.eu/rapid/pressReleasesAction.do?reference=SPEECH/04/92&format=HTML&aged=0&language=EN&guiLanguage=en (accessed August 15, 2008).

2. See "Animal Welfare: Fact Sheet" (March 2007), European Directorate for Health and Consumers, http://ec.europa.eu/food/animal/welfare/factsheet_farmed03-2007_en.pdf (accessed August 15, 2008).

3. See Bernard Rollin, *Farm Animal Welfare: Social, Bioethical, and Research Issues* (Ames: Iowa State University Press, 1995).

4. See Peter Singer and Jim Mason, *The Ethics of What We Eat* (Emmaus, PA: Rodale, 2006), chapter 12.

5. These figures are derived from Gary L. Francione, *Introduction to Animal Rights: Your Child or The Dog?* (Philadelphia: Temple University Press, 2000), xx; Matthew Scully, *Dominion: The Power of Man, the Suffering of Animals, and the Call to Mercy* (New York: St. Martin's, 2002), 30–31; and Gaverick Matheny, "Utilitarianism and Animals" in *In Defense of Animals: The Second Wave*, ed. Peter Singer (Malden, MA: Blackwell Publishing, 2006), 13. Francione and Scully both derive their data from the U.S. Department of Agriculture.

6. The Humane Society was founded in 1954. Related organizations include the Society for the Prevention of Cruelty to Animals International (SPCA) and the American Society for the Prevention of Cruelty to Animals (ASPCA). The American SPCA dates from 1866 and claims to be the first organization concerned to prevent cruelty to animals founded in the Western Hemisphere. For SPCA, see www.spca.com; for ASPCA, see www.aspca.org. The SPCA is more concerned with the care of pets, while the Humane Society is more directly involved in issues of farm animal welfare.

7. Erik Marcus reports that 80,000 pigs die each year on the trip to the slaughterhouse. Erik Marcus, *Meat Market: Animals Ethics, and Money* (Boston: Brio Press, 2005), 33.

8. This figure is according to Singer and Mason, *The Ethics of What We Eat*, 67–68. For discussions of animal slaughter see Marcus, *Meat Market*, and Rollin, *Farm Animal Welfare*.

9. A useful summary can be found in Michael Allen Fox, *Deep Vegetarianism* (Temple University Press, 1999). Before this, a seminal article was published by Phillip Devine, "The Moral Basis of Vegetarianism," *Philosophy* 53, no. 206 (1978): 481–505. For articles and vegetarian activism, see the International Vegetarian Union, http://www.ivu.org/.

10. The United Nations report is found at the Food and Agriculture Organization of the United Nations, http://www.fao.org/newsroom/en/news/2006/1000448/index.html (accessed August 15, 2008). For discussion of IPCC head Rajendra Pachauri's plea to "eat less meat," see *New York Times Magazine* (April 20, 2008).

11. The most influential argument along these lines is James Rachels, "Vegetarianism and 'the Other Weight Problem'," in *World Hunger and Moral Obligation*, eds. William Aiken and Hugh LaFollete (Upper Saddle River, NJ: Prentice Hall, 1977).

12. The best-known proponent of this point of view is Carol Adams. See Carol J. Adams, *The Sexual Politics of Meat: A Feminist-Vegetarian Critical Theory* (New York: Continuum, 1990); or Josephine Donovan and Carol J. Adams, eds., *The Feminist Care Tradition in Animal Ethics: A Reader* (New York: Columbia University Press, 2007).

13. See Descartes, *Discourse on Method*, Part V, or his letters to Henry More in *The Philosophical Writings of Descartes* (Cambridge: Cambridge University Press, 1991). Tom Regan criticizes Descartes in *The Case for Animal Rights* (Berkeley: University of California, 1983); John Cottingham offers a more sympathetic reading of Descartes in "A Brute to the Brutes: Descartes' Treatment of Animals," *Philosophy* 53, no. 206 (1978): 551–59.

14. See Immanuel Kant, "Duties to Animals and Spirits" in *Lectures on Ethics* (Cambridge: Cambridge University Press, 1997); and see Regan's discussion in *The Case for Animal Rights*.

15. Tibor Machan, *Putting Humans First* (Lanham, MD: Rowman and Littlefield Publishers, 2004).

16. Friedrich Nietzsche, *On the Genealogy of Morals* (London: Vintage, 1989), First Essay, section 13.

17. See James Swan, *In Defense of Hunting* (San Francisco: Harper One, 1995). For critique, see Scully, *Dominion*.

18. See Jan Narveson, "Animal Rights Revisited," in *Ethics and Animals*, ed. Harlan Miller and William Williams (Clifton, NJ: Humana Press, 1983).

19. David DeGrazia, *Taking Animals Seriously: Mental Life and Moral Status* (Cambridge: Cambridge University Press, 1996), 123. Also see Bernard Rollin, *The Unheeded Cry: Animal Consciousness, Animal Pain, and Science*, expanded ed. (Ames: Iowa State University Press, 1998); Donald R. Griffin, *Animal Minds: Beyond Cognition to Consciousness* (University of Chicago, 1994).

20. See Singer and Mason, *The Ethics of What We Eat*.

21. James Rachels, *Created from Animals: The Moral Implications of Darwinism* (Oxford: Oxford University Press, 1990), 5.

22. Jeremy Bentham, *Principles of Morals and Legislation* (New York: Hafner, 1948), chapter XVII, 311.

23. Peter Singer, "Ethics Beyond Species and Beyond Instincts: A Response to Richard Posner," in *Animal Rights: Current Debates and New Directions*, ed. Cass R. Sunstein and Martha C. Nussbaum (Oxford: Oxford University Press, 2004), 80.

24. Peter Singer, *Animal Liberation*, 2nd ed. (New York: Avon Books, 1990), 6. Updated discussion can be found in Peter Singer, *In Defense of Animals: The Second Wave* (Malden, MA: Blackwell Publishing, 2006).

25. For a recent discussion, see L. Wayne Sumner, *Welfare, Happiness, and Ethics* (Oxford: Oxford University Press, 1996).

26. Rollin, *The Unheeded Cry*, 285.

27. Aristotle, *On the Parts of Animals* (Whitefish, MT: Kessinger Publishing, 2004), Book 1, Section 5, 645a.

28. Martha C. Nussbaum, *Frontiers of Justice: Disability, Nationality, and Species Membership* (Cambridge, MA: Harvard University Press, 2006), 351.

29. Ibid., 402–403.

30. Regan, *The Case for Animal Rights*, 395. Regan has updated his argument in *Defending Animal Rights* (Urbana and Chicago: University of Illinois Press, 2001).

31. Regan, *The Case for Animal Rights*, 353.

32. Steven Wise, *Rattling the Cage: Toward Legal Rights for Animals* (Cambridge, MA: Perseus Press, 2000).

33. Gary L. Francione, "Animals—Property or Persons?" in *Animal Rights*, ed. Sunstein and Nussbaum, 108–142, 108.

34. See Darian Ibrahim, "The Anticruelty Statute: A Study in Animal Welfare," *Journal of Animals Law and Ethics* 1 (2006): 175.

RESOURCE GUIDE

Suggested Reading

Carruthers, Peter. *The Animals Issue: Moral Theory in Practice*. Cambridge: Cambridge University Press, 1992.

DeGrazia, David. *Taking Animals Seriously: Mental Life and Moral Status*. Cambridge: Cambridge University Press, 1996.

Machan, Tibor. *Putting Humans First*. Lanham, MD: Rowman and Littlefield Publishers, 2004.

Nussbaum, Martha C. *Frontiers of Justice: Disability, Nationality, and Species Membership*. Cambridge, MA: Harvard University Press, 2006.

Rachels, James. *Created From Animals: the Moral Implications of Darwinism*. Oxford: Oxford University Press, 1990.

Regan, Tom. *The Case for Animal Rights*. Berkeley: University of California, 1983.

Rollin, Bernard E. *Farm Animal Welfare: Social, Bioethical, and Research Issues*. Ames: Iowa State University Press, 1995.

Singer, Peter, and Jim Mason. *The Ethics of What We Eat: Why Our Food Choices Matter*. Eramus, PA, and New York: Rodale, 2006.

Singer, Peter. *Animal Liberation*, 2nd ed. New York: Avon Books, 1990.

Sunstein, Cass R., and Martha C. Nussbaum, eds. *Animal Rights: Current Debates and New Directions*. Oxford: Oxford University Press, 2004.

Web Sites

Humane Farming Association, http://www.hfa.org/about/index.html.

Humane Society of the United States, http://www.hsus.org/.

People for the Ethical Treatment of Animals, http://www.peta.org/.

U.S. Department of Agriculture, Animal Welfare Information Center, http://awic.nal. usda.gov/.

European Union Directorate for Health and Consumers Animals Welfare Site, http:// ec.europa.eu/food/animal/welfare/index_en.htm.

16

Stewardship of the Land

Eric J. Fitch

A thing is right when it tends to preserve the integrity, stability and beauty of the biotic community. It is wrong when it tends otherwise.

—Aldo Leopold, *A Sand County Almanac*[1]

Earth (Terra, Gaia) is our native world. Humankind evolved here physically, biologically, psychologically, socially, and culturally. Current understanding of the paleontological record places the emergence of the genus Homo at roughly 2.5 million years ago, and humans (Homo sapiens) emerged as a distinct species somewhere between 400,000 and 250,000 years in the past. Despite this longevity, modern society knows very little about the lives and social organization of our human ancestors beyond that of the most recent few thousand years. Written records go back five or so millennia, and the artifacts of human settlements a few thousand more. Before that, humans were organized into band, tribe, and clan, within which, in our omnivorous fashion, we hunted and gathered food and other necessities directly off the land. Ancient human numbers and ranges were limited by natural carrying capacity and interspecific competition for resources. The impact on the ecosystems we inhabited was also limited. Care for the land arose as the need for conservation of resources in their limited foraging and hunting areas. Survival needs often resulted in aboriginal peoples developing systems of "stewardship" based on spiritual kinship with the land.

The development of human ability to make tools and transform the landscape through agriculture and domestication of plant and animal species changed humans' dynamic with the land. As anthropologist Brian Fagan describes in his book *The Long Summer*,[2] climatic conditions moderated over vast sweeps of the globe's land areas, that is, the climate warmed and the areas where humans found tolerable or even ideal conditions expanded greatly. Human inhabitation and civilization spread from areas in and about the tropics to much of the land surface of the planet. As human's technological prowess and social organization increased in intensity, humans went from being one species among many in dynamic balance with their ecosystems to a species that dominates, controls, and, in some cases, demolishes delicate systems and the balances necessary for the land to sustain life. Part of this domination is from increased levels of consumption and part of this is from our sheer numbers. Both usually cause overtaxing of support resources, especially those associated with long-term intensive agriculture and animal husbandry.

A great issue for debate is whether the damage that has been done to the Earth has happened because of the lack of an "owner's manual" or the unwillingness to follow traditional wisdom of land conservation. It is clear from the worldwide damage done to the land and bioproductivity by overgrazing, farming in ways that destroy soil fertility, and other destructive land-use practices, that access to and implementation of a "planet-keeping" manual is sorely needed. This is the point at which land stewardship advocates diverge in terms of the origin of the concepts of conservation.

Some would argue that this "manual" or "land ethic" has long existed in the religious and social traditions that underlie the modern concept of stewardship, particularly stewardship of the land found in the religions and folk wisdom of indigenous peoples around the globe. Traditions of folk knowledge and ethical management of the land (i.e., stewardship ethics) arose from multiple roots. Others believe that concepts of land stewardship are exclusively science based and arise from observing the consequences of past destructive practices.

What is land stewardship and what does it entail? Is it based on theology and philosophy, science and observation, or parts of both schools? In Europe and especially America, the answer, as practiced, is all of the above.

Stewardship as a concept can be summarized as the moral-ethical responsibility to care for the land to conserve its fertility for current and future generations. Of all the essentials for human life on this world, clean air, potable water, clothing, shelter, and, of course, food, all rely to one degree or another on fertile soils and the products of life that grow within and upon them. What it takes to grow crops and raise livestock is not merely "dirt" as the uninitiated think of it, but instead is a complex dynamic matrix made up of organic and inorganic materials, water, air, and living organisms. Arable lands are comparatively rare, and prime farmland is a very rare and valuable commodity. Farmlands are often fragile and easily destroyed by abuse.

As humans increased in numbers and spread to actively inhabit and farm all but one of the Earth's continents and many of her isles, the hand of humanity and our techniques to bring forth food from the land often depleted the land of its fertility, leaving behind wasteland. In some, but not all, cultures throughout the world, observations of this began to emerge in the folktales and stories from ancient times. Included in these observations were the glimmerings of ethical and moral systems recognizing that for humans to survive and thrive in permanently settled communities, the land could not be treated as something having an infinite capacity to absorb abuse, but something that was precious and fragile and that must be cared for as we care for our own lives. The identity of persons as individuals and groups attached to a specific place that was theirs helped to generate this collective sense of duty and obligation.

This is not to say that a stewardship ethic can naturally or easily come to people as they move into systems of fixed settlement and agriculture. Evidence supports the notion that early humans and especially early human efforts at agriculture were not at all successful in maintaining long-term arability of the land. W. C. Lowdermilk in his work *Conquest of the Land through 7,000 Years*[3] documented how one ancient civilization after another, from North Africa through Asia to the Americas, fell after the destruction of their soils through over-use and abuse. Often, the concept of stewardship came about part and parcel with the establishment of some type of formalized religion with doctrine, dogma, and magisterial authority addressing the relationship(s) of humans to nature. Whether through revelation or reason, "guidelines" for ethical behavior or "right living/right action" seemed to arise first within cultures in the context of faith. In ancient polytheistic faiths, these guidelines for behavior would be tied to the lessons of faith associated with agrarian and Earth deities. In later faiths, both monotheistic and polytheistic, more reciprocal relationships between God, humans, and the rest of Creation evolved and were dispersed and accepted as wise teachings. After all, something must be able to counterbalance the normal human tendency to overtax resources as Garrett Hardin points out in his brilliant, influential, and controversial article, "The Tragedy of the Commons."[4] What better way to "encourage" people to treat the land well than through reverence for God's (the Gods') wishes?

Stewardship has been differentially defined but with similar goals in many faith traditions. To elaborate on how these traditions evolved and became actualized in faiths throughout the world would require an entire book. Here, the focus will be how the concepts of land stewardship as a religious and a secular practice evolved in Europe and North America.

Stewardship as a word in the English and French languages can be traced to roots in such earlier words as *stigward*, *stigweard*, and *seneschal*. Even today these words indicate a person with a special (royal or even divine) charge to wisely over-see, protect, and preserve something of value. One place in which one can see the import that is not directly religious is in the Arthurian legends. Sir Kay, King Arthur's stepbrother, became later in life Arthur's seneschal or steward. The role of the seneschal was a great honor with great responsibility. Not only was this knight's duty to maintain the order of the king's house, but he was to protect his lands, castle, and family when the king was abroad, especially in time of campaign (war). A poorly chosen steward could lead to tragedy, including the worst-case scenario of being outflanked by the foe and returning from war to find one's family, home, and land destroyed by a vengeful enemy. As European cultures evolved through the Middle Ages, the role of steward was less that of a warrior and more of the trusted and empowered manager of the king's estate and lands. This strain of stewardship ethic came to dominate European thinking on land stewardship in both faith and society: an honored and trusted position with duties to the land and to current and future generations depending on those lands for sustenance.

Modern Western concepts of stewardship arose in social contexts permeated by the influence of Catholicism and later by Protestant Christianity and by the social and cultural traditions of medieval through Renaissance Europe. The Christian church was meticulous in its instructions to the faithful, especially in matters that could bring it into conflict with the oversight of secular royal authority. Instruction on how to manage the lands, even those controlled by the churches, was a tricky business, especially when the teaching was based not solely on scripture but also on scholarship and insights that were being incorporated into faith tradition. When the Church did act, it did so on the highest authority in scripture and tradition so as to be perceived as being apolitical. Scholars in the church-sponsored monasteries and universities preserved, dispersed, and built on older knowledge including the practical arts of agriculture, forestry, viticulture, and so on. In the schools and churches, especially during Rogation Days and other times of prayer for the land, for crops, for harvest, and so on, there were opportunities to teach and demonstrate how to best manage the land.

Rogation Days are part are the Christian liturgical calendar, notably that of the Catholic and Anglican Faiths. They were initially a substitution for the pagan Roman festival of Robigalia during which time in the spring adherents of the old faith prayed to the gods for success planting and growing crops. In the Christian tradition, Rogation Days were observed on April 25 and the three days leading up to Ascension Thursday when the clergy blessed the fields and the congregation fasted and prayed for good crops. Rogation comes from the Latin "to ask." These liturgies and prayers created time and space where both ethical and practical management of the land could be preached and taught. Fortunately for clerics in the Middle Ages and through today, the Scriptures provide firm instructions to do this type of teaching; to paraphrase the prophet Ezekiel, "if they have but eyes to see and will to act."

Stewardship has been differentially defined but with similar goals in many faith traditions. In the Abrahamic faiths (Judaism, Christianity, and Islam), the scriptural roots of land stewardship can be traced back to Mosaic instruction laid out in the Hebrew Scriptures in the Pentateuch, the first five books of the Torah, which are also the first five books of the Christian Bible. In particular, in Exodus, Leviticus, and Deuteronomy, direct instructions are given with regard to human responsibility to the land. In Exodus 23:10-11; Leviticus 25:1-7; and Deuteronomy 15:1-11, 31:10-1, the rules and traditions of the Sabbatical years are presented to the people. Just as humanity was commanded to rest from labor every seven days, people were commanded to let the land rest every seven years. In addition to the Sabbatical years, in Leviticus 25:8-55 and Numbers 36:1-9, a further tradition of the Jubilee Year is put into the law of the people. In the Jubilee Year, every seven times seven plus one years (50), the land is to be redistributed so that justice may be met for both land and for men. These early laws set the framework linking the ideals of soil conservation and social justice.

Further examples are given throughout the Hebrew and the Christian Scriptures that draw on the agrarian cultures of the ancient Near East. God is often described in terms such as farmer, shepherd, or viticulturalist. The "goodness" of God is emphasized by his care for the land, the sheep, or the vines. The story of Exodus, the 40 years of testing in the desert, comes to a conclusion as the younger generation gets to enter the Promised Land, a land of milk and honey in the Book of Joshua. As the Hebrews became the Israelites and their identity as a people were tied to that land, religion played a key role in defining the practices that kept both healthy.

Jesus of Nazareth, as documented by his disciples, communicated his messages of faith to his followers within the context of the Jewish culture. Much of his teaching was embedded in nature-based parables, again contrasting a good and loving God who as a worker of the land cared for that land so that it would bring forth good fruit. The primary emphasis of the stories was of course the refinement of the faith, understanding the relationship between the people and God, but what was not lost was the relationship between man and nature, particularly the "good" Earth.

Parallel dogmatic and liturgical support for stewardship can be found in diverse theological and philosophical traditions throughout the world. In the Vedic scriptures of the Hindu faith, direction can be found to support land and water stewardship, especially with regard to the rivers and forests of the Indian subcontinent. In Shinto, specific lands and waters are considered sacred, as is the balancing of one's spirit with nature itself. Likewise, in Buddhism, the paths of right action are parallel to respect for the Earth. In the Aboriginal faith of Australia, few things are more sacred than the Land, and nothing is more important than learning to live wisely with nature. Although not all of these have experienced the same historical intertwining of faith and public leadership toward land stewardship, in some multicultural societies such as the United States, the traditions and beliefs of non-Christian faith with regard to land and nature have often been incorporated within the overall message of the public agencies. The teachings of First Peoples (Native Americans and Native Canadians) have been incorporation into public stewardship outreach in the United States and Canada.

In Western traditions that rest heavily on the Hebrew and Christian scriptures, religious practices and social responsibility reinforced each other. In the early Catholic Church, through the Middle Ages, and in some places even today, religious duty and land stewardship are clearly intertwined. This is not to say that good land stewardship necessarily went hand in hand with the spread of Christianity. Certain strains of theology arose that emphasized different parts of scripture and led to conflicting interpretations. This conflict was clearly delineated in historian Lynn White Jr.'s seminal article in the journal *Science*: "The Historic Roots of Our Ecologic Crisis."[5] He demonstrated that as a practical matter, scriptural, and theological arguments have been promulgated within various strains of Christianity to support a dominion or domination of the Earth's resources on the one hand and a stewardship relationship on the other hand.

A dominion-based theology (or at least practices that attempt to find some justification in theology) emphasize an interpretation of the first creation story in the Book of Genesis in which God instructs humans to "fill the Earth and subdue it" (with an emphasis on the "subdue"). Observation of the practices that have been used to cultivate croplands and pastures, especially in the last two centuries of technology-driven agriculture (mechanized, chemically saturated, industrialized, and bioengineered) would certainly seem to argue that in Europe and the United States where Christianity has been the dominant faith, the dominion model has won out.

Adding to this dominion-based view were the social phenomena of the industrial revolution and urbanization of the population. America went from being an agrarian nation to an industrial nation. The people became divorced from the land, and all too often, so did the teaching and preaching in their churches. Rogation Days began to be dropped from churches' liturgical calendars and were retained only in some rural areas. As fewer people felt and believed they had the type of connection to the land that is often part of the core identity of farmers and ranchers, priests and ministers shifted away from stewardship to other matters of theological import in teaching and preaching.

This absence of a connection to the land by more and more people in society, and the conflict between stewardship and dominion within the teaching of the broad Christian community came to a head in the United States in the first half of the twentieth century. Ongoing colonization of North America brought traditional

farming practices to places ill-suited to European and eastern U.S. norms and practices. Land destruction from soil erosion became epidemic, especially in areas of the
West that came to be called "the Dust Bowl." Even though these Western dry lands
were the focus of initial concern, they were far from being the only degraded lands.
Water-driven erosion was stripping soil from fields on steep grades throughout the
country. Southern states' streams bled red with the runoff of spring rains. New
England and Midwest farms were losing significant amounts of their "A horizon" or
topsoil to erosive forces as well. With the Stock Market Crash of 1929 and the
onset of the Great Depression, fears arose not about people being able to afford
food, but of the very ability of the nation to continue to grow the food to feed the
people. Land (soil) stewardship became a revitalized watchword in public forums
and the halls of government.

Existing research and education organizations were directed to develop techniques and disseminate information on how to continue to engage in farming, grazing, forestry, and all other production activities while preserving the integrity and
fertility of the land. The public Agricultural and Natural Colleges found at the
Morrill Land Grant Universities and their Experiment Stations and Cooperative
Extension Services led the way. Extension agents provided a key service in taking
the best soil conservation management practices and teaching them in public
forums in agricultural communities. They often worked closely with churches and
primary and secondary schools to "spread the word" as well. Churches often played
significant roles in the education process in large part because of respect for their
teaching authority and the ability to provide the faith-based component of rationale for land stewardship. Even today, Soil and Water Conservation Week program
materials contain materials for use in sermons and other prayer and teaching lessons
for Christian churches and schools produced by public agencies using public funds.

Another key contributor and cooperator in the process of creating and dissemi-
nating a foundation and practices for stewardship in the American experience in
the 1930s was the newly created Soil Conservation Service (the SCS; today called
the NRCS, the Natural Resources Conservation Service) and newly empowered Soil
and Water Conservation Districts. Along with the Land Grant Universities, they
had the responsibility to research, demonstrate, and otherwise disseminate research
on soil and water conservation. Of particular interest are two key scholars that are
prominent in the literature as providing the bridge between science and faith in the
protection of the land: W. C. Lowdermilk and Aldo Leopold, who both had their
"roots" in the SCS. Their seminal works with regard to this issue, which some point
to as books in the secular "bible" or "earthkeeping" manual, are Lowdermilk's *Conquest of the Land through 7,000 Years*[6] and Leopold's *Sand County Almanac*.[7]

Lowdermilk was the assistant chief of the SCS, and he traveled throughout
Europe, the Near East, and North Africa. He previously had spent considerable
time in China. He observed and studied soil conditions throughout these lands
and paid special attention to the social, cultural, historical, and religious milieu as
well as lands and agricultural practices. He could have written a report that was a
straightforward analysis with the central observation that civilizations that misused
their soil resources generally collapsed over time. *Conquest of the Land through
7,000 Years* went beyond that and dealt with what lessons could be learned and
what could be invoked to get farmers and others to better care for their lands.
Conquest was first published in 1939 as USDA Bulletin No. 99, and even though

it was a government publication of the then SCS, Lowdermilk spoke of the spiritual dimensions of maintenance of the land as an "11th Commandment":

> Thou shalt inherit the Holy Earth as a faithful steward, conserving its resources and productivity from generation to generation. Thou shalt safeguard thy fields from soil erosion, thy living waters from drying up, thy forests from desolation, and protect thy hills from overgrazing by thy herds, that thy descendants may have abundance forever. If any shall fail in this stewardship of the land thy fruitful fields shall become sterile stony ground and wasting gullies, and thy descendants shall decrease and live in poverty or perish from off the face of the earth.[8]

Lowdermilk himself was a practicing Christian and believed he was writing for a public audience filled with others who mostly shared his viewpoint. This "commandment" is reflective of concepts of stewardship he found in religious and secular traditions throughout the world and for him, held no contradiction with what he had discovered as a scientist. Despite being written more than 70 years ago, this document remains one of the most, if not the most, requested document ever published by the USDA. Despite some socially and culturally antiquated and even inappropriate terminology and phrasing, Lowdermilk's writing is still used today primarily because of this stunningly simple yet eloquent synthesis of theological foundations for modern scientifically based stewardship practices.

Aldo Leopold was a friend and, for a time, co-worker in the SCS with Lowdermilk. Leopold moved on from the SCS to the halls of academe. Well-published and respected in the fields of ecology, wildlife management, conservation, and related areas, his "magnum opus" is *A Sand County Almanac.*[9] Some of his key reflections in the "Land Ethic" chapter can be traced to a desire to build on his friend's idea of the "11th Commandment." Although less religious and more philosophical than Lowdermilk's work, these two pieces nonetheless represent a foundation on which an "earthkeeping" manual or "bible" has been written and acted on in the American experience and elsewhere. Leopold clearly and succinctly laid out the necessary ethical relationships and boundaries between humans and the natural environment. With or without religious underpinnings, it presents concepts of a stewardship ethic that go beyond mere self-interest and into the realms of intergenerational equity and natural justice. Leopold wrote: "A land ethic, then, reflects the existence of an ecological conscience, and this in turn reflects a conviction of individual responsibility for the health of land."[10] Boldly but without hyperbole, Leopold explained the ethical obligations of humans to the lands and nature they rely on, even though a vast portion of our modern societies live in ignorance of their essential dependence on nature's bounty. Humans are quite used to having ethical relations and boundaries within their communities. Leopold recommended pushing back the "fences" that had been built up by people who felt divorced from the land where their food, clothing, shelter, and ultimately all their material resources come from and embracing our collective ethical obligations. He attempted to redefine the concept of community back to earlier boundaries that included nature.

Leopold's work inspired many within the conservation and preservation social and political movements, as well as in the subsequent environmental movement. Today, many scholars in a vast sweep of disciplinary and interdisciplinary fields from biology to theology, philosophy to agronomy, and political science to the per-formance arts are actively attempting to flesh out the nature of these relationships. Most of the major Christian Churches, both institutionally and congregationally, promote stewardship of the land. The U.S. Conference of Catholic Bishops as well as the worldwide Roman Catholic Church promote land conservation and soil stewardship as a matter of moral obligation to the land and as a matter of social and intergenerational justice. Several branches of the Anglican and Episcopalian denominations likewise promulgate Earth ethics. From the Unitarian Universalists, through American Baptists, the Orthodox Churches, and many more large and small denominations, consensus is growing regarding the ethical obligations of humans toward the environment, and especially toward the lands and waters that support human life.[11]

The amount of lay and secular teaching about the need to be good stewards of the land is considerable. The fields of crop and soil sciences are well represented in academe, especially at land-grant universities where the knowledge of best prac-tices is not just a matter of field research and classroom teaching. Soil and water stewardship remain key missions of cooperative extension services and extension agents, the itinerant educators whose job it is to spread knowledge throughout the counties and parishes (e.g., in Louisiana) about how to best manage the land.[12]

Concepts of stewardship are being discussed in schools, churches, and commu-nity meetings, mostly in rural areas but also in some urban and suburban settings. As human population continues to grow across the planet and rates of human con-sumption of goods, pollution impacts, and in some cases the literal destruction of landscapes continue at a breathtaking pace, adoption of principles and practices of stewardship of the land has never been more important.

Theologians and philosophers continue to discuss, debate, research, write, and teach on land stewardship and environmental ethics as a standalone subject and in the larger contexts of environmental ethics and sustainability. Thomas Berry, Mat-thew Fox, H. Paul Santmire, Rosemary Radford Ruether, and an ever-increasing field of scholars continue to build on human moral and ethical relationships with the land and the Earth as a whole.[13] There are also lay ministers and teachers like the farmer-poet-philosopher Wendell Berry;[14] Wes Jackson,[15] an acknowledged leader of the sustainable agriculture movement; and renowned geomorphologist and author David Montgomery.[16] Although there remains a chasm between those who work that land and their communities, and those who live in places divorced from day-to-day exposure to farming, the concepts of stewardship have taken root throughout much of present society.

The one key question posed in this chapter has been answered: yes, a land stew-ardship ethic exists. In fact, when one broadens the scope, one would find that land stewardship, ethical, and moral principles for protecting the land, the water, and the life they nurture is found in almost all human cultures and societies. These lessons lie not only within the teaching and research of crop, soil, and other agri-cultural and related sciences, but also within the religions, philosophies, and folk wisdom of many cultures. The bigger and yet-unanswered questions are (1) can these lessons be taught and brought into practice before overuse and exploitation destroy the foundation of the human food supply? and (2) can these concepts be incorporated and adopted into an even larger endeavor, the quest to create human cultures and societies that live sustainably upon the planet?

NOTES

1. Aldo Leopold, *A Sand County Almanac and Sketches Here and There* (New York: Oxford University Press, 1949).

2. Brian Fagan, *The Long Summer: How Climate Changed Civilization* (New York, NY: Basic Books, 2004).

3. Walter C. Lowdermilk, *Conquest of the Land through 7,000 Years: AIB No. 99.* (Washington, DC: U.S. Department of Agriculture, Natural Resources Conservation Service, 1953).

4. Garrett Hardin, "Tragedy of the Commons," *Science* 162 (December 13, 1968): 1243–248.

5. Lynn White, "The Historic Roots of Our Ecologic Crisis," *Science* 155 (March 10, 1967): 1203–1207.

6. Lowdermilk, *Conquest.*

7. Leopold, *A Sand County.*

8. Lowdermilk, *Conquest*, 24.

9. Leopold, *A Sand County.*

10. Ibid., 204.

11. A few examples of these denominational statements can be found in The American Baptist "Policy Statement on Ecology," June 1989; "Creation: Called to Care," Statement of the Church of the Brethren 1991 Annual Conference; 70th General Convention of the Episcopal Church Resolution: "Affirm Environmental Responsibility and Establish an Environmental Stewardship Team," 1991; the Evangelical Environmental Network's "An Evangelical Declaration on the Care of Creation," 1994; Evangelical Lutheran Church in America's "A Social Statement on Caring for Creation: Vision, Hope, and Justice," 1993; the Mennonite Environmental Taskforce's Stewardship of the Earth, "Resolution on the Environment and Faith Issues," 1989; Message of His All-Holiness the Ecumenical Patriarch Dimitrios on the Day of the Protection of the Environment, 1989; Statement of the Friends Committee on Unity with Nature, 1987; the Reformed Church in America's "Care for the Earth: Theology and Practice," 1982; Pope John Paul II's "The Ecological Crisis: A Common Responsibility"; the United Methodist Church's "Social Principle, The Natural World"; and the General Assembly of the Unitarian Universalist Association 1997 "General Resolution Earth, Air, Fire and Water."

12. A good review of the mission of land-grant colleges and universities is Ralph D. Christy and Lionel Williamson, eds., *A Century of Service: Land-Grant Colleges and Universities 1890–1990* (Edison, NJ: Transaction Publishers, 1991). A nice example of some of the underlying research on stewardship education can be found in Gene Wunderlich, "Evolution of the Stewardship Idea in American Country Life," *Journal of Agricultural and Environmental Ethics* 17 (2004): 77–93. An excellent overview of how the missions of the Cooperative Extension Service and the Natural Resources Conservation Service shaped an American land ethic can be found in Barbara Wallace and Frank Clearfield, *Stewardship, Spirituality, and Natural Resource Conservation: A Short History* (Madison, WI: Social Sciences Research Institute, Natural Resources Conservation Service, 1997).

13. Thomas Berry, *The Great Work: Our Way Into the Future* (New York: Three Rivers Press, 2000); Matthew Fox, *Original Blessing: A Primer in Creation Spirituality Presented in Four Paths, Twenty-Six Themes, and Two Questions* (New York: Tarcher/Penguin, 2000); Paul Santmie, *The Travail of Nature: The Ambiguous Ecological Promise of Christian Theology* (Minneapolis, MN: Augsburg Fortress Publishers, 1985); Rosemary Radford Reuther, *Gaia and God: An Ecofeminist Theology of Earth Healing* (New York: HarperOne, 1994). In addition, some good sources for studying the wide spectrum of theological and

philosophical discourse on land and environmental ethics and morality are Mary Evelyn Tucker and John A. Grim, eds., *Worldviews and Ecology: Religion, Philosophy, and the Environment* (Marynoll, NY: Orbis Books, 1994); Roderick Frazier Nash, *The Rights of Nature: A History of Environmental Ethics*, (Madison: University of Wisconsin Press, 1989); Richard C. Foltz, ed., *Worldviews, Religion and Environment* (Belmont, CA: Thomson-Wadsworth, 2003); David Kinsley, ed., *Ecology and Religion: Ecological Spirituality in Cross-Cultural Perspective* (Englewood Cliffs, NJ: Prentice Hall, 1995); Roger S. Gottlieb, *This Sacred Earth: Religion, Nature, Environment*, 2nd ed. (New York: Routledge, 2004).

14. An excellent collection of some of Wendell Berry's essays on agriculture and care for the land is *The Art of the Common-place: The Agrarian Essays of Wendell Berry*, ed. Norman Wirzba (Washington, DC: Counterpoint, 2002).

15. An excellent introduction to Wes Jackson's thinking on agricultural sustainability and land stewardship is his *New Roots for Agriculture* (Lincoln, NE: University of Nebraska Press, 1985).

16. David R. Montgomery's *Dirt: Erosion of Civilizations* (Berkeley: University of California Press, 2007) presents a wonderful synthesis of current soil science as well as a synthesis of the practical ethical and moral reasoning that supports the practice of good soil stewardship.

RESOURCE GUIDE

Web Sites

Land Stewardship Project, http://www.landstewardshipproject.org/.

The Land Institute, http://www.landinstitute.org/.

The National Association of Conservation's Stewardship, http://nacdnet.org/stewardship/.

U.S. Council of Catholic Bishops Webpage on Environment, http://www.usccb.org/sdwp/ejp/.

About the Editor and Contributors

Lynn Walter is co-director of the Center for Food in Community and Culture and Rosenberg Professor of Social Change and Development at the University of Wisconsin-Green Bay, where she also teaches in Anthropology and Gender and Women's Studies. Her field research in Ecuador and Denmark focused on indigenous ethnicity and gender issues, respectively. She is editor of *Women's Rights: A Global View* and editor-in-chief of *Women's Issues Worldwide* (6 vols.) and author of *Ethnicity, Economy and the State in Ecuador*.

Patricia Allen is director of the University of California–Santa Cruz's Center for Agroecology. Her work addresses issues such as labor, gender, and access to food. She is the author of *Together at the Table: Sustainability and Sustenance in the American Agrifood System* (2004) and editor of *Food for the Future: Conditions and Contradictions of Sustainability* (1993).

E. Melanie DuPuis is professor of sociology at University of California–Santa Cruz. Her work focuses on the politics of food, agriculture, and environment. She is author of the book *Nature's Perfect Food* and more recently co-edited a special issue of *Gastronomica* on the politics of food.

Gail Feenstra is the food systems analyst at the University of California Sustainable Agriculture Research and Education Program (SAREP). SAREP's Food Systems Program encourages the development of local food systems that link farmers, consumers, and communities. Feenstra's research and outreach includes direct marketing, farm-to-school evaluation, regional food system distribution, food systems indicators, food security, food system assessments, and, most recently, food carbon footprint analysis. Feenstra has a doctorate in nutrition education from Teachers College, Columbia University with an emphasis in public health.

Andrew Fiala is professor of philosophy and director of the Ethics Center at California State University–Fresno. He is the author of numerous articles and several books: *The Philosopher's Voice*, *Practical Pacifism*, *Tolerance and the Ethical Life*, and *What Would Jesus Really Do?* His newest book is *The Just War Myth*. Fiala is also co-editor of the journal *Philosophy in the Contemporary World*.

Eric J. Fitch is associate professor of environmental science and leadership and currently director of the Environmental Science Program at Marietta College. He received his doctorate at Michigan State in Resource Development (Environmental Policy). His areas of research include water policy, coastal zone management, and religion and the environment. He is an associate editor of *Water Resources IMPACT*, and author of the "What's Up with Water?" column. He is the president of the Interdisciplinary Environmental Association, a member of the Board of Ohio River Basin Consortium for Research and Education (ORBCRE), and is a fellow of the East-West Center.

Regan A. R. Gurung is professor of human development and psychology at the University of Wisconsin–Green Bay. Born and raised in Bombay, India, Dr. Gurung received a bachelor's degree in psychology at Carleton College (Minnesota), and a master's degree and doctorate in social and personality psychology at the University of Washington. He then spent three years at the University of California–Los Angeles as a National Institute of Mental Health (NIMH) research fellow. He has received numerous local, state, and national grants and awards for his health psychological and social psychological research on cultural differences in health, body image and impression formation, and pedagogy.

Aeron Haynie is associate professor of English at the University of Wisconsin–Green Bay, where she teaches British literature and interdisciplinary humanities. She has published articles on Victorian literature, pedagogy, as well as personal essays on the profession. She is co-editor of *Beyond Sensation: Mary Elizabeth Braddon in Context* and *Exploring Signature Pedagogies: Approaches to Teaching Disciplinary Habits of Mind*.

Lisa Heldke is professor of philosophy and Sponberg Chair of Ethics at Gustavus Adolphus College, where she also teaches in the Gender, Women, and Sexuality Studies Program. She is author of *Exotic Appetites: Ruminations of a Food Adventurer* (Routledge) and editor of several books, including *Cooking, Eating, Thinking: Transformative Philosophies of Food* (with Deane Curtin). She co-edits the journal *Food, Culture and Society*.

JoAnn Jaffe is an associate professor in the Department of Sociology and Social Studies at the University of Regina in Regina, Saskatchewan, Canada. Her recent research projects include studying the effects of neoliberalization and globalization on agricultural communities in Canada and the global south and the construction of food knowledge across generations of female food provisioners. Recently, JoAnn was a review editor for the global volume of the *International Agricultural Assessment of Science and Technology for Development*. She is a former president of the Saskatchewan Council for International Cooperation and is on the board of the Saskatchewan Population Health Evaluation and Research Unit.

Esther Katz is a French anthropologist, senior scientist at the French Institute of Research for Development (IRD). She is associated with the Center for Sustainable Development of the University of Brasilia (CDS-UnB), where she is presently based. Her main research topics are ethnobiology and anthropology of food. She has done fieldwork in Mexico, the Congo, Indonesia, Laos People's Democratic Republic, and France, and is now studying agrobiodiversity and food changes in the Brazilian Amazon.

Dan La Botz is an independent scholar based in Cincinnati, Ohio. He is the author of *César Chávez and la Causa* as well as several other books on labor unions and politics in the United States, Mexico, and Indonesia. He writes frequently for *Against the Current, Labor Notes, Monthly Review*, and *Counterpunch* and is a member of the editorial board of *New Politics*. He is currently writing a history of the African American community of Cincinnati, provisionally titled *Struggle for Justice*.

Michele Micheletti holds the Lars Hiera Professorship of Political Science at Stockholm University. She has written books on corporatism, interest groups, civil society, democratic auditing, and political consumerism. Her general research focus is citizen engagement in politics. She is the author of *Political Virtue and Shopping: Individuals, Consumerism, and Collective Action* (Palgrave, 2003), was head guest editor of "Shopping for Human Rights" for the *Journal of Consumer Policy* (vol. 30, no. 3, 2007), and co-editor (with Andreas Follesdal and Dietlind Stolle) of *Politics, Products, and Markets: Exploring Political Consumerism Past and Present* (2003 and 2006). Currently, she heads a research project entitled "Sustainable Citizenship" funded by the Swedish Council of Research.

Daniel Niles is a human geographer interested in different practical and conceptual approaches to sustainable agriculture, sustainable eating, and more convivial human-environmental relationship. He received a doctorate in 2007 from the Graduate School of Geography, Clark University, in Worcester, Massachusetts, and now works at the Research Institute for Humanity and Nature in Kyoto, Japan.

Larry Smith is professor of social change and development at the University of Wisconsin–Green Bay. His professional activity focuses on issues of sustainability, and he has been active in small-scale agriculture for more than

60 years. Though trained in narrow market-admiring economics, his interdisciplinary academic career has emphasized melding anthropology, biology, sociology, and history as context for making sense of economics.

Dietlind Stolle is associate professor in Political Science at McGill University, Montréal, Canada. She conducts research and has published on voluntary associations, trust, institutional foundations of social capital, and new forms of political participation, particularly political consumerism. She is also the co-principal investigator of the unique longitudinal Comparative Youth Survey (CYS) as well as associate director of the US Citizenship, Involvement and Democracy (CID) survey. Her work has appeared or is forthcoming, for example, in the journals *British Journal of Political Science*, *Comparative Politics*, *Comparative Political Studies*, *International Review of Political Science*, *Political Behaviour*, and *Political Psychology* as well as in various edited volumes. She has also co-edited a book on social capital and one on political consumerism.

William Van Lopik is a geography and sustainable development instructor at the College of Menominee Nation in northern Wisconsin. He previously worked for an international development nongovernmental organization in El Salvador. His research interests are in the areas of political ecology, land tenure in Mesoamerica, indigenous knowledge systems, and the various perspectives of sustainability.

Jennifer Wilkins is a senior extension associate in the Division of Nutritional Sciences at Cornell University. Her work focuses on how the food and agriculture system affects public health, environmental sustainability, and community well-being. She directs the Cornell Farm-to-School Program and the Farmers Market Nutrition Program. She recently joined the Chefs Collaborative Board of Overseers and is a guest lecturer at the Università di Scienze Gastronomiche (University of Gastronomic Sciences) established by Slow Food in Pollenzo, Italy.

Index

Abalimi Bezekhaya (Xhosa), 161
Acres U.S.A., 77–78
ADM (Archer Daniels Midland), 123
African Americans, 80n24, 176, 200; food security, 4, 213; meat and poultry workers, xiii, 33–34; poverty, 33; racial discrimination, 33
agrarian populism, 9
Agricultural Justice Project, 10
Agricultural Labor Relations Act (ALRA) (California), 42
agricultural subsidies, 6, 10, 36
agriculture, alternative agriculture, 8, 19, 41, 53; artisanal agriculture, 76–78; civic agriculture, 19, 126; community-supported agriculture, 11, 12, 17, 20–22, 73, 74, 126–27, 157; corporate agriculture, 33, 41, 54, 96; export agriculture, 107, 110; industrial agriculture, 9, 13, 40, 69, 74, 76, 77, 86, 96, 110, 122, 141, 143, 150, 227–29, 229–31, 233, 235, 237, 238, 244, 247; local and regional agriculture, xv, 78, 88, 107, 127–28, 133; multifunctionality of, xiv, 11, 108, 143; organic agriculture, xiv, 8, 12, 13, 19, 23–24; peasant agriculture, 53; productionist paradigm, 68; traditional agriculture, 166, 204–6, 230, 237, 244–45; sustainable agriculture, 8, 9, 11, 40, 53, 54, 86, 184–85, 206, 250; urban agriculture, 11, 13, 73, 74–75, 130–31, 161–62

agrobiodiversity, 141, 201, 207
agroecology, vii, 54
Ahwahnee community design guidelines, 130
Allen, Patricia, 133, 219
Allen, Will, 74
alternative agrifood, 3–16, 18, 73–78; alternative agrifood movement, xii–xiv, xv, 17; alternative agrifood networks (AFN), 73–78; alternative agrifood systems, 3–16
American Farmland Trust, loss of farmland, 124
American Indians. *See* Native Americans
American Public Health Association, 123
Americans with Disabilities Act, 218
Animal Liberation Front, 228, 237
animal welfare, xxi, 90–95, 101, 113, 227–38; animal husbandry, xxi, 227–28, 230, 236, 238; animal-centered approach, xxi, 233–38; anthropocentric approach, xxi, 231–33; ethical vegetarianism, 229–31; factory farmed animals, xxi, 227–29, 238; European Union, xxi, 91, 227; "five freedoms," xxi, 91, 227; industrial agriculture, xxi, 227–28
animal welfare, animal-centered perspectives, 233–38, animal rights, xxi, 87, 91, 228–29, 237–38; Aristotelian approach, xxi, 235–37; Bentham, Jeremy, 234, 235; Darwin, Charles, 233;